Luminos is the Open Access monograph publishing program from UC Press. Luminos provides a framework for preserving and reinvigorating monograph publishing for the future and increases the reach and visibility of important scholarly work. Titles published in the UC Press Luminos model are published with the same high standards for selection, peer review, production, and marketing as those in our traditional program. www.luminosoa.org

The publisher and the University of California Press Foundation gratefully acknowledge the generous support of the Ahmanson Foundation Endowment Fund in Humanities.

# Insistent Life

# Insistent Life

*Principles for Bioethics in the Jain Tradition*

Brianne Donaldson and Ana Bajželj

UNIVERSITY OF CALIFORNIA PRESS

University of California Press
Oakland, California



Suggested citation: Donaldson, B. and Bajželj, A. *Insistent Life: Principles for Bioethics in the Jain Tradition.* Oakland: University of California Press, 2021. DOI: https://doi.org/10.1525/luminos.108

Library of Congress Cataloging-in-Publication Data

Names: Donaldson, Brianne, author. | Bajželj, Ana, author.
Title: Insistent life : principles for bioethics in the Jain tradition / Brianne Graham Donaldson and Ana Bajželj.
Description: [Oakland, California] : [University of California Press], [2021] | Includes bibliographical references and index.
Identifiers: LCCN 2020051186 (print) | LCCN 2020051187 (ebook) | ISBN 9780520380561 (paperback) | ISBN 9780520380578 (ebook)
Subjects: LCSH: Bioethics—Religious aspects—Jainism. | Medicine—Religious aspects—Jainism.
Classification: LCC R725.55 .D66 2021 (print) | LCC R725.55 (ebook) | DDC 174.2088/2944—dc23
LC record available at https://lccn.loc.gov/2020051186
LC ebook record available at https://lccn.loc.gov/2020051187

Manufactured in the United States of America

25 24 23 22 21
10 9 8 7 6 5 4 3 2 1

परस्परोपग्रहो जीवानाम्

*parasparopagraho jīvānām*

The function of living beings is to support one another.

*Tattvārtha-sūtra 5.21*

CONTENTS

# ACKNOWLEDGMENTS

Brianne and Ana would together like to thank colleagues in the Federation of Jain Associations in North America (JAINA) and Young Jains of America (YJA). We also thank Sanjeev Sogani, Kirtida Malde, Reena Shah, Atul Shah, Freya Shah, Mukul Shah, Sagar Shah, and Pradip Jain for circulating our survey, used in part 2; and the many Jain healthcare professionals who completed the survey. Special gratitude also goes to Royce Wiles, Sanmati Thole, Manoj Jain, Nitin Shah, Jina Shah, and Narendra Parson for critical assistance during the project, as well the International School for Jain Studies—especially Shugan Jain and Sulekh Jain—for bringing us together at an early stage in our careers. We are grateful to Reed Malcolm, our editor, Richard Earles, our copyeditor, and the rest of the UC Press team for all the support and help in bringing this book to light.

Brianne would like to thank the UCI Humanities Center at the University of California, Irvine, for a publication support grant; as well as the Chao Center for Asian Studies at Rice University, including Sonia Ryang, Haejin Koh, Amber Szymczyk, Hae Hun Matos, and students in Bioethics and Indian Traditions and India, Consciousness, and Science courses (2016–19). Additional thanks go to Pranav Mehta, Matthew Southey, Sunil Kothari, Saadullah Bashir, Fernando Villagómez, Jay Martin, and the Jain Society of Houston community. Special gratitude to Maple and Batmitzvah.

Ana would like to thank Tamara Ditrich, Kristi Wiley, and Knut Aukland; her colleagues at the University of California, Riverside; the donors of the Shrimad Rajchandra Endowed Chair in Jain Studies at the University of California, Riverside, and the Jain community of Southern California; the Polonsky family, Gabriel Motzkin, Shai Lavi, and the Polonsky Fellows; Yigal Bronner and David Shulman; and her students. She could not have completed this project without her friends, Matic and his family, Tilka, and Rozka.

# NOTE ON LANGUAGE AND TRANSLITERATION

Jain texts are written in several languages. For the purpose of standardization, we are using Sanskrit for most terms and titles even if they appear in Prakrits or Hindi. For primary sources in the bibliography, readers will find, where applicable, both the Sanskrit and Prakrit titles listed.

We are following standard conventions for the transliteration of words from Indic languages. Non-English terms are italicized and all technical terms are explained when they are first mentioned, for which the index will be useful.

All translations are ours unless noted otherwise.

PART ONE

# Foundational Principles

1

# Why Jainism and Bioethics?

Jainism is a religious tradition and philosophical system rooted in India whose texts and practices are perhaps more strongly focused on the ethics of life and death than any other tradition in the world. Although it does not offer a thoroughgoing "bioethics" in the modern sense, Jainism does present a detailed account of birth, life, and death; a meticulous taxonomy of diverse life-forms; a path of ethical conduct characterized by nonviolence toward all living beings; and a complex development of approaches to medical treatment from antiquity up to the present. Some of the bioethical issues faced by contemporary Jains are similar to the ethical challenges faced by Jains throughout history, while others are without precedent and have required creative ethical responses, either because they have arisen as a result of modern scientific and technological advances or because they are emerging in new social and cultural contexts.

Considering the rich history of Jain encounters with the dilemmas of birth, life, and death, the absence of a book on Jainism in relation to contemporary bioethical issues presents a significant gap in both the fields of bioethics and Jain studies. This book addresses that gap in two distinct ways, mirrored in its two-part structure. In part 1, we explore foundational Jain principles for bioethics based on rigorous analysis of primary sources and available secondary literature. In part 2, we identify provisional principles of application for modern bioethical dilemmas by examining approaches to specific ethical issues relating to birth, life, and death in primary sources and by analyzing scarce contemporary sources on Jainism and bioethics from modern lay Jains, mendicants, and Jain studies scholars, as well as data drawn from an international survey we conducted with Jain medical professionals in 2017–18. We hope that this dual approach of excavating foundational principles and deducing principles of application will make a meaningful contribution to future scholarship and clinical analysis in Jainism and bioethics.

## JAINISM AND JAINS

In this book, we refer both to "Jainism" and to "Jains." While these two terms understandably overlap, they each have their own historical derivation and they have meaningful differences in contemporary scholarship (Flügel 2005). In our attempt as Jain studies scholars to provide an *etic*, or outsider, perspective of Jainism in relation to bioethical issues, we have to account for multiple *emic*, or insider, perspectives that reflect the internal diversity of texts, sectarian disagreements, practices, and individual practitioners. The lens of bioethics unearths complexities too often obscured in a pursuit of "Jainism" or "Jains" as homogeneous realities.

The term "Jain" means one who follows a Jina ("Conqueror" or "Victor").[1] Jinas are teachers who, by their own efforts, master the disciplinary practices needed to attain liberation from the cycle of rebirths, known as *saṃsāra*. They are also called Tīrthaṅkaras or Fordmakers because they create the ford, or *tīrtha*, for others to follow across the river of *saṃsāra*.

Historical records show that Jainism has been present uninterruptedly on the Indian subcontinent for over twenty-five hundred years. Jains themselves, however, understand their tradition to be beginningless and eternal, recognizing twenty-four Jinas who, in our part of the world, appear in certain epochs of time and promulgate the same fundamental doctrine (see chapter 2). Scholars consider the last two of these teachers to be historical persons as evidenced by textual records. The twenty-fourth and last teacher of our current era, Mahāvīra ("Great Hero"), lived in the fifth century BCE, and the twenty-third teacher, Pārśvanātha, lived approximately 250 years before him.[2] Prior to their liberation, both Jinas oversaw a fourfold community of mendicant monks and nuns, as well as laymen and laywomen householders.

Mahāvīra was an elder contemporary of the Buddha, and while we do not know if they ever actually met, a Buddhist canonical text, *Sāmaññaphala-sutta*, lists Mahāvīra as one of the *śramaṇa* leaders. This indicates that at least the Buddha knew of Mahāvīra (Jacobi 1879, 1–6; Jaini 2001b, 57–60). *Śramaṇa* ("striver") was a term used for the Buddha, Mahāvīra, and other wandering non-Vedic renunciates in the Ganges plain to differentiate them from Vedic priests and renouncers (*brāhmaṇa*) (Dundas 2002, 16). *Śramaṇa*s rejected the authority of the Vedas and other sacred texts of the *brāhmaṇa*s, their gods, as well as the efficacy of Vedic rituals (Jaini 2001b; Jaini 2001/1979, 2, fn. 2).

The ethical orientation of Jainism seems to emerge hand in hand with its intricate account of living beings. As we detail in chapter 2, the Jain universe is populated by an infinite number of living beings existing in cycles of birth, death, and rebirth who are categorized in myriad ways. These sophisticated classifications indicate an effort to understand what life is and, consequently, what can be violated. Every living being possesses its own core life principle, or *jīva*, that either accumulates or sheds material karma based on activities of the body, speech, and mind. Although the Jain worldview differs considerably from modern biological taxonomies, it nevertheless presents a systematic description of living beings and provides a causal explanation through karma to explain each being's essential qualities, as well as factors of its specific embodiment.

Amid this vibrant universe teeming with a multiplicity of living beings, Mahāvīra centered his teachings on various vows of restraint that we address in chapter 3. The first and foremost of these vows is the restraint of nonviolence, often known by the Sanskrit term *ahiṃsā*. Monks and nuns take these vows fully as "great vows" during an initiation that signifies their rebirth into the houseless existence of a mendicant, while lay Jain householders fulfill them partially as "minor vows" in the context of work, family, and social life. From antiquity to the present, the fourfold community of monks, nuns, laymen, and laywomen have developed a distinct-but-symbiotic relationship (which we describe in chapter 3 particularly and which threads through the book as a whole).

In the early centuries of the Common Era, the Jain community divided into two dominant sects, due to a few key differences, one of which is the proper clothing for a mendicant, from which the sect names derive. The larger Śvetāmbara sect refers to "white-clad" mendicants, and the smaller Digambara, or "sky-clad," sect believes that male mendicants seeking liberation must practice nudity. In contrast to Śvetāmbaras, Digambaras maintain that women cannot become liberated. In addition to these two dominant sects, other subsects also split off throughout history, resulting in a diverse Jain community marked by particular differences in belief or ritual practice (Dundas 2002, 45–51; Jain 2012).[3] In spite of these differences, Jains have remained strongly united on the ethical primacy of nonviolence.

Today, Jainism is a relatively small global community. The World Religions Database (WRD) at Boston University[4] estimates that Jains make up 0.42 percent (5.85 million) of the Indian population, with approximately 285,000 Jains living in diaspora abroad (Johnson and Grim 2020).[5] These numbers almost exclusively reflect laity, rather than mendicants, since the latter would be unlikely to participate in government data collection, and fully ordained mendicants cannot travel by mechanized transport to other countries. Researchers estimate the overall Jain mendicant population in modern India as of 1999—inclusive of all sects—to be approximately three thousand monks and nine thousand nuns (Flügel 2006, 362).

The largest populations of Jains outside of India are in Kenya, the United States, the United Kingdom, and Canada, respectively, and there are smaller communities in other countries (Johnson and Grim 2020). In the United States, the WRD estimates the 2020 population of Jains as ninety-seven thousand,[6] the largest communities being in Northern and Southern California; Chicago, Illinois; Houston, Texas; and the New York–New Jersey region.

In 2014, Jainism was legally designated a distinct "minority religion" by the government of India.[7] Yet, even as a minority community, Jains have significant influence in the country. According to the National Family Health Survey taken in

2015–16, Jains have the highest rates of literacy nationally among both men (97.1%) and women (97.5%) (Ministry of Health and Family Welfare 2016, 63–65), as well as the highest levels of education.[8] Jains are the wealthiest community overall, with nearly three-quarters of the population in the top wealth division (31), resulting in a disproportionately high contribution to government tax revenue and the national charity fund.[9] Jainism has contributed widely to the social, religious, and intellectual history of India, responding to current philosophical debates, producing a vast body of literature, shaping historical trends in arts and architecture (Hegewald 2019), and adapting creative modes of monarchical rule and political participation (Dundas 2007a; Jain 2017).

Unique to this project is the examination of Jain approaches to medicine up to the present day. We provide an overview of Jain attitudes toward medicine in chapter 4, detailing accommodations for ill mendicants even in the earliest strata of the Śvetāmbara canon, followed by an increasing liberalization, including the eventual obligation for mendicants to offer aid to their sick fellow monks and nuns, and the designation of medicine as an acceptable occupation for laity to undertake. Today, Jains have high representation in medical and allied fields, especially in diaspora countries such as the United States. The prevalence of contemporary Jains in medicine, which we describe in chapter 5, provides another motivating factor for our analysis of Jainism and bioethics.

As we explore Jainism in relation to bioethics within part 1, we strive to retain the complexity of evolving concerns, changing terminologies, and textual disagreements over time—between sects and between lay and mendicant views—in order to preserve a richer account of Jainism as a multifaceted philosophical, religious, and historical tradition. In part 2, we also endeavor to represent a diverse community of "Jains" that includes mendicants and laypeople, Jains in India, Jains who migrated abroad, Jains born outside India, and Jains who retain unique regional and linguistic ties to the subcontinent that inform their identity as culturally Jain and/or as practicing Jains. The results of our research reflect these diverse personal, religious, cultural, and professional contexts, providing multiple angles from which to approach Jain interpretations of bioethical issues.

## RELIGION AND BIOETHICS

In bringing the philosophical-religious tradition of Jainism into dialogue with bioethics, it is helpful to consider the various ways in which religion and bioethics have intersected before. By many accounts, bioethics is a modern, Western, secular humanistic discipline that emerged largely in the United States in the late 1960s and early '70s as a means of addressing moral issues in contemporary medicine. Many of these dilemmas arose from advances in science and technology anachronistic to traditional Jain philosophy, religious ideals, and practices. Life-sustaining technologies, for instance, such as the positive pressure ventilator, produced twentieth-century dilemmas surrounding the definition of death and generated questions of resource allocation for bodies that could now survive previously fatal trauma. Additionally, the awareness of egregious healthcare harms required an urgent redress of informed consent principles. The cases that led to this include the Nazi medical experiments of World War II and the forty-year Tuskegee syphilis experiment on African American sharecroppers, wherein researchers failed to provide penicillin to participants after it became a known curative in the 1940s, continuing the study until 1972. Moreover, the burgeoning global pharmaceutical industry necessitated robust international regulations for review and oversight of clinical trials, subject recruitment, and patient protections.

Yet, even in addressing such distinctly modern problems, bioethics as a discipline has been pivotally shaped by enduring philosophical and religious insights that exceed the spheres of science and technology alone. Often overlooked in modern accounts of bioethics is the earliest known reference to "bioethics." Between 1926 and 1927, a German Protestant pastor and ethicist, Fritz Jahr (1895–1953), proposed "Bio-Ethik" as an ethical principle and an interdisciplinary academic discipline needed to explore relationships between the human community and nonhuman living beings (Jahr 1926; Jahr 1927).[10] Jahr looked to sources that articulated responsive relationships between humans, animals, and plants, including many religious narratives and philosophical figures, as well as Darwin's account of evolution, and the physical and psychological similarities between various forms of life assumed by animal research and revealed in plant studies (Goldim 2009, 378; Sass 2014, 221–22).

Based on these, Jahr proposed the "Bioethical Imperative": "Respect every living being in general as an end in itself and treat it, if possible, as such!" (2013, 21).[11] Jahr issued this imperative, which included all living beings, as a critical response to Immanuel Kant's influential concept of the Categorical Imperative that articulated three unconditional moral obligations solely among "rational persons": (a) to act in such a way that the action could become universal law; (b) to treat others as their own end, and not merely as a means; and (c) to respect the self-determination of oneself and others. To reconfigure Kant's commitments beyond "rational persons," Jahr envisioned a moral partnership between humans, animals, and plants that pursued appropriate, though not necessarily equal, consideration of the flourishing of all living beings. Despite some fundamental differences, Jahr's broad understanding of life and expansive moral obligations stemming from it bear significant resemblances with Jain ethics.

It is important to note that Jahr was at least somewhat familiar with religions of India and their ethics, and it is perhaps no coincidence that in his 1927 introduction of the term *bioethics*, he specifically references a religious tradition that seems to be Jainism. He calls it "Yoga":

> The yoga repentant [Jogabüßer] under no circumstances is allowed to live at the cost of co-creatures; above all, he shall under no circumstances kill any animal, and only

> under certain settings enjoy vegetable foods. He has to wear a veil over his mouth in order not to inhale even a small living being; for the same reason he has to filter drinking water and shall not take a bath. (Jahr 2013, 25)

While Jahr seems to consider this position too extreme, he nevertheless aims to transcend the widespread ethical approach driven solely by human interest, in favor of all life.

The second known use of the term *bioethics* came from the American biochemist and oncologist Van Rensselaer Potter (1911–2001), who was, for a considerable period, credited with coining the term in his 1970 article "Bioethics, the Science of Survival"[12] and with founding the field of bioethics. In the text, Potter described bioethics as a new form of interdisciplinary ethics that would integrate biological knowledge and human values, aimed at supporting the survival of the whole ecosystem (Potter 1970, 127–28). He found inspiration for his ideas in the humanities and social sciences, such as the work of the cultural anthropologist Margaret Mead, the philosopher and Jesuit priest Pierre Teilhard de Chardin, and the pragmatists, as well as in the work of the pioneers in environmental ethics, such as Aldo Leopold.[13] In his later publications, Potter expressed disappointment about the overemphasis that modern bioethicists placed on short-term issues, individual needs, and medical concerns, and he reiterated the need for a wider perspective that he designated as "global bioethics," a discipline that would address and correlate medical, environmental, and social issues as well as adopt a long-term approach (Ten Have 2012, 75–77).[14] He later included even religious ethics under the umbrella term *bioethics* (79).

These early visions of bioethics express distinct metaphysical sensibilities inclusive of various life-forms, a future of collective thriving, and the assertion that personal experiences and values are an important part of ethical debate and social development. With a wide-ranging notion of who counts as a moral subject that in several ways resembles Jain ethics, they provide an additional precedent for a Jain engagement with modern bioethics.

As we have highlighted, religious ethics played a formative role in the development of modern bioethics. This means that since its inception as a discipline, bioethics has been shaped by both secular and religious principles. Religious sources were influential even in the case of the more narrow understanding of bioethics as medical bioethics that eventually became predominant. Protestant ethicist Paul Ramsey, Catholic moral theologian Richard A. McCormick, and Jewish theologian Immanuel Jakobovits were but a few of the visible figures who applied their respective traditions' insights on life, death, suffering, and justice to moral issues in medicine. Religious ethicists were key members of early governmental policy committees that issued federal reports and guidelines for human subjects research, forgoing life-sustaining treatment, healthcare access, and the definition of death. Religious authors wrote academic literature[15] and helped initiate organizations that would later become the Kennedy Institute of Ethics at Georgetown University[16] and the Hastings Center in New York.[17]

Non-Western traditions began to engage the field of Western bioethics in the 1990s. The Dalai Lama was a key figure in opening dialogue between Buddhist philosophy of mind and Western scientists in a series of publicized conversations beginning in 1989. Many books exist today on Buddhist social or ecological ethics, but only a few address bioethics, such as Damien Keown's *Buddhism and Bioethics* (1995) or Peter Harvey's *An Introduction to Buddhist Ethics: Foundations, Values and Issues* (2000). Likewise, Hindu bioethics has modest representation, with only a few notable titles: *Hindu Ethics: Purity, Abortion, and Euthanasia* (1989), edited by Harold Coward, Julius Lipner, and Katherine Young; *Dilemmas of Life and Death: Hindu Ethics in North American Context* (1995) and *Hindu Bioethics for the Twenty-first Century* (2003) by S. Cromwell Crawford; and *Magical Progeny, Modern Technology: A Hindu Bioethics of Assisted Reproductive Technology* (2006) by Swasti Bhattacharyya.

While contemporary Jains encounter the same bioethical issues as everyone else, usually as healthcare users and sometimes as providers, there are no books specifically exploring Jainism in relation to Western bioethics. As noted above, this leaves a gap in the fields of bioethics as well as Jain studies. Several writings exist on Jain ethics generally (Bhargava 1968; Jain 1934; Sethia 2004; Sogani 1967; Williams 1963) as well as on Jain ecology (Chapple 2002; Rankin 2018; Rankin 2019) and, to a lesser extent, Jain business ethics (Shah and Rankin 2017). Bioethics, however, is treated minimally in only a few academic articles, book chapters, and online reflections by contemporary lay Jains or Jain studies scholars (these sources are discussed below).

## METHODOLOGY

As authors, our methodology reflects the approach that would have served us well as younger scholars who came to Jain studies by a circuitous route, often seeking to understand Jain philosophy alongside its textual and historical complexity.

In part 1, we explore foundational principles related to bioethics drawn from in-depth analyses of a wide range of Jain primary sources in Sanskrit and Prakrit. We offer a comprehensive examination of the Jain understanding of birth, life, and death, based on the complex and rarely addressed karmic relationship between material bodies and living, immaterial selves. Further, we offer a distinctive investigation of the development of central Jain ethical principles, including nonviolence, that, in contemporary representations, are too often depicted one-dimensionally, divorced from their wider soteriological framework and historical contexts. Lastly, we trace the Jain attitudes to medicine and medical treatment from the early canon up to the medieval period.

In part 2, we provide basic overviews of modern bioethical issues and explore Jain principles of application for these dilemmas. Drawing upon several years of teaching courses in multicultural bioethics at the graduate and undergraduate levels, we define key bioethical terms (e.g., *autonomy, beneficence, nonmaleficence*) and identify key legal precedents, relevant philosophical commitments of other religious communities, and (to a lesser extent) Western normative ethical theories that feature in bioethics debates (e.g., deontology and utilitarianism). Where debates are especially polarized on controversial topics such as abortion or animal research, we map a continuum of ethical positions in order to contextualize contemporary Jain views.

Our research in part 2 is cross-cultural and interdisciplinary, analyzing primary sources in relation to specific bioethical issues as well as scarce contemporary sources on Jainism and bioethics from modern lay Jains, mendicants, and Jain studies scholars. In this portion of the book we also include analyses from two Jain medieval medical treatises—the *Kalyāṇa-kāraka* and *Taṇḍula-vaicārika*—heretofore largely untranslated into English. Further, we investigate how Jain teachings inform the attitudes and practical decisions of contemporary Jain medical professionals, utilizing data from an original international survey we conducted with Jain medical professionals in India, as well as in diaspora communities of North America, Europe, and Africa. The details and demographics of this survey are introduced in chapter 5. This is the first time, to our knowledge, that such a systematic survey on bioethical attitudes and practices has been attempted among Jain medical practitioners. (Readers interested primarily in the Jain principles of application for bioethical issues can move straight to part 2 of the book.)

Our aim is to provide a comprehensive resource for future scholarship that does not simplify Jain philosophy or ethics for the sake of a surface comparison with modern bioethics or a formulation of a fixed code of conduct for bioethical issues, and the arguments we advance throughout the book are primarily descriptive and analytic. While our work is not prescriptive and aims to highlight the complexity of the approaches within the Jain tradition, we do synthesize and summarize key insights of our description and analysis. In part 1, we conclude each chapter by identifying foundational principles related to bioethics that reflect that chapter's multivalent content. Likewise, in part 2, we conclude each chapter by identifying provisional principles of application that emerge from the interface between traditional textual sources and diverse contemporary Jain views related to modern bioethical dilemmas.

## CONSIDERING CONTEMPORARY JAIN VIEWS ON BIOETHICS

There are very few contemporary sources exploring Jainism and bioethics. Because bioethics is a modern phenomenon, it is outside the purview of traditional textual sources. It is also largely outside the realm of Jain mendicants. While some mendicants do offer opinions on social debates and provide guidance to lay Jains, few such sources are widely available. That said, where we have found any relevant mendicant views, we have included them. As a result, the contemporary Jain views presented in part 2 come primarily from lay Jains or Jain studies scholars. Jain studies scholar Christopher Chapple, for instance, has written articles on bioethical themes such as death, synthetic life, and animal research (2010, 2013, 2016a). We also draw upon several other contemporary scholars who have written generally on Jain attitudes toward death and human-animal relations.

Additionally, some literature on bioethics exists from Jain-sponsored conferences or events. These include three international conferences addressing the theme of Jainism and bioethics (in 2012, 2016, and 2017)[18] and an annual conference hosted by the Gyan Sagar Science Foundation exploring Jainism and science.[19] Other helpful sources include Jain-created guidelines for hospital staff in the United States and United Kingdom who encounter Jain patients,[20] reports about a successful political campaign among global Jains to reverse the Indian Supreme Court's decision banning the Jain end-of-life fast known as *sallekhanā* or *saṃthāra* ("SC Stays" 2015), and a nascent selection of Jain-created responses to bioethical issues—often found on online forums—that we utilize throughout part 2. Because of the dearth of contemporary resources, we also designed the aforementioned survey for Jain medical professionals.

## CHAPTER SUMMARIES

Part 1 analyzes doctrinal foundations for bioethics in Jainism and includes four chapters. Following this introduction, chapter 2 examines the fundamental assertions of what "exists" in the Jain understanding of reality. We particularly focus on the relationship between life and nonlife that comprises embodied living beings. We lay out the taxonomy of life-forms by way of explaining the distinctions, similarities, continuities, and entanglements between humans, animals, plants, and the unique Jain description of earth-bodied, water-bodied, fire-bodied, and air-bodied beings. We explore how Jains understand (re)birth, life, aging, and death in a given bodily form in relation to multiple varieties of material karma, a technical topic rarely addressed substantively in Jain studies scholarship, especially scholarship for Western audiences less familiar with karmic frameworks. In this context, we delineate, among other things, the Jain conceptions of pain, sentiency, vitalities, instincts, and the violability of life.

Chapter 3 investigates the complex foundations and the development of the Jain notion of right conduct, particularly in relation to nonviolence. We identify underexplored concepts that form the ethical guidelines of the canonical and postcanonical textual sources, such as nonpossession, passions, intention, and "careful" action. We move beyond the general account of the five Jain vows, locating the vows as one part of the broader soteriological context described in the fourteen stages of decreased karmic bondage and less harmful action, which present an essential theoretical framework for understanding Jain practice among mendicants and laity.

Chapter 4 explores the Jain approaches to illness and medicine. Given that Jainism originated as an ascetic tradition in which mendicants aimed to transcend the body, the central question of this chapter is whether illness is an occurrence that should be transcended through endurance or whether it can/should be treated. Is medical treatment a transgression of mendicant religious commitments or does a healthy body have a function in such a rigorous ascetic context? The chapter draws from diverse primary sources to identify the meaning of physical and mental illness, Jain attitudes toward the medical treatment of mendicants, and the regulations and exceptions regarding who can receive treatment, who can provide it, and what kind of medications they can use.

In part 2, consisting of three chapters, we identify provisional principles of application deduced from multiple sources expressing Jain views of birth, life, and death.

Chapter 5 introduces our 2017–18 survey methodology and Jain respondents' basic demographics. Following this, we look at the Jain understanding of conception, embryology, fetal life, and maternal connection against the wider backdrop of traditional Indian medicine, including two extant medieval Jain medical treatises. We then examine several bioethical issues related to taking/preventing nascent life (abortion, population control, contraception), facilitating nascent life (IVF, cloning, stem cell research), and altering nascent life (sex selection and genomic editing). We outline current Western bioethical terms, precedents, and debates, followed by various Jain perspectives on these issues. We conclude by identifying provisional Jain principles of reproductive ethics that emerge from the analysis.

Chapter 6 first explores the Jain views of surgery, antibiotics, and vaccinations, highlighting the unique Jain concern for living beings beyond the human community. This is followed by a descriptive overview of clinical bioethical issues related to the physician-patient relationship, research trials, and access to care, including Jain responses to these issues. We pay special attention to how autonomy and truth inform Jain views of clinical practice and research obligations to individual patients and advancing medical knowledge. We outline various ways that contemporary Jain medical professionals maintain their Jain identity alongside competing values of science and society, and conclude with a focused examination of Jain views on using animals for biomedical studies. As before, we close out the chapter by summarizing tentative principles for patient approaches to bioethics and clinical medical practice.

Chapter 7 explores the critical transition of death as an essential ethical moment in the Jain account of rebirth or liberation. Death's certainty figures prominently in Jain texts, which offer detailed descriptions of various kinds of death, alongside guidelines for achieving the best death possible. In this chapter we explore ongoing bioethical debates over defining death in modern medicine, its relation to organ donation, and key legal decisions related to refusing life-sustaining treatment and other advance directives. We introduce the Jain practice of voluntary death, exploring its compatibility with and/or distinction from various end-of-life options with varying legal standings globally, including suicide, euthanasia, physician aid-in-dying, terminal sedation, and the voluntary refusal of food and fluids. To close, we identify Jain values that inform a principled approach to death.

The book ends with an epilogue in which we revisit key themes, aims, and methods, highlighting the inherent multiplicity of "Jain" views and identifying possible future areas of research we hope this work might contribute to.

## JAINISM AND BIOETHICS: PERSPECTIVES OF A "CUMULATIVE TRADITION"

We do not advance a single Jain view of bioethics in this book. On the contrary, we have tried to account for the complexity of Jainism as an evolving philosophical system, ethical path, and living religious tradition. Jain studies scholar John Cort has previously argued that Jainism should not be viewed as a set of fixed doctrines across time, but rather as "the sum total of the practices and beliefs of all the people who called themselves Jain throughout the centuries," akin to what Wilfred Cantwell Smith has termed "cumulative tradition" (Wiley 2002, 65).

In line with this, any Jain view of bioethics must contend with fluid foundational principles and varied, open-ended modes of application. As noted above, we have tried to account for a diverse community of Jains from antiquity to the present and in particular historical moments and geographic locales: mendicant and lay Jains, those living in India and those living abroad, distinct diaspora generations, those with diverse sectarian commitments, and those who are professionally employed in medical fields and those who are not, among many other distinctions.

Taking in these multiple views, however, does not mean that we can say nothing overall about Jainism and bioethics. The foundational principles and principles of application we have identified capture distinctive themes, philosophical doctrines, historical and contemporary concerns, and ethical orientations that are uniquely Jain. We hope this work will provide a framework for further scholarship and clinical discourses in many ethical arenas through which to bring Jainism and Jains into critical conversation.

2

# Life, Nonlife, and Karma

In this chapter, we introduce the Jain understanding of life as it exists in and interacts with the various aspects of the nonliving reality. Since the karmically produced, material body is considered to be nonliving and perishable, while life itself is eternal, understanding this interaction is essential for determining the principles for Jain bioethics. We first explore the foundations of Jain cosmology and metaphysics, after which we closely examine the doctrine of karma. We then outline the various classifications of living beings, as well as the Jain conceptions of birth, aging, death, rebirth, and liberation. We conclude the chapter by identifying four foundational principles when considering what exists according to the Jain view of reality.

## THE JAIN COSMOS

The interactions between the living and nonliving reality all take place in the Jain cosmos (*loka-ākāśa*, "space with worlds"). The cosmos is understood to be uncreated and eternal, without temporal beginning or end. While it is deemed to be very large, its specific shape indicates that it has a finite size. Within their canonical texts, Jains imagined the cosmos as being narrow in the middle and wide at the top and bottom.[1] As the Jain cosmological teachings became more complex, their depictions of the cosmos also became increasingly elaborate, and the cosmos commonly came to be rendered in the shape of a human being (*loka-puruṣa*), narrow at the waist, with legs standing wide apart and arms bent at the elbows, resting at the hips (see figure 1).[2]

Even though they are highly technical, the Jain doctrines of the cosmos are importantly intertwined with the Jain soteriology, which is why they are well known and widely circulated not only among Jain mendicants but also in the lay circles.[3] In fact, reflecting on the nature of the cosmos is taken to be an important spiritual practice for all Jains.[4] Since there is order in the cosmos, one can use the

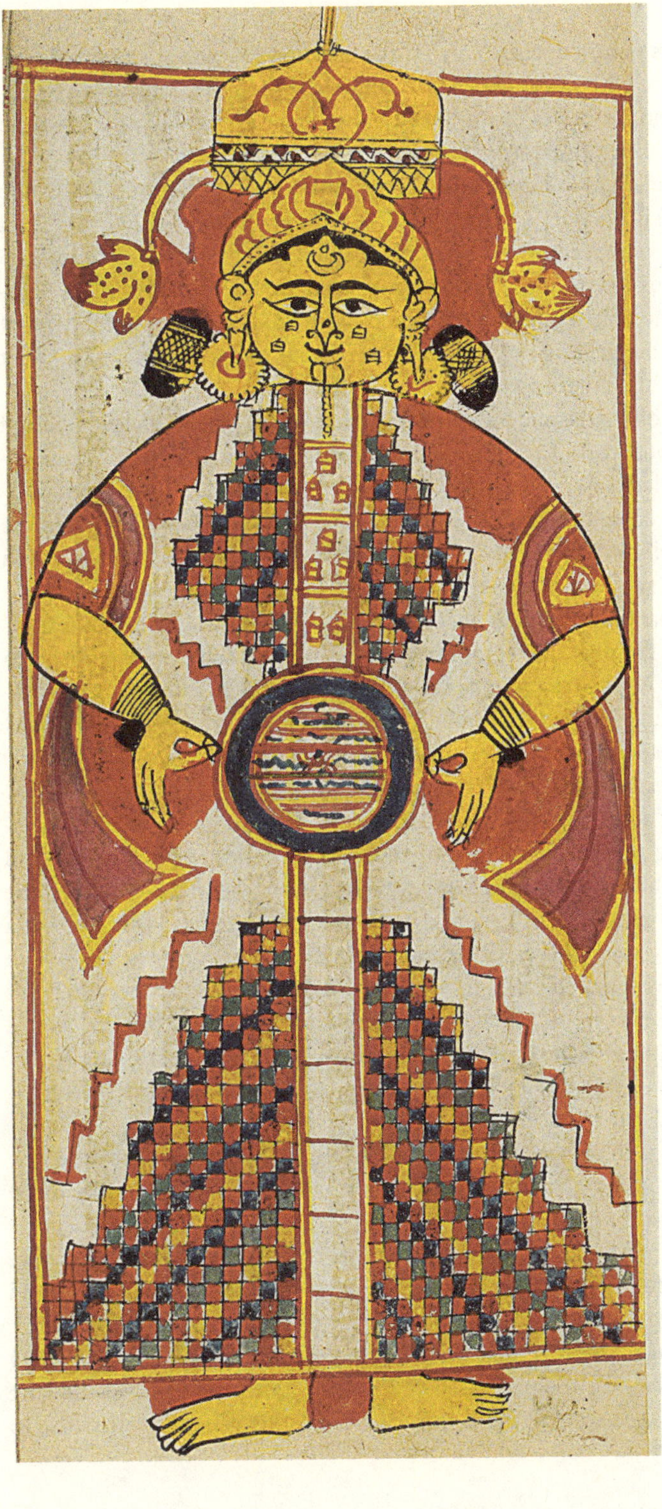

FIGURE 1.
Depiction of the Jain cosmos as a human being, from a seventeenth-century manuscript of Śrīcandrasūri's *Saṃgrahaṇī-ratna* (Pkt. *Saṃghayaṇa-rayaṇa*), composed in Prakrit with a Gujarati commentary. This twelfth-century text explains the structure of the cosmos and the living beings that occupy it, and the manuscript contains a large number of rich visual representations of the various aspects of the cosmos. Credit: British Library.

knowledge about its nature to anticipate future situations as well as carve out a life course in accordance with what one deems valuable, and it is only by understanding the structure and processes of the cosmos that one can hope to take the right steps on the path to liberation (see chapter 3).

The Jain cosmos is said to be enclosed in an infinitely vast and empty acosmic space (*aloka-ākāśa*) but is itself completely filled with living and nonliving entities (US 36.2). Jains not only recognize a great diversity of living entities, but they also have a remarkably expansive understanding of what "counts" as life and is therefore considered inviolable. Different embodied life-forms exist in specific parts of the cosmos, which means that some of them are likely to encounter and interact with one another while others are not.

The upper body of the cosmic human being, shaped somewhat like an inverted pyramid, is the upper world (*ūrdhva-loka*) that consists of a number of heavenly realms and is populated by heavenly beings or gods (*deva*). The lower, pyramid-shaped part of the cosmic human is the lower world (*adho-loka*), which is the abode of various hell-beings (*nāraka*).[5] The world in between is the middle world (*madhya-loka*), the smallest one of the three. It is often visually represented as a circle in the navel part of the cosmic being, even though it is described as a horizontally positioned flat disk that contains a central island called the Jambū-dvīpa (Island of the Rose-Apple Tree). This island is surrounded by numerous concentric oceans and islands, and while animals (*tiryañc*, "going horizontally") can exist throughout the whole of the middle world, human beings (*manuṣya*) occupy only two-and-a-half innermost islands (TS 3.7–9, TS[Śv] 3.14[6]).

This small living space highlights how scarce the human presence in the cosmos is, underlining the exceptionality of the human condition, which we will return to below.[7] While the abode of human beings is by far the most limited, the living regions of animals, hell-beings, and heavenly beings are also restricted to a central, cylindrically shaped area called the mobile channel (*trasa-nāḍī*), which reaches from the lowest hell to the highest heaven. In contrast to this, certain types of living beings can exist in all parts of the cosmos, including beyond the central cylinder. These are plant- (*vanaspati-kāyika*), earth- (*pṛthvī-kāyika*), water- (*āpo-kāyika*), fire- (*tejo-kāyika*), and air-bodied beings (*vāyu-kāyika*), which are commonly classified under the fourth category together with animals.

Some living beings in the cosmos are easily recognizable, while others occupy subtle and elusive bodily forms. In accordance with this, the *Ācārāṅga-sūtra* (Pkt. *Āyāraṃga-sutta*),[8] a Śvetāmbara canonical text, describes Mahāvīra's practice of carefully examining the surroundings in order to prevent causing harm to any, even minute, life-forms whose animacy may not be apparent, such as mold (*panaka*), seeds (*bīja*), (minute) plants (*harita*),[9] as well as earth-, water-, fire-, and air-bodied beings. The text states that Māhāvīra's realization of their being alive came after observing them closely, and consequently, he avoided injuring them (ĀS 1.8.1.11–12). As we will discuss in chapter 3, this general instruction to pay attention to the minutest of living beings gradually evolved into detailed rules for mendicants, including exercising great care when performing daily activities (*samiti*) as well as a regular inspection of clothes and implements for any small life-forms.

The ethical aspiration not to harm the abundant life that exists in the cosmos represents one of the core endeavors constituting the Jain path to liberation. As will be explained in detail in chapter 3, Jain practitioners realized that violence caused to other living beings is in fact violence caused to oneself, preventing one from attaining the ultimate goal of the religious path. This not only resulted in restrictive practical rules for mendicants and laity, such as those mentioned above, but also contributed to the development of complex metaphysical doctrines (cf. Johnson 2014, 135). Jains endeavored to delineate the boundary between life and nonlife with meticulous care, provide detailed taxonomies of life-forms, and thoroughly understand how they are born, live, and die.

## THE "REALS"

Jain texts often put forward the distinction between the living and the nonliving in the context of the broader outlines and considerations of that which exists or is real. A common method of organizing reality is to list the so-called "reals" (*tattva*), or fundamental categories, of which texts frequently enumerate seven or nine. They include (1) living entities (*jīva*); (2) nonliving entities (*ajīva*); (3–6) the influx (*āsrava*), bondage (*bandha*), stoppage (*saṃvara*), and removal (*nirjarā*) of karma; (7) liberation from the karmic cycles of rebirth (*mokṣa*); and sometimes (8–9) nonmeritorious types (*pāpa-prakṛti*) and meritorious types (*puṇya-prakṛti*) of karma.[10] While the Śvetāmbara canonical texts tend to record nine "reals,"[11] a commonly mentioned reference for the list of "reals" is the *Tattvārtha-sūtra* 1.4 in which Umāsvāti (c. fourth century CE) lists seven of them. His Digambara commentator Pūjyāpada (sixth century) explains that the nonmeritorious and meritorious types of karma are already implied in karmic influx and bondage (SSi 1.4§19).[12] John Cort suggests that the exclusion or inclusion of the last two "reals" may relate to disagreements with regard to the relative moral value of the meritorious types of karma. He writes:

> If *puṇya* and *pāp* are considered only within the framework of karmic bondage, then they are viewed in a wholly negative light. If they are considered as universal principles independent of their classification under bondage, then action that is karmically binding yet morally valuable is not viewed so negatively. In other words, an ontology of just seven *tattvas* accords value only to the *mokṣa-mārg* goal of liberation from the world by eliminating all karmic bondage; whereas an ontology of nine *tattvas* allows room for positive valuation of action within the world by distinguishing among forms of karmic bondage, and therefore accords some importance to wellbeing. (2001a, 192)

We will be returning to this distinction between action that is aimed at the ultimate goal of liberation and action that is directed at well-being in the next chapters of the book.

While the list of "reals" is primarily concerned with metaphysical principles and processes, it came to be associated with epistemological, ethical, practical, and soteriological considerations by connecting them with the triple path to liberation or the so-called "Three Jewels" (*ratna-traya*): right worldview (*samyag-darśana*), right knowledge (*samyag-jñāna*), and right conduct (*samyak-cāritra*) (cf. Ohira 1982, 56).[13] From the late canonical period onward, the "reals" were defined as the content of the right worldview (Ohira 1982, 56).[14] Right knowledge came to include various means of attaining valid knowledge about the "reals." Right conduct, to which is sometimes added asceticism (*tapas*),[15] relates to the ethical and practical aspects of the path that are aligned with the first two "jewels," which we will discuss in detail in chapter 3.

Connected with the triple path to liberation, the list of "reals" indicates that in philosophical and practical respects, living and nonliving entities interact with one another and remain intractably bound together in the world of embodied living beings. The rest of the present chapter will explore the complexities of this relationship, particularly concerning the living entities and karma.

## LIVING AND NONLIVING ENTITIES

The first two "reals" represent a basic categorization of everything that exists, recognizing that some things that exist are alive while others are not.[16] The "reals" that are listed after this initial statement of fundamental ontological dualism represent various aspects of the operation of nonliving karma, including its complete elimination and the *jīva*'s consequent attainment of liberation. Knowledge of metaphysics is therefore placed at the very foundation of the soteriological path.[17]

### *Structure and Dynamics of Existents*

Jains consider everything that exists to be expressed through substances (*dravya*) and their qualifiers.[18] They posit a multiplicity of eternal substances, five kinds of which are considered nonliving and one kind of which is living. The living kind of substance is called *jīva* or *ātman*, often translated as the self, living substance, living entity, or soul.[19] Nonliving kinds of substances include matter (*pudgala*),[20] medium of motion (*dharma*), medium of rest (*adharma*), space (*ākāśa*), and, according to some Jain authors, time (*kāla*).[21] Among these six living and nonliving kinds of substances, Jains regard space, which is single in number, as the only one that is infinite. The media of motion and rest are two single substances that enable entities to move and come to a stop, and their size, which is vast yet finite, determines the boundary between the above-mentioned finite cosmic part of space and the infinite acosmic part that stretches beyond it. The other substances, including an infinite number of *jīvas*, exist only inside the boundary of the cosmic space.

All substances, no matter what type, have the same basic structure.[22] They all possesses essential qualities (*guṇa*), some of which are unique to each kind of substance and represent criteria by which substances can be differentiated from one another. All the qualities undergo continuous, momentary, beginningless, and endless modifications in the form of a series of modes (*paryāya*).

A simple example of this may be to consider the material substance of a leaf changing in its quality of color from green to red to yellow to brown, which represent its modes. Like the leaf that persists through its various changes, all entities in the Jain conception of reality are understood to be permanent in one aspect and changing in another. They are permanent when considered from the perspective of the substance and its qualities, and they are changing when considered from the perspective of the modes. This emphasis on taking into account a multiplicity of perspectives when exploring an object is present already in the canonical period,[23] and it gradually develops into sophisticated metaphysical, epistemological, and logical doctrines of non-one-sidedness (*anekānta-vāda*). These include (1) *nikṣepa-vāda* and *naya-vāda*, or the doctrines of various standpoints (*nikṣepa*)[24] and viewpoints (*naya*) from which an object can be considered; and (2) *syād-vāda*,[25] or the doctrine of conditional assertion, which expresses that something exists in a specific way "in some respect" (*syāt*), and is formalized in the list of seven kinds of predication (*sapta-bhaṅgī*) that can be made about an object (Balcerowicz 2001; Balcerowicz 2003; Jaini 2001/1979, 90–97; Koller 2000; Long 2009, 141–54; Matilal 1981).[26]

With these doctrines, Jains carved out a space for themselves in the South Asian philosophical arena. The non-one-sided approach allowed them to illuminate the competing doctrines that did not follow their methodology as one-sided (*ekānta*) and only partially true, and to distinguish their own doctrines from them (Bajželj 2020).

In line with this, it is important to note that the non-one-sided approach traditionally does not represent a form of philosophical pluralism or relativism, since it is clear that for Jains their own view of reality is absolutely, and not only relatively, true. As we will see below, a perfectly developed comprehension of reality involves a complete capturing of all existing objects in their infinite complexity, which represents absolute truth that transcends all partial perspectives. Truth is relative and confined to its specific contextual parameters only for a limited cognizer, and taking a limited truth to be the whole truth is what constitutes a wrong view (*mithyā-dṛṣṭi*). In line with this, the doctrines of non-one-sidedness do not correspond to intellectual nonviolence, as some have suggested. Jain texts unambiguously promote their doctrines as the only truth and usually do not spare their opponents when engaging with them, even while recognizing that they too put forth comprehensive philosophical systems (Cort 2000; Johnson 1995b; cf. Barbato 2017).

### *The Relationship between Living and Nonliving Entities*

Jains deem all *jīva*s that we encounter in our lives to be embodied, and it is in the embodied condition that their non-one-sidedness is commonly referred to.[27] Each *jīva*, which is a living substance, inhabits a body (*kāya* or *śarīra*) that is a material and therefore nonliving substance. This means that embodied beings are understood to be living in some respect and nonliving in another.

What, then, is the mark by which life can be detected and distinguished from nonlife? In his *Tattvārtha-sūtra*, Umāsvāti describes the active use (*upayoga*) of consciousness as the defining characteristic of the *jīva* (TS 2.8; Soni 2007). In fact, Jains consider consciousness to be an essential and inalienable quality of all *jīva*s, which means that no *jīva* can ever lose conscious awareness no matter what its state or material form. In his Digambara commentary to the *Tattvārtha-sūtra*, Akalaṅka (eighth century) describes it as the beginningless inherent nature (*svabhāva*) of the self (*ātman*), in the same way that gold has its inherent nature that persists through its various modifications into a bracelet, a ring, or some other object (TVā 2.8.1).

Consciousness operates in two aspects: (1) perception (*darśana*) and (2) knowledge (*jñāna*). The two other essential qualities that are unique to a *jīva* are (3) energy (*vīrya*) and (4) bliss (*sukha*), with the former animating different levels of perception and knowledge and the latter representing the degree to which a *jīva*'s desire is self-contained (*svabhāva-sthita*) rather than grasping at external objects (Jaini 2001/1979, 104–5). This basic structure indicates that all *jīva*s are essentially equal in their qualities of and capacity for perception/knowledge, energy, and bliss, varying only in the modal aspect of each quality.[28] These inherent qualities of *jīva*s, according to Jainism, therefore define life and distinguish it from all nonlife, including the body.

As a way of highlighting the *jīva*'s complex relation to nonlife, Pūjyapāda instructively describes four different kinds of earth in his *Sarvārtha-siddhi*. The first kind is earth as *nonliving material* (*pṛthivī*), which is devoid of consciousness. This is just matter and is not presently associated with a *jīva*. The second kind is earth as a *body* (*pṛthivī-kāya*) that has been abandoned by the *jīva* present in it, similar to the dead body of a human being. The third is earth as an *embodied being* (*pṛthivī-kāyika*), which is a *jīva* that has earth for its body and presently occupies it. The fourth is earth-*jīva* (*pṛthivī-jīva*), a *jīva* that has discarded its previous bodily form and is in transit toward a new earth body based on past karma (SSi 2.13§286).

The mention of these four types of earth is significant, because it means that not everything material that a Jain practitioner encounters is violable, but also that identifying what is violable can be challenging. The first two kinds of earth,

earth as matter and discarded earth-body, are not conscious (*acetana*), not living, and, therefore, cannot be violated. The fourth kind, earth-*jīva* in transit, is also considered nonviolable, since it does not yet occupy a gross material body,[29] the only form in which an immaterial entity can experience harm. Out of the four, only the third kind of earth, a *jīva* that presently occupies an earth body, is violable (Wiley 2002, 39–40). The case of these four types of earth is particularly suggestive, since it is much more difficult to differentiate between living and dead earth than, for example, between a living and a dead body of a human, insect, or flower. It draws attention to the fact that *jīva*s in bodily forms that are difficult to distinguish from material forms that may not or no longer house a *jīva* can easily be unrecognizable as living beings, and are thus more vulnerable to violation.

### *Inhabiting a Succession of Bodies*

In the case of *jīva*s that are presently embodied, the duality between life and nonlife is also somewhat misleading because, even though essentially different from it, the *jīva* cannot really be separated from the body until the attainment of liberation. Pūjyapāda compares the relationship between a *jīva* and the body that it occupies to a mixture of silver and gold. Just as the two metals remain distinguished by their color, and so on, even though they are combined together, so can the *jīva* be differentiated from the body by its property of consciousness even when in bondage (*bandha*) (SSi 2.8§271). Here, Pūjyapāda alludes to one of the central facets of the Jain doctrine, namely, that the occupation of bodies is an entrapment. This condition has no beginning and possibly no end,[30] unless an individual rigorously adheres to an ascetic life of nonviolence, including the purification of bodily, verbal, and mental activities (described in greater detail in chapter 3). The continuity of the entrapment is considered to be uninterrupted, since upon death in one particular body, a *jīva*—as will be detailed below—almost instantaneously migrates to another body, and is enclosed by subtle bodily forms even during the migration. A *jīva* successively occupies a multiplicity of bodies, and even though particular embodiments form a continuum, they are all necessarily impermanent, because every occupied body—while real and significant in the journey of each *jīva*—is transitory in nature.

In his twelfth-century *Triṣaṣṭiśalākāpuruṣa-caritra*, Hemacandra, a Śvetāmbara Jain mendicant leader and polymath, compares the migrations of *jīva*s between bodies to the experience of traveling, with bodies representing temporary stops for the travelers: "Not even the body is one's own. There is nothing but a halt in one place of those who have come here from different places, like that of birds in a tree. Then people go elsewhere to different places, like travelers who have slept in one place at night departing at dawn" (TC 2.1.61–62, trans. Johnson). Throughout their migrating journeys, *jīva*s are then merely borrowing bodies—places to temporarily inhabit. As indicated above, these bodies that the *jīva*s occupy are of a wide variety, and the connection between a *jīva* and the specific body it inhabits is not arbitrary. Jain philosophy explains each particular embodiment through the doctrine of karma.

## THE CAUSE AND EFFECT OF KARMIC MATTER

The complex and remarkably detailed Jain doctrine of karma far exceeds any popular notion of "what goes around comes around" determinism.[31] It is essential for understanding how Jains view the bond between bodies and *jīva*s; the events of birth, life, and death; and the temporal, physical, and moral entanglements between living beings; as well as the motivations and goals of Jain ethics. As such, it is central for the exploration of Jain bioethics. Jains understand the process of migration from one birth to another to be driven and operated by karma that each *jīva* accumulates throughout its lives. This karmic deposit determines the nature of all of its embodied existences and defines other aspects of its bondage in the cycle of rebirths (*saṃsāra*). This means that knowledge about karmic processes provides insight into the intricate mechanism of the entrapment, one's specific circumstances in it, and the possible methods of transcending them.

### *Karma as Material*

Among the religious traditions of India, Jainism is rare in understanding karma to be material.[32] However, only a portion of matter is deemed to be karmic. The substance of matter exists throughout the entire cosmos, and its most basic units are indivisible particles (*aṇu*), which like *jīva*s also possess their own set of essential qualities. For particles, these qualities are color (*varṇa*), taste (*rasa*), smell (*gandha*), and touch (*sparśa*). The quality of touch constantly undergoes modal change in the different degrees of dryness (*rūkṣatva*) and viscosity (*snigdhatva*). The greater the degree to which particles differ in their quality of touch, the stronger the attraction between them. For example, a very dry and a very viscous particle will be drawn to each other, whereas two very dry particles will repel each other. This dynamic causes the material particles to continuously integrate and disintegrate, and results in the formation of numerous kinds of material compounds or aggregates (*skandha*) (TS 5.23–27, TS$^{Dig}$ 5.33–36[33]). Some very subtle types of aggregates are capable of interacting with *jīva*s, and in accordance with this, one of the Jain classifications divides them into two categories: (1) those that are karmically bondable (*yogya*), meaning being able to bind to the *jīva*; and (2) those that are not bondable (*aprayogya*) (PS 2.76).[34]

How does this interaction between material aggregates and *jīva*s occur? It is the bodily, verbal, and mental activities of embodied *jīva*s themselves that trigger the matter to flow to them. Some of this matter is karmically bondable aggregates (Wiley 2003, 338–39). Pūjyapāda compares the channeling function (*praṇālikā*) of the activities through which karma flows to a *jīva* to streams by means of which water flows into a lake (SSi 6.2§612).[35] However, as Umāsvāti states, it is passions (*kaṣāya*) that fasten these inflowing karmic aggregates to a *jīva:* "Because of the state of having passions (*sakaṣāyatva*), the *jīva* grasps the bondable (*yogya*) material substances (*pudgala*) of karma. This is bondage (*bandha*)" ($TS^{Dig}$ 8.2;[36] Schubring 2000/1962, 174).[37]

While earlier Jain texts place particular emphasis on the passions of aversion (*dveṣa*) and attachment (*rāga*),[38] the classification of passions gradually becomes more detailed and systematized, with anger (*krodha*) and pride (*māna*) listed as two kinds of aversion, and deceitfulness (*māyā*) and greed (*lobha*) as two kinds of attachment, each having four subtypes in accordance with the degree of their intensity.[39] If *jīva*s engage in bodily, verbal, and mental activities that are guided by any one or a combination of these passions, the attracted karma is firmly bound to them for a long time (*sāmparāyika*), constituting the constricting bond between *jīva*s and matter and strengthening the bondage in *saṃsāra*.[40] Accordingly, the *Daśavaikālika-sūtra*[41] describes the four passions as watering the roots (of the tree) of rebirth (*punar-bhava*) (DVS 8.39).

As will be explained in detail in chapter 3, in the absence of passions, matter is drawn to a *jīva* but does not attach to it, producing short-term karmic bondage (*īryāpatha*) (Jaini 2001/1979, 112–13; Schubring 2000/1962, 174). A passionless *jīva*, says Akalaṅka, is like a dry wall to which nothing sticks (TVā 6.4.7). Indicating that passions, on the other hand, act like glue, Akalaṅka compares karma that gets attracted to a passion-driven *jīva* to dust attaching to a wet cloth, which also accentuates the idea that karma is a polluting agent (TVā 6.2.5; Glasenapp 1999/1925, 184–85).[42] In this way, a *jīva* surrounds itself, as Hemacandra states, "by self-made snares of karma, like a spider with webs made from its own saliva" (TC 2.1.53, trans. Johnson). Walther Schubring points out that matter is not yet karmic while being attracted to the *jīva*. Only once it penetrates the *jīva* does it attain karmic character. "All other matter," Schubring states, "pertains to the soul but externally" (2000/1962, 173).[43]

Jain philosophers mostly maintain that no one can affect another person's karma, which means that everybody is solely responsible for the karma they have accumulated (Jaini 2010b, 136–37). This, however, does not mean that practices contrary to this idea did not develop within Jainism, and Cort records a number of instances based on inscriptions, texts, rituals, and his fieldwork that demonstrate the presence of the idea of karmic transfer within the tradition. Common examples are donations of images, donations for manuscript copies, and temple constructions, accompanied by information about the persons for whose welfare they are intended.[44] Even some mendicant leaders, such as Devendrasūri, the second leader of the Śvetāmbara Mūrtipūjaka Tapā Gaccha,[45] and the great Tapā Gaccha philosopher Mahopādhyāya Yaśovijaya, are shown to have promoted these ideas, which indicates that they did not develop only in lay circles and in isolation from mendicancy. One of the examples that Cort mentions in support of his argument is the story of King Śrīpāla and his wife Mayaṇāsundarī, in which Mayaṇāsundarī uses the merit accumulated through worship[46] to cure her husband and a community of seven hundred of leprosy by pouring water that she used for worship over them (2003).[47] While the notion of karmic transfer was clearly not absent from the Jain tradition, the predominant methods of influencing one's own karma prescribed by the doctrine have been arduous practices of restraint and asceticism. These will be discussed in detail in chapter 3.

### *Kinds of Karma*

Bondable material aggregates that are ready to interact with a *jīva* exist in an undifferentiated state while still unattached, but once interaction with a *jīva* occurs, they modify into specific kinds of karma (Jaini 2001/1979, 112).[48] Jain texts distinguish 148 kinds (*uttara-prakṛti*) of karmic matter that bind *jīvas*, with their names indicating the sorts of effects they produce. Different types of karma are directly related to the types of activities that attracted karmic matter in the first place, reflecting both the type of activity (bodily, verbal, mental) and its nature (meritorious or nonmeritorious) (Jaini 2001/1979, 113, 115; Schubring 2000/1962, 292–93).[49] Jain texts classify them into two main groups. The first group—called *ghātiyā*—describes four kinds of karma that are *destructive* of the four essential qualities of the *jīva*. The second group—called *aghātiyā*—includes four kinds of karma that are *nondestructive* to the *jīva*, but instead determine the kinds of embodiments the *jīva* will experience.[50] These two groups together represent the eight main kinds (*mūla-prakṛti*) of karma, described in detail below (GKK 7–9).[51]

*Destructive Karma.* As indicated above, destructive types of karma are considered "destructive" because they weaken the operation of *jīvas*, preventing the total and potentially infinite manifestation of their essential qualities. They are divided in accordance with the quality of the *jīva* they impede: (1) perception-obscuring (*darśana-āvaraṇīya*), (2) knowledge-obscuring (*jñāna-āvaraṇīya*), (3) energy-obstructing (*vīrya-antarāya*), and (4) bliss-defiling (*mohanīya*)[52] types of karma (Glasenapp 1942/1915, 6–11, 18–19; Jaini 2001/1979, 117–23). We will address the relation between the qualities of the *jīva* and their respective destructive karmas in turn.

Perception- and knowledge-obscuring karmas inhibit the arising of omniscience or perfect knowledge (*kevala-jñāna*) of every existing substance and all of its infinite modes, which is an innate capacity of *jīvas*.[53] This form of knowledge is a precondition for release from the cycle of rebirths, and the people who attain it are called *kevalins*, a category that includes the Jinas. The destructive karmas affect the changing modes of the quality of consciousness and consequently determine how "conscious" each living being is. While all living beings are equal from the perspective of possessing consciousness, since consciousness is not an alienable characteristic, as indicated above, they differ from the perspective of the degree of its modal manifestation. For example, depending on how much knowledge- and perception-obscuring karma is active, the quality of consciousness of some embodied beings, such as plants, is heavily impaired, while it is much more operative in some other living beings, such as humans or animals that possess a mind (see "Classification of Living Beings" below).

Like the quality of consciousness, the quality of energy cannot be completely terminated by karma. It can, however, be severely diminished by it, and it is the weakening of the energy-quality that is instrumental for karmic influx. Helmuth von Glasenapp explains that in its restricted condition, the energy-quality operates through material media in the form of the body, the organ of speech, and the mind, producing activities (*yoga*) that we mentioned above. These three kinds of activities bring about vibrations (*parispanda*) of the space-points of the *jīva* or the self (*ātma-pradeśa*).[54] As noted above, passions cause karma to bind, but it is these vibrations produced by the bodily, verbal, and mental activities of *jīva*s that cause karmic influx in the first place (Glasenapp 1942/1915, 45; Jaini 2001/1979, 112; Wiley 2000a, 42; cf. Soni 2016). Furthermore, because the energy-quality powers perception and knowledge, these two qualities function less effectively when energy is obstructed by karma. In line with this, Wiley mentions that apart from impeding physical energy and willpower, the energy-obstructing karma inhibits mental powers and concentration (2012, 190). Energy-obstructing karma also hinders generosity to others, accepting gifts, and enjoyment of things that can be taken once (such as food or drink)[55] or repeatedly (such as a dwelling or clothes) (Glasenapp 1942/1915, 18–19).

Unlike karma's partial impact upon the other three qualities, bliss is the only quality of *jīva*s that can undergo true defilement (Jaini 2001/1979, 117). Jaini notes that this transformation (*vibhāva-pariṇāma*) of the quality of bliss represents a proper change of state, similarly to the transformation of a liquid state into a solid state (2001a, 137).[56] It is important to note that bliss is not a pleasant sensory or mental feeling, since both senses and the mind are material as will be discussed in detail below. Moreover, pleasant feelings are a product of nondestructive feeling-producing karma. Instead, in its pure manifestation bliss represents precisely independence from all the various material media of experience like all the other essential qualities, and refers to a state of self-contained desire that is not grasping at things "out there," as mentioned above (137). In contrast to this, bliss-defiling karmic matter results in delusion (*moha*) and passions (*kaṣāya*).[57] It is accordingly divided into two types: (1) worldview-deluding (*darśana-mohanīya*) and conduct-deluding (*cāritra-mohanīya*). These factors enact a cycle of karmic capture wherein worldview-deluding karma hinders right worldview of the true nature of reality (*samyag-darśana*), which attracts more worldview-deluding karma, sustaining a wrong view of reality (*mithyātva*). Conduct-deluding karma results in nonobservance of right conduct (*samyak-cāritra*), which, in turn, attracts more conduct-deluding karma, leading to further damaging actions. Passions represent a key factor in karmic bondage, so removing the karma that produces them is essential on the path to liberation, as will be detailed in chapter 3.

According to the Jain doctrine of destructive karma, each embodied living being is, therefore, enlivened by a unique, authoritative *jīva* whose inherent qualities are always present and operational. These qualities are obscured to various degrees, but never permanently so. This means that a snail is similar to other living beings in that it houses a *jīva*; it is also radically singular since the *jīva* is characterized by, among other things, perpetually fluctuating degrees of perception, knowledge, energy, and bliss conditioned by the ongoing karmic dynamics. As will be demonstrated below, the levels to which the qualities of living beings are polluted by the destructive kinds of karma provide the basis for the Jain classification of living beings as well as their hierarchical categorization.

*Nondestructive Karma.* Whereas destructive karma affects the inherent qualities of *jīvas*, nondestructive karma determines the characteristics of their embodiments. Nondestructive karma is also subdivided into four types: (1) name-determining karma (*nāma-karman*),[58] (2) longevity-determining karma (*āyu-karman*), (3) status-determining karma (*gotra-karman*),[59] and feeling-determining karma (*vedanīya-karman*)[60] (Glasenapp 1942/1915, 8, 11–18; Jaini 2001/1979, 124–27).[61] We will describe each of these types here.

Name-determining karma, which is subdivided into ninety-three different kinds, determines into which birth state (*gati*) a *jīva* will be born, as well as the subclass (*jāti*) of the birth state, and each *jīva*'s particular body (*śarīra*) for every embodied existence. According to Jain texts, there are 8,400,000 possible birth states,[62] which fall into four main groups that were mentioned above in the section on the cosmos: (1) humans; (2) heavenly beings; (3) hell-beings; and (4) a group of beings that includes animals, plants, and earth-bodied, water-bodied, fire-bodied, and air-bodied beings (SSi 8.23§778; Glasenapp 1942/1915, 11). By determining the specific bodies that the *jīvas* occupy, name-determining karma defines their particular sense-faculties, the specific ways in which their bodily parts are formed, their mobility, and so forth.

Apart from the principal gross physical body (*audārika-śarīra*), which is unique to humans and living beings with one to five senses, name-determining karma generates other kinds of bodies as well. The luminous body (*taijasa-śarīra*) contains fiery matter, and its function is to sustain the temperature of living beings and digest food for the gross physical body.[63] The karmic body (*kārmaṇa-śarīra*) represents all the subtle karmic matter that adheres to *jīvas*. Glasenapp highlights that this body "changes every moment, because new *karman* is continually assimilated by the soul and the already existing one is consumed" (1942/1915, 12; TVā 2.36.17). It is through this body, explains Akalaṅka, that all the other bodies are formed (TVā 2.36.12). There are an additional two bodies that may be formed, namely the transformational body (*vaikriya-śarīra*), which can perform various supernatural functions,[64] and the translocational body (*āhāraka-śarīra*), which allows humans to travel to those places in the cosmos where Jinas teach, while leaving the gross physical body behind (PS 2.79; TS$^{Dig}$ 2.36; Glasenapp 1942/1915, 12). Of these various bodies, the gross physical body is the least subtle and the karmic body is the most subtle, with subtlety being related to the density of material units (TS$^{Dig}$ 2.37–39)[65] (Glasenapp 1942/1915, 12; Schubring 2000/1962, 139; Tatia 2010, 287–88). Umāsvāti states that all living beings trapped in *saṃsāra* have the karmic and the luminous body (TS$^{Dig}$ 2.42).[66] While most Jain authors agree that the connection between a *jīva* and its karmic and luminous bodies is beginningless, the fifth-century *Tattvārtha-bhāṣya* 2.43 mentions that some Jain thinkers viewed only the association between a *jīva* and its karmic body to be beginningless.

All four kinds of nondestructive karma can manifest either in a meritorious (*puṇya*) or a nonmeritorious (*pāpa*) form. Meritorious name-determining karmas will result in the formation of bodies of humans, heavenly beings, or highly complex animals that have a pleasant voice, gait, color, taste, touch, odor, and so on. Nonmeritorious name-determining karmas, on the other hand, will result in the formation of bodies of hell-beings and less complex animals, plants, and earth-, water-, air-, and fire-bodied beings that have an unpleasant voice (if they can utter voices), gait (if they can move), color, taste, touch, odor, and so on (Wiley 2000a, 117–18).

Longevity-determining karma establishes the length of a *jīva*'s embodied lives. A distinctive feature of longevity-determining karma is that it is bound only once in a given lifetime and is activated in the subsequent embodied existence. This is unlike other forms of karma that are continuously attracted and bound to the *jīva* and can come to fruition in either the present life or one of the future ones (BhS 5.3§214a; Wiley 2000a, 88; Wiley 2003, 337). In spite of this difference, *āyu-karman* is closely related to *nāma-karman*, since embodied existences are restricted to specific life spans (TVā 3.27.3; Wiley 2003, 337). If *āyu-karman* determines that the next life will last a certain span of time, the *jīva* will have to be reborn in a bodily form that allows it. Accordingly, the longevity-determining karma has four subtypes, each relating to one of the four birth states (*manuṣya-āyus, deva-āyus, nāraka-āyus,* and *tiryañca-āyus*) (Glasenapp 1942/1915, 11; Wiley 2003, 340). Nevertheless, this karma does not determine the exact number of years an embodied being will live, but rather an overall "quantity of life." Glasenapp explains: "For as the quantity of water in a sponge is definite, but not the period in which it drains it, the quantum of life is also definite, but not the period in which it is used up" (1999/1925, 188; see Schubring 2000/1962, 185).[67] This will be relevant for our discussion on shortening the life span through illness, injury, and other factors in chapter 7.

Conversely, specific birth states define the types of *āyu-karman* that can be bound to the *jīva*. The *āyu-karman* of a human being, for instance, cannot be bound by a fire-bodied or air-bodied being (Jaini 2003, 4). While the justification for this limit is not absolutely clear, Wiley suggests that "it might be that fire-bodied beings and air-bodied beings are thought to cause more *hiṃsā* [violence] than earth-bodied beings, water-bodied beings, and vegetable life because they can move quickly from place to place with no restriction or without assistance" (2000a, 72). Whatever the reason, this particular prohibition demonstrates the close link between nondestructive karmas associated with body and longevity.

Status-determining karma determines the family, environment, or status of embodied existences, with *ucca-gotra-karman* occasioning more favorable and *nīca-gotra-karman* less favorable conditions (Jaini 2001/1979, 125; $TS^{Dig}$ 8.12[68]). The two subtypes of status-determining karma cannot be bound and come to fruition at the same time (Wiley 1999, 114). As Wiley emphasizes, Jain texts define status in different ways, "including family lineage, conduct, or internal modifications of the soul" (124). She also points out that Śvetāmbara texts she is drawing from tend to emphasize family lineage and external manifestations of this karma, such as bodily strength, appearance, power associated with wealth, and performance of austerities. Digambara texts, on the other hand, place more emphasis on internal qualities, spiritual conduct, and even associating with virtuous people. Virtuous conduct is sometimes highlighted as binding *ucca-gotra-karman* (118–20). Some texts, further, clearly state that status-determining karma can change throughout one's life. *Nīca-gotra-karman* can, for example, change to *ucca-gotra-karman* upon the assumption of total restraint, indicating progress in spiritual conduct (124; see chapter 3).

*Vedanīya-karman*, the fourth and last type of nondestructive karma, controls whether the embodied lives of *jīvas* have pleasant (*sat*) or unpleasant (*asat*) feelings (*saṃvedana*) about their environment, and thus conditions the degree of happiness or unhappiness inherent in any individual. *Sātā-vedanīya-karman* (also *sad-vedya*) gives rise to pleasant and *asātā-vedanīya-karman* (also *asad-vedya*) to unpleasant feelings (Wiley 2000a, 272). As *vedanīya-karman* is closely related to the experience of pain and illness, it will be discussed in more detail in the section on pain and sentiency below and in chapter 4.[69]

An important point to note is that no type of karmic matter, be it destructive or nondestructive, is bound to embodied *jīvas* eternally, but only for a limited duration (*sthiti*). After a period of dormancy (*ābādhā-kāla*), the attached karma rises (*udaya*) and comes to fruition with a particular degree of intensity (*anubhāva/anubhāga*), and then breaks away (*nirjarā*) from the *jīva* (Wiley 2003, 339). Due to the fact that *jīvas* are usually engaged in one or another kind of passion-informed activity, the karmic matter that has fallen off is ordinarily replaced by newly bound karma.[70] Furthermore, the complex karmic mechanism expands beyond the present life. The karma that the *jīva* has accumulated in the past reaches fruition in the present, and the karma that it accumulates in the present will shape the possibilities of the future. The *jīva*, through its relation to karma, therefore maintains a thread between (a) the temporal past, present, and potential future; and thereby (b) between bodies occupied in the past, its current body, and rebirths yet to come; and (c) between the moral insights and actions of the past that determine its current understanding and conduct, and shape what capacities it might develop or diminish, in this lifetime or the next.

## CLASSIFICATION OF LIVING BEINGS

As noted above, Jain texts state that all living beings share certain basic qualities, such as consciousness. Despite this inherent similarity, living beings are also greatly diverse, mostly owing to their karmic bondage. Jains developed detailed taxonomies of the different varieties of life-forms, drawing from a wide range of criteria. Some of these taxonomies eventually came to be understood as hierarchical classifications that have been used to inform ethical decisions, as described in chapter 3. It suffices to say at present that early Jain mendicants were guided by ethical ideals that were fairly uncompromising, rooted in the equal value of all life-forms. In time, harm caused to the less complex living beings came to be understood as less karmically burdensome than harm caused to more complex living beings. This accommodation enabled the Jain lay community to live their lives as householders and still abide by the Jain ethical principles, only to a lesser degree than the mendicants for whom stringent ideals more or less remained the norm.

### *Bound and Liberated Beings*

The broadest classification organizes living beings into those that are trapped in *saṃsāra* (*saṃsārin*) and those that are liberated (*mukta*) (TS 2.10; US 36.49). While liberated living beings, which always remain individual, are differentiated mainly with reference to their past lives ($TS^{Dig}$ 10.9;[71] US 36.50–55), most classifications relate to nonliberated beings. These *jīva*s are divided into "an infinity of possible birth-states," according to Jaini. "It is not only said that a given soul *can* be born into uncountable states of every type, but that indeed it already *has* done so and will carry on in virtually endless repetition of these experiences" (2001/1979, 108). Even though the states of embodiment that *jīva*s migrate between are infinite in number, Jain texts find numerous ways of classifying them.

### *Beings in the Four Birth States*

The most common classification of nonliberated embodied living beings is the already mentioned distinction between four birth states:[72] (1) humans; (2) heavenly beings; (3) hell-beings; and (4) animals, plants, and earth-bodied, water-bodied, air-bodied, and fire-bodied beings. As this book deals with bioethics, we will predominantly focus on human beings, but where applicable to bioethical issues, we will also refer to living beings that we as humans encounter most frequently in our part of the cosmos. As indicated in the section on the cosmos, these are mainly beings belonging to the fourth category.

### *Beings with Various Bodies*

We noted above that living beings in *saṃsāra* possess various bodies. One of them is the gross physical body, which describes the familiar "enfleshed" body of humans, animals, and plants, as well as the less familiar bodies of earth-, water-, air-, and fire-bodied beings. The gross physical body is the principal body (*pradhāna-śarīra*) of these beings, and it is the foundation on which their further classifications are primarily based. Along with plants, earth-, water-, air-, and fire-bodied beings are subdivided into two kinds: those with a subtle (*sūkṣma*) body and those with a gross (*bādara*) body. Whereas the latter are restricted to living in the middle world, the former can occupy any part of the cosmos (GJK 184).[73] Subtle-bodied beings are imperceptible, both when they exist individually and when collected into groups, and they can pass through matter. They do not obstruct, violate, or kill other forms of life, nor can they be obstructed, violated, or killed by them.[74] This means that they always die naturally when their longevity-determining karma runs its course. Drawing from Devendrasūri's *Karmagrantha* (thirteenth century), Wiley points out that individual *gross* bodies of earth-, water-, air-, and fire-bodied beings are also imperceptible, even though they are described as "gross." They become visible only in larger collections (Wiley 2000a, 120).

The *Uttarādhyayana-sūtra*[75] helpfully lists the different kinds of these subtle and gross embodied lives, revealing an astounding variety of matter that may be concealing life apart from the more apparent living forms. Highlighting that these lists do not have merely a taxonomic purpose, the text says that a mendicant has to know the division of living and nonliving things (*jīva-ajīva-vibhakti*) in order to practice restraint (*saṃyama*) (US 36.1). As few contemporary Jain studies scholars address the great details provided in Jain taxonomy, it is worth outlining some brief examples to demonstrate the rich observation of (even minute) life-forms upon which Jain ethics is based. Whereas subtle bodies are identical in the case of each one of the groups of living beings that possess them, their gross bodies vary a great deal. This is true even for earth-, water-, fire-, and air-bodied beings. Gross earth-bodied beings, for instance, are divided into two categories: smooth (*ślakṣṇa*) and rough (*khara*), with the former having seven and the latter thirty-six subcategories. Smooth gross earth-bodied beings include black, blue, red, yellow, white, pale dust, and clay. Rough gross earth-bodied beings include, among others, earth (i.e., soil), gravel, sand, stones, rocks, rock-salt, iron, copper, tin, lead, silver, gold, diamond, orpiment, vermilion, realgar, antimony, coral, hyacinth, natron, crystal, emerald, sapphire, red chalk, sulfur, and lapis lazuli (US 36.71–77). The life duration of earth-bodied beings, both subtle and gross, ranges from less than a *muhūrta* (forty-eight minutes)[76] to twenty-two thousand years (US 36.81). Gross water-bodied beings include pure water, dew, fog, and ice. Water-bodied beings, subtle and gross, live anywhere between less than a *muhūrta* and seven thousand years (US 36.85–88). Gross fire-bodied beings include, among others, coal, burning chaff, fire, flame of fire, meteors, and lightning. Life durations of subtle and gross fire-bodied beings range from less than one *muhūrta* to three days (US 109–113). Gross wind-bodied beings include squalls, whirlwinds, thick winds, high winds, and low winds, as well as hurricanes, and so on. Subtle and gross wind-bodied beings can live from less than one *muhūrta* to three thousand years (US 36.118–22). The *Uttarādhyayana-sūtra* adds that there are, further, thousands of varieties of all these living beings, based on their color, smell, taste, touch, figure, and place (US 36.84, 36.92, 36.117, 36.126).[77] This holds also for the other categories of embodied life.

*Individual or Communal Beings*

Another important criterion of classification is whether living beings live as individual bodies (*pratyeka-śarīra*) or communal bodies (*sādhārana-śarīra; sāmānya-śarīra*) (GJK 185). The *Uttarādhyayana-sūtra* states that plants that lead individual lives include trees, shrubby plants (where many stalks spring from the same root or bulb), shrubs (where twigs or stems spring from the same root or bulb), big plants such as lotuses, creeping plants such as gourds, grasses, palms, plants with knotty stems or stalks such as sugarcane, mushrooms, water plants, annual plants such as rice, and herbs. On the other hand, communal forms of plant life have more than one *jīva* occupying a single physical body, such as elephant foot yam, radish, ginger, onion, garlic, plantain-tree, red waterlily, turmeric, and many others (US 36.95–100).

*Nigodas and Their Hosts.* According to the Śvetāmbaras, the communal-bodied plants listed in the *Uttarādhyayana-sūtra* are plants that act as hosts (*pratiṣṭha/ sapratiṣṭha*) to a minute kind of plant life called a *nigoda*. Jaini describes *nigodas* as being located at the very bottom of their birth category, "hence comprising the lowest form of life" (2001/1979, 109). *Nigoda*s are themselves a communal type of plant life, with an infinite number of *nigoda-jīva*s functioning in a single coordinated *nigoda* body or cluster (*golaka*) (Jaini 2010b, 127). The *Gommaṭasāra-jīva-kāṇḍa* (ninth century) states that *nigoda*s take nourishment, breathe, die, and are born together in the same body, at the same time (GJK 191–93). Even though the plants whose bodies they occupy may live a long time, the existence of *nigoda*s is the briefest among all living beings.

*Nigoda*s are divided into those that contain *jīva*s who have fallen to the state of *nigoda* from one of the higher birth states (Dig. *itara-nigoda;* Śv. *vyāvahārika*),[78] and those who have always been born only into the birth state of a *nigoda* (Dig. *nitya-nigoda*; Śv. *avyāvahārika*)[79] (GJK 197; Jaini 2010b, 127–28). Jaini points out that the category of the *nitya-nigoda* is how Jains have dealt with the problem of potentially exhausting the number of living beings trapped in *saṃsāra* due to their constant attainments of liberation. If living beings continue getting liberated, will the cycle of rebirths eventually run out of embodied lives?[80]

> The Jainas deal with this problem by means of the *nitya-nigoda*. These beings are, unlike those of any other category, said to be *infinite* (*anantānanta*) in number, and thus to provide an inexhaustible reservoir of souls; as we might suspect, the rate at which members of the *nitya-nigoda* class leave their dismal condition and enter higher states for the first time is either equal to or greater than that at which human beings in various parts of the universe attain *siddha*-hood [i.e., liberation]. (2010b, 128)

*Nitya-nigoda*s can be reborn into any of the higher birth states. The Śvetāmbaras believe that Marudevī, the mother of Ṛṣabha, the first Jina of our time, was a *nitya-nigoda* before her life as Marudevī in which she attained liberation as the first person to do so in the current cycle of time (Jaini 2003).[81]

According to the Śvetāmbaras, communal-bodied plants that function as hosts contain innumerable *nigoda* bodies and, thus, infinities of *nigoda-jīva*s. They maintain that plants that are listed as having individual bodies cannot act as hosts (*apratiṣṭha*) to *nigoda*s. The Digambaras dispute this claim, asserting that only *nigoda-jīva*s possess a communal body. All the other plants have a single body only, but they are divided into those that can and those that cannot host *nigoda*s (GJK 186). Host plants are classified as *ananta-kāyika*s, that is, those with bodies that hold an infinite number of *jīva*s. The difference between the Śvetāmbara and the Digambara understanding of the relationship between *nigoda*s and their hosts is merely in classification, but for both, defining certain plants as hosts has an ethical significance. In karmic terms, destroying a plant that acts as a host has a much higher karmic cost than destroying a plant that does not (as further discussed in chapters 3 and 6). It should be pointed out that similarly to earth-bodied, water-bodied, fire-bodied, and air-bodied beings, *nigoda*s are also categorized into those with a gross and those with a subtle body; only the gross-bodied *nigoda*s can be violated. As in the case of the others, the subtle-bodied *nigoda*s can exist anywhere in the cosmos, whereas the gross-bodied *nigoda*s exist in specific locations that are the bodies of other plants. Harming a plant that is a host, therefore, harms not only the host plant itself but the gross-bodied *nigoda*s within it as well (Wiley 2000a, 122–24). This led Jains to avoid using host plants for dietary and medical purposes (see chapters 3 and 6). Importantly, Jaini notes that *nigoda*s inhabit not only other plant-bodied beings, but also the flesh of animals and humans, where they "tend to become especially concentrated" (Jaini 2010b, 127; Jaini 2001/1979, 109).[82] In line with this, cutting into flesh could be considered a violent action, even if for the sake of healing, an ethical limit that has implications for medical treatment and bioethics.

### *Pain and Sentiency*

Jain texts demonstrate a deep awareness of the fact that the type of body that a living being possesses affects its experience in the world. A central hinge in Jain taxonomy in relation to bioethics is living beings' experience of pain. There is a recognition of the universal experience of pain and, thus, of a basic similarity of all forms of life as a motivation for refraining from causing harm to other beings (Vallely 2020). Already the earliest extant texts state that all living beings are the same in the sense that they want to live (*priya-āyus*) rather than be killed (*apriya-vadha*) as well as experience pleasure (*sukha-svāda*) rather than pain (*duḥkha-pratikūla*) (ĀS 1.2.3.4).

As noted above, the type of karma that produces the feeling of pain is *asātā-vedanīya-karman*, one type of nondestructive karma.[83] Jaini emphasizes that feelings of pleasure and pain that are produced by *vedanīya-karman* accompany living beings throughout their lives. As long as *jīva*s are embodied, they are "never free from pleasant and unpleasant feelings" (Jaini 2001a, 135; see also Wiley 2000a, 272). In fact, the state of liberation from karma, he explains, is not described as characterized only by the perfect manifestation of the *jīva*'s four essential qualities, but is also characterized by one specific "negative" quality called the *avyābādha*, which represents the "absence of restlessness or hurt." "In the notion of *avyābādha*," Jaini points out, "the Jainas seem to be emphasizing . . . that the restlessness associated with the presence of feeling—even pleasant feeling—is at some level alien and painful to man [*sic*]" (2001, 136). In line with this, he points out delusion (*moha*)—resulting from deluding karma, which transforms the quality of bliss—as a central factor of all of our experience of pain and suffering, comparable to the Buddhist concept of *saṃskāra-duḥkhatā*.

> Like the latter it represents the *a priori* condition for all our ordinary experience, and, hence, for our experience of pleasure and pain. It stands, then, in opposition, not to pleasure as we ordinarily understand it, but to an absolute state of bliss, which is realized precisely in the absence of both pleasure and pain. . . . In this sense *moha* might be called a metaphysical kind of suffering—the instability and internal contradiction of a being whose actual state is a denial of his [*sic*] true nature. (2001, 137–38)

Living beings experience ordinary pain through their bodies, but not all of the five bodies that we discussed above allow their occupants to feel pain. The transformational and gross physical bodies both permit the experience of pain, while the karmic and fiery bodies do not (TVā 2.44; Wiley 2000a, 158). The transformational body, for example, allows the great suffering of hell-beings, and the gross physical body enables living beings to feel pain through the senses (*indriya*) and/or the mind (*manas*). Since the operation of the senses and the mind is driven by consciousness, the degree to which consciousness is karmically obstructed affects the complexity of living beings' sensory and mental capacities and, consequently, their experience of pain. It is important to note that sense cognition has two aspects: (1) the sense organ (*dravya-indriya*), as the physical aspect; and (2) the sense faculty (*bhāva-indriya*), as the internal aspect (TS 2.16–2.18).[84] Nathmal Tatia explains them as "senses as clusters of matter" and "senses as modes of the soul" (2011, 43), a distinction we will revisit in chapter 5 in relation to embryology.

*One-Sensed Beings.* All beings that occupy a gross physical body according to Jainism possess at least one sense (*eka-indriya*), that is, the sense of touch (*sparśana*), and living beings that possess this single sense are considered the least complex forms of life. These are plants and earth-, water-, fire-, and air-bodied beings ($TS^{Dig}$ 2.22). However, despite a severely obstructed quality of consciousness and a single sense of touch through which they come into contact with the world, Jain texts maintain that they still experience pain. The *Bhagavatī-sūtra* states that all of them experience pain (*vedanā*) in the same way, indeterminately (*anirdhārita*), since they do not possess reflective awareness (*asaṃjñi-bhūta*)[85] (BhS 1.2§39a).[86] It seems that it is in line with this that the *Bhagavatī-sūtra*, further, compares the pain of an earth-bodied being to that of an "old decrepit man whom a young strong man gives a blow on the head" (BhS 19.3§766b, Deleu 1996/1970, 250). The same holds for other one-sensed beings. While these beings experience pain differently from more complex living beings like humans, and are not able to be aware of it in a reflective manner, they nevertheless experience it, and comparing them to an elderly person highlights their frailty. Furthermore, one-sensed beings are not devoid of agency, and are stated as being capable of performing harmful activities and attracting karma like all other embodied lives (BhS 9.34§491b; SKS 2.4.9–10).

*Two- to Five-Sensed Beings.* As indicated above, the greater the number of senses that living beings experience the world with, the greater their complexity. There are five senses in total: the already mentioned sense of touch, along with the senses of taste (*rasana*), smell (*ghrāṇa*), sight (*cakṣus*), and hearing (*śrotra*). Two-sensed beings include animals such as worms, conch shells, pearl mussels, snails, and leeches. They possess the senses of touch and taste (TBh 2.24). "The ability to taste indicates that these beings have a mouth," says Wiley, "through which they consume 'morsel food' (*kavala-āhāra*) and by means of which they produce sounds (i.e., they have the ability of 'speech')" (2000a, 126). Three-sensed animals experience the world through the senses of touch, taste, and smell; this group includes ants, bugs, fleas, lice, weevils, centipedes, springtails, and termites. Four-sensed animals, which have an additional sense faculty of sight, include bees, flies, gnats, mosquitos, scorpions, spiders, butterflies, and moths. Five-sensed beings, which in addition have the sense of hearing, include human beings and animals such as fish, snakes, birds, and quadrupeds, as well as heavenly beings and hell-beings (TBh 2.24). Living beings are further divided into those that have a mind (*samanaska*)—and can, therefore, reflect on and discriminate between merit and demerit[87]—and those that do not have a mind (*amanaska*) (TS 2.11, $TS^{Dig}$ 2.24[88]). Hell-beings, heavenly beings, human beings born from a womb, and some five-sensed animals born from a womb belong to the group that have a mind (TBh 2.25), as discussed below in a section on birth in a womb. As in the case of sense cognition, the mind has two aspects: (1) the organ, which is the physical aspect (*dravya*) ("clusters of matter"); and (2) the faculty (*bhāva*), which is the internal aspect ("modes of the *jīva*"). Despite these many differences, all living beings that have two or more senses have an individual, gross body that they experience the world around them with (Wiley 2000a, 126).

### *Mobility and Immobility*

The distinction between cognitive abilities of living beings serves as a helpful foundation for another classification that groups them into those that can move (*trasa*) and those that cannot (*sthāvara*). Digambaras and Śvetāmbaras agree that all living beings that have two or more senses are mobile. The Digambaras designate all one-sensed living beings as immobile (TS^Dig 2.13–14; TVā 2.12.5), which means that, as stated by Tatia, "the automatic movement for the maintenance of life does not qualify a being as 'mobile'" (2010, 42). Akalaṅka, further, indicates that despite not being able to move, living beings in the womb (*garbha*) still count as mobile beings (TVā 2.12.2). In fact, he says, mobility and immobility do not really depend on whether a living being is in motion or stationary; it rather relates entirely to the arising of particular karmas that determine mobility and immobility (TVā 2.12.5). These are *trasa-nāma-karman* and *sthāvara-nāma-karman*, respectively.

In contrast to the Digambaras, the Śvetāmbaras classify air-bodied and fire-bodied beings as mobile, along with all living beings that possess two or more senses (TS^Śv 2.13–14). The *Tattvārtha-ṭīkā* (ninth century) complicates the Śvetāmbara position on the status of air-bodied and fire-bodied beings by stating that—even though they move—they are not capable of moving voluntarily, which distinguishes them from the rest of the mobile beings (TṬ 2.14; see also Tatia 2010, 42). Pandit Sukhlalji indicates that while fire-bodied and air-bodied beings are characterized by the manifestation of the *sthāvara-nāma-karman* like all the other one-sensed beings, they are mobile in a figurative sense because their motion is like that of mobile beings (Sanghvi 2000/1974, 87). In line with this, Wiley points out that, despite the difference in classification, "Śvetāmbaras and Digambaras agree that the bodies of fire-bodied and air-bodied beings are formed through the operation of *sthāvara nāma karma*" (2000a, 125). The prevailing criterion for classification seems to be the underlying karma for the Digambaras and the manifested motion for the Śvetāmbaras.

### *Ability to Develop a Body's Capacity*

Another important classification divides living beings into those that are capable or incapable of completely developing their main physical body. This relates to, as Glasenapp explains, the "complete development of the organs (*karaṇa*) and capacities (*labdhi*) of nourishment, of the body, of the senses, of breathing, of speech, and of thought" (1942/1915, 17), which will be discussed in more detail later in the chapter. The ability to attain complete development is decided by the arising of a specific kind of *nāma-karman*, called *paryāpta-nāma-karman*; its opposite is *aparyāpta-nāma-karman* (17–18). Beings that experience the arising of the latter pass away very soon after their birth[89] (a trait we will revisit in regard to reproductive ethics in chapter 5). On the other hand, Wiley explains, "if *paryāpta nāma karma* comes into rise, then all of the capacities appropriate for a specific type of being will develop to completion, and death will not take place until this process is finished" (2000a, 129). Based on their cognitive capacities, subtlety, and ability to fully develop, the *Gommaṭasāra-jīva-kāṇḍa* lists fourteen classes of living beings (*jīva-samāsa*): (1) subtle one-sensed beings; (2) gross one-sensed beings; (3–5) two-sensed, three-sensed, and four-sensed beings; (6) beings without a mind;

(7) beings with a mind; with each of them (8–14) either having a capacity for full development or not (GJK 72).

As noted, the meticulous taxonomies that we have discussed serve a better understanding of what in the world is violable and what is not. Furthermore, the diversity of life gradually came to function as a foundation for drawing hierarchical distinctions between living beings. This enabled the thriving of the lay community, who were permitted to harm one-sensed beings (see chapters 3 and 6).

## TRANSITIONS FROM BIRTH TO LIBERATION

We conclude this chapter by describing various aspects of the different stages of existence, including birth categories, vitalities, capacities, and instincts of life; phases of aging; causes of death; the mechanisms of rebirth; and characteristics of liberation. This background demonstrates the comprehensive, and often technical, nature of Jain philosophy as it informs the ethical applications we will explore in part 2 of this book.

### *Birth Categories*

Jains do not understand the processes of conception, growth of the body, and birth to be defined solely by material factors. All of them are determined by the arising of specific kinds of name-determining karma that have been accumulated as a result of various past activities performed by the embodied immaterial *jīva*. Since these activities vary greatly, the types of accumulated karma and their effects do as well. This means that living beings differ in how they are conceived, in how they grow, and in how they are born. Embodied life-forms are understood to be born (*janma*) in three different ways: (1) by agglutination or coagulation (*sammūrcchana/sammūrcchima*), (2) by the womb (*garbha*), or (3) by descent (*upapāda*) (GJK 83; TS$^{Dig}$ 2.31$^{90}$). Heavenly beings and hell-beings are born by descent, meaning that they appear without having any need for a mother and a father (Jaini 2001/1979, 110), "with lightning-like suddenness without any material basis" (Schubring 2000/1962, 139; GJK 84). Living beings born by agglutination, which refers to matter joining together to form the *jīva*'s body, include some five-sensed animals and humans, and all beings with fewer than five senses. Wiley describes birth by agglutination in the following way: "When the soul arrives at the place of birth, which contains matter suitable for forming the gross physical body (*audārika-śarīra*), it begins to assimilate matter present there, which can be living, nonliving, or both" (Wiley 2000a, 134).

The rare class of human beings who are born through agglutination potentially has some bearing on bioethical calculations in Jainism (SthS 6.20). The birth of these agglutinated humans is not attributed to sexual reproduction between a mother and father (Wiley 2000a, 136). Rather, as Tatia explains, they "originate in human excreta such as faeces, urine, sputum, mucus, vomit, bile, pus, blood, semen, etc." (2010, 54). Citing a passage from the *Prajñāpanā-sūtra*,[91] Wiley writes that these humans can be found "in matter that has been made damp with semen before it has dried, in a corpse, in the union of males and females, and in sewers or holes where bodily wastes are deposited" (2000a, 137–38; see also Glasenapp 1942/1915, 57). These agglutinated beings are very small, and their life spans are extremely short, as they do not have the ability to fully develop their bodily capacities (*aparyāpta*) (GJK 92). Unlike other human beings, they do not even have a mind (Wiley 2000a, 136–41). Understood in this way, the category of humans born by agglutination has ethical significance for the understanding of sexual union, masturbation, and menstruation, as well as the practice of medicine, given that substances such as blood, mucus, vomit, bile, pus, and other matter all potentially contain minute kinds of agglutinated human beings. For example, an idea emerged that nine hundred thousand living beings are killed during sexual intercourse, most likely referring to the type of living beings discussed here (see chapter 5). Wiley is skeptical, however, about the violability of these beings, pointing out that "if one accepts the view that the life span of these beings is always the minimum possible, then it cannot be cut short by any action whatsoever" (2000a, 139). She continues:

> Perhaps a possible explanation for "killing" here might be that of causing harm (*hiṃsā*) by providing a medium in which these *sammūrcchima* humans can take birth, whether it be in the body of a woman following intercourse or in other unclean substances mentioned above. By providing a place for their birth, a person would cause massive numbers of these beings to suffer on account of the inevitable rise of *asātā-vedanīya-karma* and to suffer the pain and fear that are associated with their nearly simultaneous death. (140)[92]

Five-sensed beings that are not born by agglutination are born by the womb and are the result of a sex act between a woman and a man.[93] Unlike those born through agglutination, five-sensed beings born by the womb have a mind. The *Tattvārtha-sūtra* divides womb-born animals into viviparous with placenta (*jarāyu*), viviparous without placenta (*potaja*), and oviparous (*aṇḍaja*), meaning those born from an egg (TS$^{Dig}$ 2.33[94]). Humans belong to the viviparous with placenta class, and their new embryonic form is developed in the womb as a combination of nonliving matter from their parents (semen and blood) and their own *jīva* (to be discussed further in chapter 5, on reproductive ethics). While ordinary human beings are usually born in a womb that is shaped like a bamboo leaf (*vaṃśapatra-yoni*), texts claim that Jinas are born in a tortoise-shaped womb (*kūrmonnata-yoni*), signifying their special status (GJK 81–82; Wiley 2000a, 221).

### *The Vitalities, Capacities, and Instincts of Life*

In the beginning of this chapter, we noted that in the Jain tradition, consciousness is the mark by which living stuff is distinguished from nonliving stuff. Jain texts also propose another set of criteria by which to recognize life in matter, that is, through the so-called vitalities or life-forces (*prāṇa*). Ten vitalities are listed, including (1–5) five sense vitalities (*indriya-prāṇa*), (6) vitality of respiration (*ucchvāsa-prāṇa* or *ānapāna-prāṇa*), (7) vitality of life span (*āyu-prāṇa*),[95] and (8–10) strength vitalities (*bala-prāṇa*) of body, speech, and mind (GJK 130; Glasenapp 1999/1925, 198–99). Nemicandra states that only beings that are capable of attaining complete development have the vitality of respiration, and only beings possessing two or more senses have the vitality of speech. Moreover, five-sensed beings with a mind possess the mind vitality. All living beings, both those capable and those incapable of attaining complete development, possess the life span vitality, the vitality of the body (referring to bodily strength or energy), and at least one sense vitality (GJK 132; Wiley 2000a, 188).[96] This includes human beings who do not have the capacity to fully develop their bodies.

This indicates that vitalities are closely connected with the capacities of the physical body for attaining complete development (*paryāpti*), which were mentioned above.[97] There are six such capacities: (1) *āhāra-paryāpti* (capacity for assimilating matter that builds the body), (2) *śarīra-paryāpti* (capacity of accumulated matter to form into the body's essential parts),[98] (3) *indriya-paryāpti* (capacity for developing the senses), (4) *prāṇāpāna* or *ucchvāsa-paryāpti* (capacity for developing the faculty of respiration), (5) *bhāṣā-paryāpti* (capacity for developing the faculty of speech), and (6) *mano-paryāpti* (capacity for developing the mind). One-sensed beings that are capable of development (*paryāpta*) possess the first four *paryāpti*s, and all living beings with more than one sense possess the additional capacity of speech, and the five-sensed animals and humans with a mind also possess the capacity of mind (GJK 119). While vitalities (*prāṇa*s) and capacities for attaining complete development (*paryāpti*s) seem to closely resemble one another, Jain texts do distinguish between them. In his comment on the *Gommaṭasāra-jīva-kāṇḍa* 129, J.L. Jaini explains the difference between them in the following way: "*Paryāpti* is the attainment of the capacity of developing body, mind, speech, and the five senses, while *prāṇa* is the activity of those functionaries" (GJK 90; Wiley 2000a, 187).

Instincts (*saṃjñā*) are another defining feature of all living beings. They include craving for food (*āhāra-saṃjñā*), fear (*bhaya-saṃjñā*), desire for reproduction (*maithuna-saṃjñā*), and accumulation of things for future use (*parigraha-saṃjñā*) (GJK 134–38; Jaini 2010e, 284). Among these, craving for food is the root instinct. It should be noted that living beings possessing a mouth consume food voluntarily, whereas those without a mouth absorb food through the surface of their whole bodies involuntarily (Wiley 2002, 42). For example, in the case of womb-born living beings, a *jīva* entering the womb is said to consume the father's semen, the menstrual blood of the mother, as well as various other liquids (Wiley 2000a, 191; see chapter 5). Because its body is not fully developed, it cannot use its mouth to take food, but rather absorbs it through the entire body. We will address the significance of the food instinct in several later chapters, with special attention in chapter 6. The instinct for reproduction will be discussed further in chapter 5.

*Phases of Aging*

The aging process of an embodied being is not explicitly dealt with in Jain texts. Rather, texts describe the decline of bodily strength, the weakening of sense-faculties, and symptoms of deterioration, such as trembling or cough. The *Sthānāṅga-sūtra*[99] describes these processes within ten stages (*avasthā*) of human life, corresponding to one hundred possible years of existence:

(1) 1–10 years: the stage of a child (*bāla*)
(2) 10–20 years: the stage of play (*krīḍā*)
(3) 20–30 years: the stage of being slow in understanding or enjoying pleasures (*manda*)
(4) 30–40 years: the stage of strength (*bala*)
(5) 40–50 years: the stage of knowledge (*prajñā*)
(6) 50–60 years: the stage of the weakening of the senses (*hāpana*)
(7) 60–70 years: the stage of developing trembling and cough (*prapañca*)
(8) 70–80 years: the stage of walking with a stoop (*prāgbhāra*)
(9) 80–90 years: the stage of wishing for liberation or the end of life (*unmukha*)
(10) 90–100 years: the stage of lying down (*śayana*) (SthS 10.154)[100]

In line with this, a human body will start weakening from the age of fifty onward.

Illness will be described in more detail in later chapters, but it is important to note here that not all humans in the Jain cosmos age and suffer from illness in the same way. Humans who live in the so-called "lands of action" (*karma-bhūmi*), which is also our geographically bound part of the cosmos, do undergo stages of decline. However, humans who live in the so-called "lands of enjoyment" (*bhoga-bhūmi*) never undergo the physical decline described above and they all die a natural death (on which more below). All wishes and needs are fulfilled without any effort by wishing-trees in the "lands of enjoyment," and suffering is hardly present there. Consequently, liberation is not attainable in those lands, since people are unmotivated to pursue the path of purification, and Jinas are not born there to spread the Jain teaching. On the other hand, living beings must always strive to survive in the "lands of action." Since suffering abounds, they are motivated to seek the path to liberation, which is attainable in these parts of the cosmos, and Jinas are born in these lands to teach the Jain doctrine.

*Death and Its Causes*

Just as birth is a beginning of one particular embodied existence rather than the beginning of life itself, Jains "regard death as a transition, not a finality" (Chapple 2010, 189). Life in the form of *jīva* is indestructible, with only its embodied forms being finite. As indicated in the section on karma, the life duration of an embodied living being is determined by a type of nondestructive karma, called longevity-determining karma (*āyu-karman*). This karma arises prior to death and determines the duration of the next bodily form. As long as the previously bound longevity-determining karma is active, the living being's life continues. The extinguishment of longevity-determining karma marks the death of the living being. This means that the time between the first activation of longevity-determining karma and its cessation represents the life span of an individual embodied living being. Life spans of embodied beings vary greatly, as we described above regarding the longevity of plant-bodied, earth-bodied, water-bodied, fire-bodied, and air-bodied beings. Humans born in our current part of the cosmos, whose life spans extend approximately one hundred years, exemplify a duration of life measured in countable numbers (*saṃkhyāta*). Some humans who live in the "lands of enjoyment," however, are said to live so long that their life spans are measured in uncountable numbers (*asaṃkhyāta*) (Wiley 2000a, 48).

These numbers all represent the ideal amount of time that a living being can exist if nothing intervenes. In other words, if a living being were to die "naturally," it can live up to the full amount of years that are ascribed to it. As we will discuss in chapter 7, a "natural," uninterrupted death is considered to be a *timely death* (*kāla-mṛtyu*). Those humans residing in the "lands of enjoyment," whose life span is measured in uncountable years, always die "naturally." However, in our part of the cosmos, life can be terminated early due to external efficient causes (*nimitta*), such as weapons, poison, illness, natural disasters, and accidents. Digambaras also articulate one efficient cause that pertains to death as a result of self-injury or accident, known as *upaghāta-nāma-karman*, a subclass of *nāma-karman*. While Śvetāmbaras do not associate this type of karma with death, Digambaras assert that it motivates people to hurt themselves and provides an object or substance that can harm them, such as a poison or weapon (Wiley 2000a, 171–72). This kind of karma, according to Glasenapp, also "produces that the parts of the body of a being (e.g., the uvula in the throat) cause its death" (1942/1915, 17).

In the case of living beings whose longevity-determining karma is bound very firmly, even the operation of an external efficient cause will not bring about premature death. This is especially true for Jinas, who are described in Jain stories as surviving all manner of mortal attacks and injuries that would typically kill an ordinary person. Ordinary human beings, whose longevity-determining karma is bound loosely, more easily succumb to external efficient causes, and so their lives may result in premature or *untimely death* (Wiley 2000a, 49–51; see chapter 7). When a living being dies prematurely, all the remaining longevity-determining karma is experienced simultaneously.

Jains place great value on one's mental attitude and conduct in the face of death, be it timely or untimely, which plays a significant role in the Jain ethics of dying. We will explore this more fully in chapter 7.

*Mechanisms of Rebirth*

As indicated above, *jīvas* have always been trapped in *saṃsāra*, and, as Pūjyapāda explains, the cycle of continued births (*bhava-antara*) is sustained because of the fruition of karmas (*karma-vipāka-vaśa*) (SSi 9.7§801). The type of karma that supports the migration of the *jīva* from one form of embodied existence to the next is name-determining karma. Glasenapp explains that a specific type of name-determining karma, called the *ānupūrvī-nāma-karman*, "causes that the *jīva*, when one existence is finished, goes from the place of death in the proper direction to the place of his [*sic*] new birth" (1942/1915, 16; see also Wiley 2000a, 160). This karma has four subtypes in accordance with the four birth states that it can lead the *jīva* to.

The aforementioned subtle bodies (karmic body and luminous body) enable *jīvas* to easily and nearly instantaneously pass from one type of principal physical body to the next. These subtle bodies function as a protective vehicle of sorts during the transition. "At the moment of death, the *aghātiyā* [nondestructive] karmas have preprogrammed, as it were, the particular conditions of the coming embodiment," says Jaini (2001/1979, 126). "This information is carried in the *kārmaṇa-śarīra* [karmic body], which, together with the *taijasa-śarīra* [luminous body], houses the soul as it leaves its physical body" (126). The nature of *jīvas* themselves is not affected in these transitions. Because they extend in space, *jīvas* can adapt to the size of all the bodies that they occupy and are therefore coextensive with them (*sva-deha-parimāṇa*) (DS 2).[101] Other than that, the Jain doctrine does not offer much more detail about the transitions between various embodiments. Jaini says that, for example, "Jaina texts make absolutely no mention whatsoever of how a soul actually enters the body of the mother-to-be" (2010b, 124; cf. Wiley 2000a, 162–63). This lack of detail is perhaps owing to the fact that transitions occur so quickly. As indicated above, Jain texts are committed to the idea that the transition (*antar-gati* or *vigraha-gati*) happens in a single moment, so long as there is a direct line between the previous and the current life. If the *jīva* needs to make turns to reach its destination, the travel takes a few additional moments (Wiley 2000a, 154–56). Such a fast transition results from the fact that *jīvas* possess an innate ability to move upwards at great speed, though when embodied, this upward movement is corrupted in various ways, causing *jīvas* to move in different directions. The *Tattvārtha-bhāṣya* explains that "worldly beings (*saṃsārin*), owing to the ties of *karman*, [move] downwards, sidewards, and upwards" (TBh 10.6). It is only in the disembodied state of liberation that this innate upward movement can be completely manifested. According to the *Tattvārtha-bhāṣya*, "one who is liberated from ties (*saṅga-vinirmukta*) has the motion of one being liberated (*sidhyamāna-gati*), which is upwards, owing to the upward gravitation (*ūrdhva-gaurava*)" (TBh 10.6). We will look at the state of liberation in the next section.

### *Characteristics of Liberation*

The ultimate Jain goal of liberation is also linked to the karma doctrine. We explained above that nondestructive karmic matter determines the *jīva*'s body and birth state, but not its inherent qualities. Consequently, a *jīva* may perfect all of its qualities—such as perception, knowledge, energy, and bliss—while still embodied. Only a human *jīva* is capable of achieving that, which differentiates it from the rest of embodied beings. As noted, the perfection of consciousness is often described as the perfect knowledge of all existing substances with all of their modes, but has alternatively also been interpreted as the perfect knowledge of the self (Jaini 2001/1979, 266–67; NSā 158). Once the embodied *jīva* attains perfection, it has fulfilled the necessary condition of attaining liberation and will exit the cycle of rebirths upon death. This means that the body the *jīva* occupies when it reaches perfection is its final body.[102] It is important to emphasize that the *jīva* does remain in its body even after reaching perfection until its current embodied form ceases—that is, until all the nondestructive karmas determining its body, longevity, status, and feeling run their natural course and expire (Dundas 2002, 104).[103] This "exhaustion of all karma is liberation" (TS$^{Dig}$ 10.2;[104] see also TBh 10.3). Although a human being that has attained perfect knowledge (*kevalin*) stays in the cycle of rebirths until death and continues to occupy a material body due to the operation of the remaining nondestructive karmic matter that determines its embodiment, its inherent qualities remain perfectly functional until and throughout liberation.

Uniquely, the disembodied liberated being can be viewed as both *free from* yet *still connected to* its previous karmically determined body. It is free insofar as the elimination of all karma results in the *jīva* moving, in a single moment, "upwards to the border of the cosmic space (*loka-anta*)" (TS 10.5), which is an inverted-umbrella-shaped part of the cosmos where liberated *jīva*s remain.[105] A classical Jain example compares this event of the *jīva*'s transformation from bondage to liberation to a gourd that sinks in water when covered with clay, but floats to its surface as soon as the clay is removed (TBh 10.6). Just as the gourd rises when freed from the clay weighing it down, so liberated *jīva*s, which have been detached from their bodies and the heavy entanglement with karmic matter, move upwards because that is their natural direction. Once they reach the very top of the cosmos, they stay there forever, never again to be tainted by karmic matter and completely out of reach for *jīva*s that remain embodied and trapped in the cycle of rebirths.

At the same time, these bodiless *jīva*s remain connected to their karmic life through the "shape" of their liberated, nonbodied existence. Since the Jain teaching asserts that liberation is only possible from the human birth state, as noted above, the visual image of the liberated *jīva*, called the *siddha*, depicts an outline of a hollowed-out, nongendered human form, highlighting its immateriality (Dundas 2002, 105; figure 2). *Siddha*s are said to retain the size and shape of the body they occupied at the moment of liberation, or rather two-thirds of it (Schubring

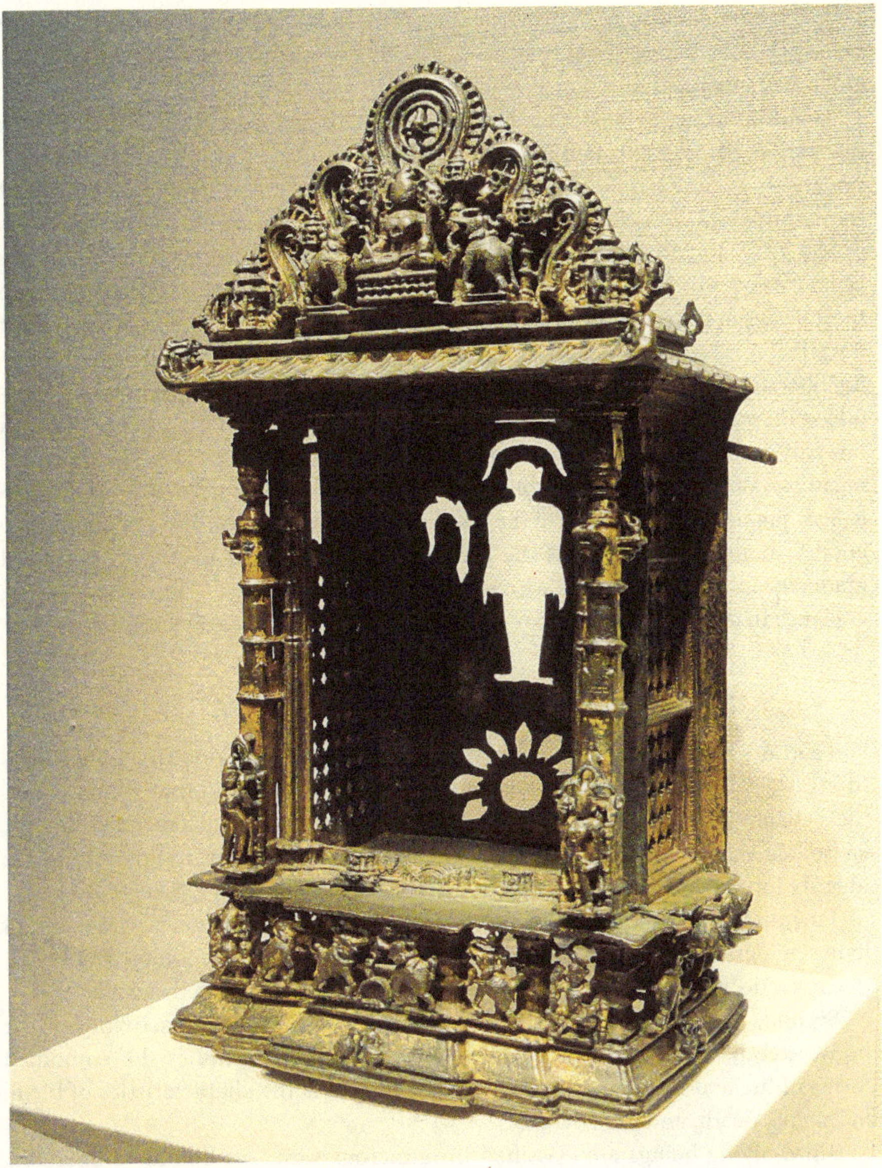

FIGURE 2. This fourteenth-century bronze shrine depicts the outline of the liberated *siddha*. Credit: Freer Gallery of Art.

2000/1962, 329; SSi 10.4; Jaini 2010b, 122).[106] This hollow shape, without flesh or organs, echoes the materiality of its last body even as it is no longer limited by embodied form and function (Donaldson 2015, 79).

It is important to note that liberation is at present not actually possible in our part of the cosmos. Jain cosmology asserts that our specific "land of action" undergoes cycles of time in which conditions improve and decline. Our part of the cosmos has entered a time of general decline (*avasarpiṇī*) after the death of Mahāvīra, and no Jinas will be born here until the conditions eventually improve again (*utsarpiṇī*). However, there are other "lands of action" that do not undergo these cycles of time where liberation is always possible and Jinas always teach their doctrine. A rebirth there as a human being would represent a possibility of attaining liberation. This means that liberation—and the characteristics of the *siddha*—offer a theoretical rather than a practical ideal for the present life of all humans in our part of the cosmos, even among contemporary Jains themselves. Nevertheless, regardless of the geographical context, living beings can still strive toward the perfected qualities exemplified by the *siddha*, as well as toward other "penultimate goods" (Long 2009, 112). It is the ideal of the *siddha*—this possibility activated gradually and in penultimate ways—that guides the actions of Jains, encouraging vigilance in a world full of embodied living beings that are easily harmed.

## JAIN FOUNDATIONAL PRINCIPLES OF WHAT EXISTS

Jain authors have propounded a truly complex metaphysical doctrine that defines in great detail the difference between that which is living and that which is not, the violable and nonviolable, and further explains the karmic mechanisms for embodied encounters that so often result in the violation of life. In this section, we identity four key principles related to the Jain account of what exists.

First, life and nonlife are distinct, but entangled, phenomena, in the realm of living beings. To fully understand the structure and dynamics of a living being, one must decipher how life and nonlife entwine within embodied existence.

Second, karma is a material substance that results from the activities of the body, speech, and mind among all living beings. It determines the embodied forms of life and their cognitive capacities, as well as the characteristics of birth, life, aging, death, and rebirth.

Third, living beings are classified in numerous ways—as bound or liberated, according to birth state, by type of body, as individual or communal, by their experience of pain, by sentience, mobility, vitalities, capacities for development, and instincts—but all possess a *jīva*, characterized by the qualities of consciousness, energy, and bliss. Where life is more difficult to distinguish from the nonliving matter or its nonliving previous material body, it is even more vulnerable to injury.

Fourth, even after liberation, a liberated *jīva*, or *siddha*, remains associated with its bodily existence in bearing the physical outline of its final embodied form.

The ultimate goal of liberation, though seeming to transcend the realm of karmic bondage and its resultant embodiment, remains an expression of both.

The technical details of these principles inform the wider approach to Jain ethics and, thus, provide an essential foundation for considering or developing a Jain approach to modern bioethics. The Jain account of life, nonlife, and karmic causality is presented with an almost mathematical precision. As any such system permits, Jainism allows one to no longer generate causes that result in predictable effects, if the latter become undesirable.

# 3

# Nonviolence and the Framework of Jain Ethics

A defining feature of the Jain tradition is its emphasis on ethical behavior that emulates the twenty-four Jinas. These liberated teachers showed the path of right worldview, knowledge, and conduct needed to free oneself from repeated births in *saṃsāra*. In popular presentations of the tradition, the path of conduct is frequently summarized through the five Jain vows. The first and most primary vow is *ahiṃsā*, or nonviolence. The term signifies the opposite of *hiṃsā*—violence, a derivative from the Sanskrit verbal root *han-*, meaning to hit, strike, or kill (Monier-Williams 1899, 1287).[1] It is signified visually in the contemporary Jain symbol of an open palm raised in the *abhaya-mudrā* of peace and fearlessness (figure 3). As the first vow, nonviolence provides the basis for the other four vows: truthfulness (*satya*), nonstealing (*asteya*), sexual restraint (*brahmacarya*), and nonpossession (*aparigraha*). These vows are to be practiced fully, as great vows (*mahā-vrata*), by mendicants; and partially, as minor vows (*aṇu-vrata*), by lay Jains.

These five vows might appear to be the logical starting point in our effort to examine the Jain foundations for bioethics. However, the understanding of right conduct has evolved a great deal in the Jain tradition from the earliest mendicant texts to the contemporary practices of modern lay Jains, such that the vows alone do not paint a sufficient picture. In order to understand the complex foundations of Jain conduct, and its relation to nonviolence, we will move beyond the traditional account of the vows and excavate the philosophical layers that have shaped Jain practice among mendicants and householding laypeople.

In this chapter, we examine the ethical doctrines in the earliest layers of the Jain canon, as well as emerging accommodations for mendicants and lay Jains. These accommodations include a growing emphasis on the motivations that inform actions, as well as a developing doctrine of beneficial karma and good rebirth.

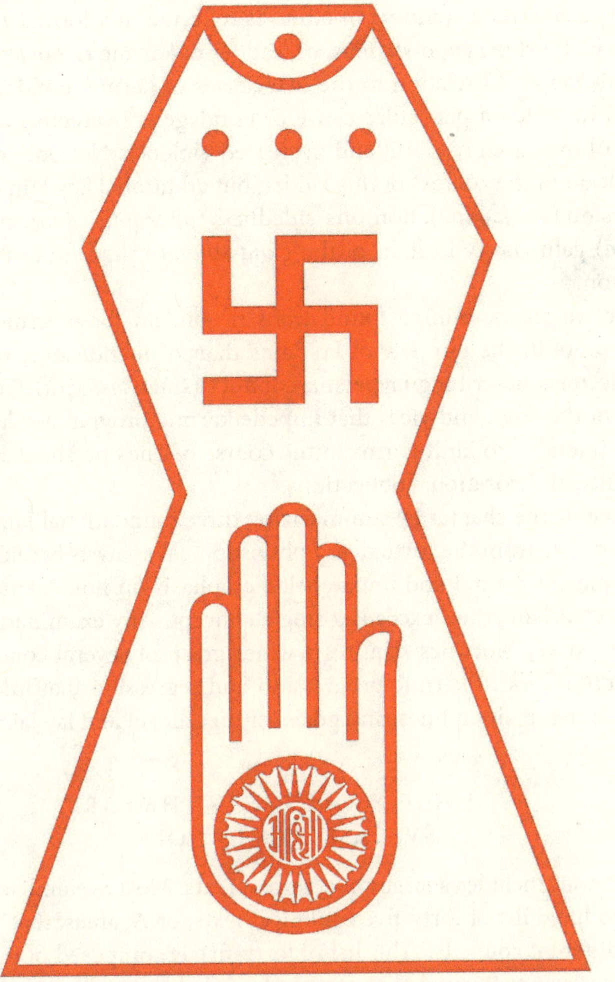


FIGURE 3. Various Jain groups adopted this hourglass-shaped cosmos as an emblem (*pratīka*) of their tradition in 1975 in celebration of the 2,500th anniversary of Mahāvīra's attainment of liberation. It includes several other Jain symbols, from top to bottom: a liberated *siddha* atop the universe; the "Three Jewels" of right worldview, knowledge, and conduct; the *svastika*, denoting four birth states within the cycle of rebirths, as well as the community of monks, nuns, laymen, and laywomen; the symbol of *ahiṃsā* in Jainism—an open palm in the *abhaya* position, dispelling fear, with the word *ahiṃsā* in the *devanāgarī* script at the center. Finally, the bottom phrase *parasparopagraho jīvānām* describes the mutual support of living beings (TS 5.21). See also Jaini (2001/1979, 316).

The evolving Jain understanding of ethics is reflected in a formalized framework known as the fourteen *guṇa-sthānas*, or "ladder of karmic removal." We show the logic of this ladder in relation to the five causes of karmic bondage, noting key milestones in which a particular cause of bondage is overcome, advancing one on a path of increased restraint and decreased violence. Not only must the vows be understood in the context of this ladder, but additional key Jain concepts such as compassion (*anukampā*), non-one-sidedness (*anekānta-vāda*), and carefulness (*apramāda*) gain clarity in light of the *guṇa-sthāna* framework of advancement or regression.

Because we are examining foundations in Jainism for bioethics, which is a discipline more in the purview of lay Jains than of mendicants, we pay special attention to texts describing layperson conduct (*śrāvaka-ācāra*). The texts detail violations of the vows and vices that impede karmic progress for laity, including guidelines intended to limit harms in the course of one's personal activity, family responsibility, and vocational obligations.

We conclude the chapter by summarizing three foundational Jain ethical principles that derive from the textual and philosophical analysis herein. While these principles place a central and unparalleled emphasis on nonviolence, a comprehensive view of Jain ethics exceeds a single concept. Any examination of Jainism and contemporary bioethics requires a wider grasp of several concepts within a dynamic framework of karmic progression and regression that informs the distinct ways of living, disciplines, and goals for mendicant and lay Jains.

## AVOIDING VIOLENCE IN THE EARLY ŚVETĀMBARA CANON

The Jain "canon" includes a large collection of texts. Most Śvetāmbara Jains accept a full or modified list of forty-five canonical texts, or Āgamas, that were codified at several different councils.[2] This list of forty-five is composed of the Aṅgas (and the no longer extant Pūrvas) that contain knowledge passed directly from a Jina to students. Later texts within this list were composed by mendicant leaders, often as practical commentaries on the early Āgamas. Digambaras, however, reject the authenticity of this collection, believing that the canonical texts were lost, and that only some contents of the canon were remembered and passed on. Consequently, the Digambara sect has a collection of texts that are primarily postcanonical expositions composed by mendicant leaders (Jaini 2001/1979, 47–87; Wiley 2009, xix–xxvi). We primarily consider Śvetāmbara canonical texts here as they provide a unique window into the development of the early Jain ethical doctrines.

### Parigraha *and* Ārambha

The first parts (*śruta-skandha*) of the *Ācārāṅga-sūtra* and *Sūtrakṛtāṅga-sūtra* (*Ācārāṅga-sūtra* I and *Sūtrakṛtāṅga-sūtra* I, respectively), which are considered to represent some of the earliest surviving portions of the Śvetāmbara canon,[3] place absolute primacy on renouncing harmful activities through the mendicant way of life. In his book *Early Jainism*, K.K. Dixit notes that although the five great vows appear jointly in the *Sūtrakṛtāṅga-sūtra* I, their treatment is "almost perfunctory," and they are not mentioned together in the *Ācārāṅga-sūtra* I (1978, 7; see also Ohira 1994, 8–9).[4] A greater emphasis is placed, in these early canonical strata, on possession (*parigraha*) as one of the worst vices for an ascetic who has renounced the world. Possession is linked with violence (*ārambha*)[5] to form a pair of the two main kinds of harmful activities that sustain one's entrapment in the cycle of rebirths (Dixit 1978, 5; Ohira 1994, 8).

Dixit explains that in the early portions of the canon possession, or *parigraha*, primarily refers to attachments to material objects and familial/social relations (Dixit 1978, 5, 19).[6] Due to the pursuit of enjoyment or necessities for oneself or others, these attachments lead to violence, or *ārambha*, toward living beings. As described in chapter 2, living beings range from beings in water and fire (etc.) to plants, animals, and humans.[7] Dixit describes the intractable relationship between attachment and violence this way: "[A]ll attitude of *parigraha* towards one must involve—directly or otherwise—an attitude of *ārambha* towards another," meaning that every accumulation of a material good or pleasure enacts a harm on a living being (5). In this dynamic, notes Dixit, *ārambha* functions as an immediate cause of a harmful activity and *parigraha* as its proximate cause (5).

The term *ārambha* is derived from the verbal root *rabh-*, with the prefix *ā-*, meaning to undertake, commence, or begin (Monier-Williams 1899, 150).[8] William Johnson explains that the term evolved a sense of physical violence or killing, perhaps through the Jain account of a cosmos permeated with living beings, in which "beginning," "commencing," or "undertaking" *any action* would inevitably cause harm to some living being. Hence, he states, the two meanings of the term—to undertake an action and to kill—were probably understood to be synonymous (1995a, 38–39). Suzuko Ohira points out that in such a view of the world, one could not escape committing violence: "In breathing, speaking or stretching out his [*sic*] hand, he cannot but kill wind-beings. In extinguishing fire he murders fire-beings, in walking a street he harms earth-beings, and in shaking a water pot he hurts water-beings" (1994, 5). In line with this, any action would result in accruing karma and one's continued entrapment in the suffering cycle of rebirths,[9] though the precise mechanisms for how karmic bondage occurs were not yet formalized (Dixit 1978, 9).[10] Therefore, the only way to liberation was considered to be, at least theoretically, nonaction (*akarman*) by which one could lead a life of nonviolence (*anārambha*) (1994, 6, 10).

Already in these early portions of the canon, action—often in relation to causing some kind of harm—is understood to be threefold: (1) one can perform it directly, (2) cause another to perform it, or (3) approve of another performing it. As stated succinctly in the first teaching of the *Ācārāṅga-sūtra*, the three types of actions are "I did it," "I caused another to do it," and "I shall approve of[11] another doing it" (ĀS 1.1.1.5).[12] All three are understood as resulting in karmic retribution. The earliest canonical strata also hardly distinguish between deliberate and nondeliberate actions. The *Ācārāṅga-sūtra* 1.5.4.3, for example, describes a monk who harms living beings, even though virtuous and observant in conduct. It states that the result of such action will come to fruition in the present lifetime. On the other hand, if harm occurs that is due to not observing the rules, the text states that a monk needs to perform an atonement (*viveka*).[13] While there is an acknowledgment of a difference between the two actions, they are both understood as generating karmic cost. One of the main ways that mendicants are instructed to circumvent both attachments and violent activity in any of the three ways is by avoiding the preparation of their own food or the purchase of any needed goods. Rather, these items must be collected as alms from householders, ideally, without forming any attachment to what is collected or to householders themselves, who are described quite negatively in the *Ācārāṅga-sūtra* I as careless, greedy, and violent, among their many other undesirable traits. A mendicant should, further, lead a wandering rather than a sedentary life.

### *Solitary Mendicancy, the Goal of Liberation, and Violent Householders*

It is not entirely clear what the state of the mendicant community was at the time that the *Ācārāṅga-sūtra* I reflects. Several sections of the text mention students being taught by teachers, but the text also asserts that those who have realized the truth do not need a teacher at all and may live as solitary mendicants. This possibly indicates that mendicants either lived in small groups comprising a teacher with junior mendicants as students, or—in the case of highly developed wandering mendicants—led a solitary life (ĀS 1.6.2.3), with the student period likely functioning as a preparatory stage for the latter. Solitary life and a stringent emphasis on nonaction are certainly highlighted as an ideal lifestyle, promoting a mendicant path that emulates the asceticism and self-reliance of Mahāvīra and other Jinas. Drawing on the *Ācārāṅga-sūtra* 1.8, Ohira describes Mahāvīra's arduous asceticism in the following way:

> He went alone stark naked, without using cold water, not bathing, not cleaning his teeth, not using fire and not scratching his body. He slept little, was always vigilant, and wandered around carefully without speaking much. He bore all the hardships . . . , ate coarse food and often fasted. He exposed himself to the heat and sat squatting in the sun. He often practised meditation. . . . He might have eaten only once a day, because food, necessarily obtained by killing living beings, should be cut down in frequency, quantity and quality. Likewise using medicine which is acquired by grinding herbs, roots, etc., of living beings would have been avoided by him. He had a mission to spread his message and train his disciples, but otherwise he would probably have refrained from unnecessary speech, for speaking involves violence to subtle beings. (1994, 10)

*Ācārāṅga-sūtra* I speaks, further, of liberation as an immediately attainable goal for one who adopts the correct practices, and sharply contrasts liberation as the only worthwhile aim with every other possible outcome. These portions of the canon do not speak of a good rebirth; on the contrary, any path that does not lead to liberation is a wrong path that should be avoided (ĀS 1.2.3). This means that there is no consideration of a good householder life, since the stringent understanding of violence to living beings as a result of attachments functionally excludes laity from the possibility of liberation. Laypeople, who by definition participate in social and family life, are viewed as intrinsically attached to the activities of doing, causing, and approving of harm. Unsurprisingly, then, the behavior of householding lay Jains is described as a direct contradiction to the mendicant ideal (Dundas 2002, 42).

The question arises: if the Jain ethic of nonviolence is only for mendicants, ideally removed from society, and laypeople are innately unable to practice it, how can we examine any Jain foundations for bioethics, a discipline shaped by social and institutional activities? To answer this, we have to note that the early textual references that we are studying tend to represent ideal types of practitioners. However, even these texts are nuanced and record deviances from the arduous ideals, as evident in the next section. Furthermore, various shifts in the understanding of the doctrine and goals of practice seem to have occurred early on that enabled the development of Jainism as a fourfold community of monks, nuns, laymen, and laywomen with two distinct but related paths toward nonviolence and purification.

## EMERGING ACCOMMODATIONS FOR MENDICANTS AND LAITY

As is becoming clear, the content of the Jain canon is not uniform. Rather, texts record important shifts among an evolving religious tradition. This includes accommodations for mendicants who are less disciplined, as well as for laypeople.

### *Failure on the Path and Bad Reputation*

While the *Ācārāṅga-sūtra* I emphasizes the ideal of the solitary ascetic life, it indicates that some mendicants, despite understanding the nature of *saṃsāra* and their own bondage within it, are not able to follow the path to the same extent as others. Some of these "weaker" individuals may give up the mendicant life, it states, and in so doing gain a bad reputation (ĀS 1.6.4.3). While householders are generally shunned, as noted above, this statement seems to indicate a concern with how mendicants are perceived, possibly by the broader, householding community. The *Sūtrakṛtāṅga-sūtra* I, similarly, upholds the ideal of mendicants that lead solitary lives, but also records the difficulty of the ascetic path and failure upon it. The text identifies mendicants, for instance, who may be too weak to handle difficult austerities and return to their homes, like elephants who have been broken down with arrows (SKS 1.3.1.17). Further, it reprimands students for all sorts of unsuitable behavior toward their teachers and urges them to obey and serve the teachers (SKS 1.9.33), with one teaching even stating that only one who lives with their teacher will reach the end in liberation (SKS 1.14.4). The *Uttarādhyayana-sūtra*, a later text from the early portion of the canon, also celebrates the solitary mendicant (US 2.18, 15.16), yet describes one who does not serve and stay with the teacher as a bad mendicant (US 11.14, 17.5, 17.17) (Dixit 1978, 23–25).

These references could be interpreted as reflecting a gradual establishment of more stable groups of mendicants beyond the smaller groups of students living with their teachers during their education mentioned above,[14] or even the existence of several possible modes of mendicancy. Paul Dundas suggests the possibility of a coexistence of two alternative mendicant lifestyles already in the early phases of the development of the Jain community:

> The early medieval scriptural commentaries and texts on monastic law . . . bifurcate Jain monastic life into two modes (*kalpa*), namely the *jinakalpa*, the solitary and highly ascetic way of life corresponding to that of the Jinas in which indifference towards oneself and others is cultivated, and the *sthavirakalpa*, "the way of the elders" which was followed by those monks living in groups. This is arguably similar to the model which some scholars have identified as existing in the early *śramaṇa* tradition when at the outset there was the simultaneous possibility of two types, complementary as much as contrasting, of renunciatory life, one being more radically isolationist in style and located in the "forest", the other more communal in orientation and connected with town and village. (1997, 498; cf. Dixit 1978, 28)

### *Good Rebirth and Nonviolent Householders*

The *Sūtrakṛtāṅga-sūtra* I also records the emergence of the possibility of a good rebirth. It states: "Having heard the doctrine, which was proclaimed and established by the Arhat [i.e., Mahāvīra], and which is supported with arguments, believers will either come to an end of their [worldly] life or become like Indra, king of the gods" (SKS 1.6.29). While the *Ācārāṅga-sūtra* I sees only liberation as a worthy result of religious practice, the *Sūtrakṛtāṅga-sūtra* I contends that the path outlined by Mahāvīra will lead to either liberation or the other good option of being reborn in the heavenly realm while staying in *saṃsāra*.[15] In line with this expanded goal of the religious path, the *Sūtrakṛtāṅga-sūtra* I explains that a nonviolent householder will be reborn in the heavenly realm (SKS 1.2.3.13).

The above-mentioned concern about the reputation of mendicants—as well as such an early inclusion of laity in the spiritual path—suggests that mendicants and laity were most likely more intertwined than some passages from these early canonical strata might lead us to infer. Dundas notes that the Buddhist texts that discuss the early Jain community would most likely have mentioned that Jain mendicants were not associated with laypeople if this were the case (1997, 504). Without them, he asks, "how . . . could such a community adequately reproduce itself? How did a corpus of teaching come to be organised and expanded?" (496).

While later texts in the early canon continue to focus on mendicants rather than laity, the possibility of a good rebirth for virtuous householders remains. For example, the *Uttarādhyayana-sūtra*[16] differentiates between the "death of the unwise," who is violent and attached to pleasures, and the "death of the wise," who is nonviolent and controls the senses (see chapter 7). The text states that both virtuous mendicants and householders fall under the second category, with the latter being reborn as heavenly beings and the former attaining either liberation or rebirth in the heavenly realm (US 5.24–25). Dixit points out that this is a "position maintained by all later Jaina authors" (1978, 22). This section of the *Uttarādhyayana-sūtra* also points out that there are even householders who are more advanced in self-control than some mendicants (US 5.20).

As indicated above, the possibility of meritorious karma is not a feature of the earliest canonical strata. Karma—as a factor responsible for binding living beings in *saṃsāra*—is considered to be a result of any action, and has an inherently negative quality. Mendicant restraints can stop the karmic accrual but cannot positively influence it. By the early common era, however, the Jain doctrine accepted that liberation was no longer attainable in our part of the cosmos, owing to the weakened presence and strength of Mahāvīra's teaching in the centuries after his death.[17] With that change, practice was no longer focused only on annihilating karma, but also on gaining beneficial karma through meritorious actions that could lead to a good rebirth. Dundas highlights the significance of the notion of meritorious and nonmeritorious actions as providing "an ethical dimension which was meaningful not just for ascetics but for a community which as a whole also contained lay people" (2002, 96–97).

As the mendicant community grew, it became increasingly dependent on its lay supporters (Dundas 2002, 187). One way this is reflected in the texts is in detailed rules for mendicants' interactions with laity. The *Ācārāṅga-sūtra* II, for instance, enumerates many regulations guiding mendicants in their encounters with laypeople and, in effect, "training" laity how to properly provide for mendicants' basic needs within very circumscribed limits. In order to maintain strong lay support, mechanisms of mutual benefit evolved. The *Sūtrakṛtāṅga-sūtra*, for example, references a minimal exchange between laity providing food and mendicants providing teaching (SKS 1.7.24–27). Beyond serving practical purposes, the value of this arrangement was expanded to include karmic benefit such that a layperson's disciplined effort to feed a mendicant and the mendicant's proper reception of food, both according to detailed rules meant to minimize harms, could earn them karmic *merit* (DVS 5.1.100; see also Johnson 1995a, 30–31).

### *Activities, Motivations, and Karmic Retribution*

The notion of collectively assuming the five great vows, together with the sixth vow of refraining from eating at night, seems to have been developed by the time of the *Daśavaikālika-sūtra*[18] (Dixit 1978, 28–29; Ohira 1994, 9). In the text, as Ohira points out, the vows are explained in the form of the so-called *trividhaṃ trividhena* formula (1994, 9). This represents the threefold notion of action (*karaṇa*) explained above, along with the notion that activities (*yoga*) can be performed with the body, speech, and mind.[19] In line with this, the observance of the first great vow is, for example, explained as refraining from violence by not performing a violent act oneself, not causing somebody else to do it, and not approving of somebody else's violence, all three either with the body, speech, or mind (DVS 4.11). This triple formulation—or what Dixit calls "a triple evil act committed in a triple manner" (1978, 89)—becomes standard in later canonical texts (Ohira 1994, 154). Ohira points out that between the third and first centuries BCE the term *yoga* came to encompass all actions committed by living beings, replacing the earlier *karman* as the term for action in general.[20] *Karman* gradually developed into a specific technical term signifying karmic matter (1992, 7–8, 19, 141, 175).

Johnson suggests that in the formulation of the three different methods of violence—doing, causing, or allowing/approving of—the last term may have evolved from a prohibition of *physically allowing* harm in the earliest canon, to a prohibition of *mentally approving of* harm in the later canon. He argues that initially at least some Jains may have understood the third element—"to fully permit, or allow or consent to, wholly acquiesce in, or approve of" (Skt. *samanujānīyāt*)—as "one should not allow others to commit violence *if one is aware of their action*" (1995a, 9; emphasis added).[21] The physical character of intervention, Johnson argues, eventually diminished as the canon gradually "*internalised* the idea to a matter of [mental] attitude, of approval or disapproval" (1995a, 9; emphasis added).

The early canonical strata do not seem to give much weight to the motivations behind activities when it comes to karmic retribution. As indicated above, the *Ācārāṅga-sūtra* I is uncompromising in its understanding that every action draws karma. The *Sūtrakṛtāṅga-sūtra* I, further, attributes the distinction between mental intent and physical action to the wrong view of the *kriyāvādins*. This view distinguishes between (a) intentional violent action that is carried out, (b) nonintentional violent action that is carried out, and (c) mere violent intention. The first, according to this wrong view, accrues the most karma. The text states: "One who intends [to harm a living being] but does not do it by [an act of] the body, and one who harms it unknowingly, both are affected through a contact [with the act], but the demerit [in their case] is not very developed" (SKS 1.1.2.25). To put it another way, this passage suggests a twofold significance of mental action: first, that the mental willingness to harm, even when not accompanied by physical action, still accrues modest karma; second, physical harm that is *not* accompanied by mental action, also accrues modest karma. The first assertion seems to expand karmic accrual to encapsulate mental formations; the second assertion seems to provide a way to diminish karmic accrual if physical actions that cause harm lack mental intention. The text clearly positions itself against such a view.

Accordingly, the *Sūtrakṛtāṅga-sūtra* II mocks Buddhists for emphasizing the importance of intention. In line with their thinking, the text claims, someone who pushes a spit through a gourd, mistakenly thinking that it is an infant, is a murderer. On the other hand, a person who intends to roast a gourd but accidentally roasts an infant is not considered a murderer (SKS 2.6.26–28). The idea that the absence of intention to harm could in any way karmically redeem the action that results in harm is vehemently rejected. Nevertheless, the differentiation between deliberate and nondeliberate actions with regard to karmic accrual gradually took hold in the Jain teachings, and increasingly more emphasis was placed on motivations behind actions.

The *Daśavaikālika-sūtra* seems to be the text to start using the umbrella term *kaṣāya* to jointly refer to the four passions of anger, pride, deceitfulness, and greed mentioned in chapter 2, which, according to Dixit, suggests a relatively late date of the text (1978, 28–29; Ohira 1994, 8). While the term *kaṣāya* does not feature in the earliest portions of the canon, all the components that this term eventually comes to represent do. Apart from attachment (*parigraha*) as the main cause of violence, attraction (*rāga*), aversion (*dveṣa*), anger (*krodha*), pride (*māna*), deceitfulness (*māyā*), and greed (*lobha*) are also mentioned as causes of violence (*ārambha*) in the *Ācārāṅga-sūtra* I and the *Sūtrakṛtāṅga-sūtra* I (Ohira 1994, 8). Another cause of violence and karma that is listed in the early canon is carelessness (*pramāda*) (SKS 1.8.3). These terms were important in developments related to foregrounding the significance of motivations behind actions. The *Bhagavatī-sūtra/Vyākhyāprajñapti-sūtra* (Pkt. *Bhagavaī-sutta/Viyāhapaṇṇatti-sutta*)[22] states that a disciplined mendicant who observes his duties *carefully*, performs his actions in line with religious duties (*īryāpatha-kriyā*), because his passions have been extinguished and he acts in accordance with the vows (BhS 7.7§309b). While such actions still accrue karmic cost, they attract only short-term karma (BhS 3.3§182b).

> [A] disciplined monk who performs *īryāpatha kriyā* binds karma at the first moment, experiences it at the second moment and purges it at the third moment, inasmuch as a bundle of hay burns as soon as it is thrown into fire, drops of water on red hot iron dry up instantly, and a boat with a hundred holes can float when the holes are closed. (Ohira 1992, 145)

This holds, for example, even if a monk accidentally kills a living being while walking carefully (BhS 18.8§754b). The *Bhagavatī-sūtra* also describes the opposite kind of behavior, which is not in line with the vows (*sāmparāyika-kriyā*) (BhS 7.7§309b). This is understood as careless conduct because of passions and not observing the vows. It attracts long-term karma. The distinction between actions that accrue short-term and long-term karma serves to differentiate mendicants who are very disciplined from those who are lax in belief and practice.

All the different shifts in conceptual frameworks and practical goals that we have discussed in this chapter so far opened the way for various efforts to systematize a path of karmic progression and regression for both mendicants and laity.

## A PATH OF KARMIC REMOVAL: THE FOURTEEN *GUṆA-STHĀNAS*

The *guṇa-sthānas*, or "stages of qualities/virtues," is a term for a formal ladder of spiritual purification that constitutes the Jain path toward liberation. It consists of fourteen stages, or rungs, in which a *jīva* "exhibits different virtues (*guṇa*), indicative of increasing independence from karmic bondage" (Cort 2001a, 25). Jérôme Petit identifies several Śvetāmbara and Digambara texts that describe these steps of progress, noting that the first complete list of fourteen stages is found in the Digambara *Ṣaṭkhaṇḍa-āgama* (c. third century CE) though with few details (2015, 110). Nemicandra's *Gommaṭasāra*[23] likely offers the first full formalization of the framework (110–11), and, as John Cort points out, "the text through which most contemporary ideologues study and understand the *guṇasthānas* is the second chapter of Devendrasūri's *Karmagrantha*" (2001a, 214, fn. 24).

The path of every being in our part of the Jain universe is karmically located somewhere upon this ladder, including the whole of humanity, both Jain and non-Jain, mendicant and laity. In theory, this means that every individual *jīva* can progress on parts of the ladder to some degree. However, only humans who assume the five great mendicant vows may pursue the higher rungs. It is important to note that the *guṇa-sthānas* do not represent only a path of progression. Regression is likewise possible. Helmuth von Glasenapp notes that the order of the fourteen rungs is logical rather than chronological, and that the actual path can vary from one living being to another. "This becomes still more comprehensible," he states, "if we call to mind the fact that in the morning one can be on a high level, sink down from it at noon, and climb up to it again in the evening" (1942/1915, 69). The ladder thus represents a formal succession of stages that need to be passed if one is to attain liberation. Within this fourteen-stage framework, there is a second, smaller ladder—known as the *pratimās*—specific to laypeople. We will address both ladders in detail in the following sections. The two ladders locate nonviolence, and the rest of the vows, within a larger framework of Jain social relations and soteriological action (Kirde 2011, 85–86), illuminating many of the ethical terms discussed above.

### *The Causes of Karmic Bondage in the* Guṇa-sthānas

As already stated, Jain doctrine gradually came to consider passions, careless conduct, and conduct not aligned with the vows as affecting the nature of karmic bondage whenever bodily, verbal, and mental activities in any of the three ways are performed. Efforts to systematize the diverse threads from earlier sources eventually incorporated these factors into a scheme of five primary causes (*mūla-hetu*) of karmic bondage (*bandha*): (1) wrong worldview (*mithyā-darśana*); (2) nonrestraint (*avirati*); (3) carelessness (*pramāda*);[24] (4) passions (*kaṣāya*); and (5) the activities (*yoga*) of the body, speech, and mind (TS 8.1). These causes of bondage are each responsible for binding specific kinds of karma.[25]

The overcoming of the five primary causes of bondage marks key points of progress along the ladder of karmic removal. As we show below, the first cause of bondage (wrong worldview) is overcome at rung 4; the second cause (nonrestraint) is overcome partially at rung 5 when a layperson takes the minor vows, and fully at rung 6 when a mendicant takes the great vows; the third cause (carelessness) is overcome at rung 7; the fourth cause (passions) is gradually eroded in rungs 4 through 11 and completely overcome at rung 12; and the fifth cause (activities of body, speech, and mind) is overcome at rung 14.

*Rungs 1–4: From Wrong Worldview to Right Worldview*

The first major move along the ladder is getting from the first to the fourth rung, from wrong worldview (*mithyā-darśana, mithyā-dṛṣṭi, mithyātva*) to right worldview (*samyag-darśana, samyag-dṛṣṭi, samyaktva*). Banārsīdās describes the shift to the fourth rung as moving from "deluded" (*mūḍha*) self to "clear-sighted" (*vicakṣaṇa*) self (AA 1–4, trans. Petit), and in line with this, Nathmal Tatia compares it to a person who was born blind gaining sight, an experience accompanied with joy (1951, 273). Because right worldview is the necessary condition to achieve right knowledge and right conduct (see the "Three Jewels" in chapter 2), its importance cannot be overstated. As Jaini puts it, "the significance of *samyak-darśana* in the life of the soul is second only to that of attaining Jinahood itself" (2001/1979, 144). Its attainment is neither an easy nor a linear task.

At the first rung of wrong worldview, all five causes of karmic bondage operate. Glasenapp lists specific activities that attract worldview-deluding karmas (*darśana-mohanīya-karman*), resulting in a fundamentally mistaken worldview: "The teaching of a false [teacher], the hindrance of the true religion, the blasphemy of the Jains, of the saints, of the images of gods, of the community, of the canon, the rape of sacred objects" (1942/1915, 63). The delusion (*moha*) that is characteristic of this stage and consists of inadequate knowledge of the "reals" or the fundamental categories of existence (*tattva*), including the nature of karmic bondage, karmic removal, and liberation (GJK 15–18; see chapter 2), means that all *jīva*s—from one-sensed beings to humans—"who either have never heard the Jain teachings or else have consciously rejected them" reside here (Cort 2001a, 26).

The capacity to take the initial step of leaving this state rests in the *jīva*'s innate qualities that can never be fully subsumed by karma (see chapter 2). According to Jaini, the *jīva* "possesses a sort of built-in advantage, an everpresent tendency to develop its qualities and temporarily reduce the influence of the karmas" (2001/1979, 141). From this arises a universal urge toward self-development, present even in the smallest life-forms, to combat the passions and deluding karmas that prevent it (143), often—but not exclusively—in combination with various external factors that encourage this development (Tatia 1951, 268). The initial confrontation with one's bondage (*yathā-pravṛtta-karaṇa*)[26] may be followed by two other processes, *apūrva-karaṇa* and *anivṛtti-karaṇa*. Through these, respectively, (1) the duration and intensity of all karmas that are bound are reduced (continuing the process started during the *yathā-pravṛtta-karaṇa*) and (2) the worldview-deluding karmas are temporarily suppressed, enabling a brief experience of right worldview at the fourth rung (Jaini 2001/1979, 144, cf. 146; Tatia 1951, 269–73).

Jaini describes this brief glimpse as a "first awakening" of right worldview at the fourth rung, before—as is most common—the suppressed karmas assert themselves again and the *jīva* falls back to the third and possibly second rung,[27] from where it returns to the beginning of the ladder (2001/1979, 134, 145). But the glimpse is transformative as it eradicates a great amount of already bound karmas, weakens other karmas, as indicated above, as well as limits future influx of karmas, thus generating longer durations of right worldview. Jaini states that a *jīva* that retains right worldview at death will not be reborn as a hell-being or any of the lower life-forms of the *tiryañc* birth state (see chapter 2), and its path to total karmic removal, while still of an immense duration, will be considerably shortened, with liberation guaranteed (144–45).

The fourth rung of right worldview is considered the first official step toward liberation. Glasenapp writes that this stage belongs to those "who believe renunciation worthy of being striven after" (1942/1915, 79). According to Jaini, "it is said that only one who has undergone such an experience [in the fourth stage] should be called 'Jaina,' for only he [*sic*] has truly entered upon the path that the Jinas have followed" (2001/1979, 146). Both five-sensed humans and five-sensed animals with a mind can reach this stage (SSi 2.3§258; Glasenapp 1942/1915, 70; Wiley 2006b, 252). Since right worldview is the prerequisite step for greater advancement along the ladder, it is important to note that many beings in the universe who have not reached the fourth rung are not actually considered to be on the path toward liberation at all. Likewise, one who falls below the fourth stage, in effect, slips off the path, and must again strive to regain right worldview.

While a living being may lapse back many times to lower stages after reaching the fourth rung, the permanent attainment of the right worldview signifies a complete overcoming of the first cause of bondage, that of wrong worldview (*mithyā-darśana*). All of the worldview-deluding karmas as well as the gross forms of passions—called "pursuers from the limitless past," or *ananta-anubandhī* passions, which express themselves in extreme kinds of attachment and aversion—are conquered on this occasion (Jaini 2001/1979, 118–19). A living being that attains it will never again regress below the fourth rung and will reach liberation in no more than four lives (146).

In spite of attaining right worldview, however, a *jīva* at this stage still lacks right conduct. As Tatia states, "It has the requisite vision and knowledge and wisdom. It has the right will. But the energy for self-control is wanting" (1951, 277; see also Glasenapp 1942/1915, 79). While overcoming deluding karmas and gross passions enables the *possibility* for right conduct in later stages, nonrestrained actions and associated passions still characterize this rung.

*Changing Attitudes and Behavior: The Development of Compassion.* Glimpsing the fourth stage, even momentarily, transforms individuals who have had this experience, and Jains maintain that the results of this change are not only internal (*bhāva-samyaktva*), but are evident also externally (*dravya-samyaktva*). Jaini details a foundational realignment of consciousness regarding the attitude toward oneself, from being a "self" that identifies with external factors, objects, and results (e.g., body, wealth) and aims to actively intervene in the world, to gaining a focus on the internal self. This reorientation results in a state of bliss (*sukha*), "hardly imaginable to an ordinary person," and tranquility (*praśama*), as well as fear of and disillusionment with the worldly existence (*saṃvega*), sometimes leading to renunciation (2001/1979, 147–49; see also YŚ 2.15; Brekke 2005, 75–75; Williams 1963, 42). The experience of right worldview produces confidence (*āstikya*) in the Jain teachings, particularly the "reals," preventing skepticism, nihilism, and the dogmatism of non-one-sided views. A clear understanding of the true relation between eternal substances (*dravya*) and their constantly changing modes (*paryāya*) (see chapter 2), further, "generates a feeling of great compassion (*anukampā*) for others"(Jaini 2001/1979, 150). We address this important ethical concept briefly here.[28]

The role of compassion (*anukampā, dayā, kāruṇya*), its precise meaning, and its relation to nonviolence and karmic bondage in Jain ethics are not always clear. In the early Śvetāmbara canon, for example, one of the motivations for not pursuing violence (*ārambha*) seems to be a recognition that all beings are universally vulnerable to pain, akin to oneself. In those same early texts, however, attachments (*parigraha*) to social relationships are also a cause of violence and subsequent karmic bondage (see chapter 2). If the ultimate goal is to avoid attachment and escape from the world of suffering, does that mean that orthodox mendicant practice is incompatible with a thoroughgoing sense of and/or acting from compassion?

Jaini states that the experience of right worldview provides an insight into the nature of bondage and through it a deep awareness of and a sense of identity with all the other living beings trapped in the cycle of rebirths (2001/1979, 149–50), much like the awareness of the universal experience of pain mentioned above. However, he also notes that compassion gained in right worldview signifies something different than its typical social meaning: "Whereas the compassion felt by an ordinary [hu]man is tinged with pity or with attachment to its object, *anukampā* [compassion] is free of such negative aspects; it develops purely from wisdom, from seeing the substance (*dravya*) that underlies visible modes [*paryāya*], and it fills the individual with an unselfish desire to help other souls towards *mokṣa*" (150).[29] A moderate experience of compassion at the fourth rung, Jaini says, "brings an end to exploitative and destructive behavior, for even the lowest animal is now seen as intrinsically worthwhile and thus inviolable" (150). On the other hand, a strong desire to help others who are suffering in the cycle of rebirths may accumulate the auspicious karmas that produce the birth of a Jina (150; see also Wiley 2006, 447). The fundamental assertion articulated in the *Tattvārtha-sūtra* that "[the function] of living beings is to support (*upagraha*) one another" (TS 5.21) highlights the importance of such help. The *Tattvārthādhigama-bhāṣya* understands this support as offering advice: "The support of *jīvas* is advice to one another with regard to that which is beneficial and that which is unbeneficial (*hita-ahita-upadeśa*)" (TBh 5.21), which Siddhasenagaṇin glosses as helping others in attaining that which is beneficial (*hita-pratipādana*) and preventing that which is unbeneficial (*ahita-pratiṣedha*) (TṬ 5.21).

The relationship between attachment and compassion in relation to the different stages of the ladder of karmic removal, including those beyond the fourth rung, is addressed in various postcanonical texts. Wiley notes that Digambara commentaries to the *Tattvārtha-sūtra* distinguish between two kinds of right worldview: (1) right worldview *with* attachments (*sarāga-samyag-darśana*) and (2) right worldview *without* attachments (*vītarāga-samyag-darśana*). The external characteristics (including compassion) of a person who has experienced the fourth rung, which were listed above, fall under the right worldview *with* attachments. The right worldview *without* attachments, on the other hand, "is characterized only by the purity of the soul itself (*ātma-viśuddhi-mātra*)" (2006a, 440; see also PS 2.65–67). According to these texts, compassion arises in association with the right worldview when individuals are still influenced by conduct-deluding karma that produces passions in the form of attachment or aversion (see chapter 2). It is maintained through the twelfth rung—described shortly—and relinquished with all other attachments thereafter (Wiley 2006a, 441).

In line with this, the *Tattvārtha-sūtra* describes compassion (*anukampā*) as a cause that binds *sātā-vedanīya-karman*, a non-destructive type of karma that gives rise to pleasant feelings (see chapter 2), thus perpetuating one's entrapment in *saṃsāra* ($TS^{Śv}$ 6.13;[30] Wiley 2006a, 439, 441–42). The *Tattvārtha-sūtra*, further, lists compassion (*kāruṇya*) as one of the contemplations (*bhāvanā*), that is, supporting practices that strengthen the vows: "Friendliness (*maitrī*) toward all living beings (*sattva*), delight (*pramoda*) with those whose qualities are superior (*guṇa-adhika*), compassion (*kāruṇya*) for the afflicted (*kliśyamāna*), and equanimity (*mādhyastha*) toward the ill-behaved (*avinaya*) [should be contemplated]" ($TS^{Śv}$ 7.6;[31] trans. Wiley 2006a, 443). Compassion, then, seems to be a factor that can aid progress on the path to liberation, but since it still produces karma, it must eventually be transcended at the highest levels of the spiritual path.

How have such complex teachings on compassion been reflected in the understanding and practices of the Jain communities? In her research on Jains in diaspora, Anne Vallely argues that young, second-generation lay Jains frequently interpret compassion, not only as recognition of shared vulnerability, but also as a positive injunction to protect living beings, though she recognizes that this interpretation conflicts with the orthodox goal of overcoming all attachments (2002b, 205–13). While certain scholars see the outreach of diaspora Jains as a "neo-orthodox" revision of earlier restraints (Banks 1991, 244–57), there are certainly sectarian examples of active compassion among lay Jains. The Sthānakavāsī sect of Śvetāmbara Jains, for instance, distinguishes itself by venerating mendicants and encouraging merit-making activities of householders, which include not only gifting (*dāna*) mendicants with proper donations, but also compassionate service toward humans and animals (Wiley 2009, 203–4). Sthānakavāsī monk Ācārya Suśīlkumār (1926–94) exemplified modern social outreach by traveling in 1975 by plane—a form of travel generally forbidden to mendicants—to the United States, where in 1983 he developed a religious center called Siddhācalam for US Jains and non-Jains (Dundas 2002, 254). He actively worked to bring peace in the Punjab region of India during the 1980s, and promoted dialogue between Hindu and Muslim parties during the Ayodhya dispute in 1992.[32]

The Terāpanthī sect of Śvetāmbara Jains, on the other hand, originally strictly distinguished between worldly compassion (*laukika-dayā*) in the form of social activism and merit-making acts, and spiritual compassion (*dharma-dayā*) in the form of religious instruction. They viewed only the latter as part of the path to liberation (Wiley 2006a, 445–47). However, that changed in the 20th century, particularly with Ācārya Tulsī (1914–97), the ninth leader of the Terāpanthī sect, who promoted civic engagement through the Aṇuvrat Movement for laity, which he established in 1949. In 1980, he also initiated an intermediary class of Jain mendicants known as *samaṇ* (male) and *samaṇī* (female), who have greater flexibility with their vows and can use mechanized transport, travel abroad, and handle money in order to support Jains living in diaspora countries (Wiley 2009, 217; see chapter 5).

If anything can be deduced here regarding the role of compassion in relation to nonviolence and a Jain approach to bioethics, it is that the Jain concept of compassion indicates a comprehension of shared vulnerability and suffering, and not merely a sense of impassioned sympathy (Vallely 2018). Even if compassion is an attachment that must be ultimately overcome, as most scholars and texts seem to suggest, its experience can be a catalyst for advancement up to that point, and perhaps nurture qualities of Jinahood at an early stage.

### *Rung 5: Lay Restraints: The* Pratimās *and the Minor Vows*

Having overcome the first cause of bondage of wrong worldview in the previous stage, one becomes an "active member" of the Jain community in the fifth *guṇa-sthāna* (Petit 2015, 99). This rung is called "partial restraint" (*deśa-virata*), since the second cause of bondage—that of nonrestraint (*avirati*)—is *partially* overcome. It results from the elimination of the *apratyākhyāna-āvaraṇa* passions, or "obstructors of partial renunciation," and represents Jain laity accepting limited restraints. Tatia defines the attainment of the rung as a shift to "right vision with capacity for partial abstinence" (1951, 277), while Glasenapp describes it as "partial self-control" (1942/1915, 81).

As with the previous stage, one can experience the fifth *guṇa-sthāna* for a brief or lengthy duration, and with greater or lesser intensity. In order to experience the stage fully, a layperson can undertake a series of eleven steps, called *pratimās*,[33] which function as a smaller ladder for laity within the larger ladder of the *guṇa-sthānas*. These steps are intended to help laypeople progress from the fifth to the sixth *guṇa-sthāna*, and they accordingly provide them with religious commitments that increasingly resemble those of mendicants. Once a layperson accepts a specific *pratimā*, the commitment is considered to be lifelong. Although Śvetāmbara and Digambara sources have some variation in the order, names, and content of the eleven steps (GJK 477; SSN 13.56–58; ŚĀ 4; Kirde 2011, 11; Williams 1963; 173–74), all sources affirm that the *pratimā* ladder involves laity taking the vows. They are taken partially, as minor vows (*aṇu-vratas*), under the guidance of a teacher.[34] It is important to understand where these minor vows fit into this stage more broadly.

*Pratimā* 1: Accepting Fundamentals. The first step in the *pratimā* path, called *darśana-pratimā*, or "the stage of right views," comprises acts of devotion and preparatory restraints demonstrating the right worldview gained in the fourth stage and the commitment to Jain "fundamentals" (Jaini 2001/1979, 161). The acts of devotion express the acceptance of the Jinas as objects of worship, the Āgamas as sacred texts, and Jain mendicants as the sole proper teachers (162). One of the central devotional practices is the recitation of the foundational Prākrit mantra, called the *pañca-namaskāra-mantra*, which pays homage to the five supreme beings (*pañca-parameṣṭhin*): (1) the Jinas (*arhat*), (2) the liberated beings (*siddha*), (3) the mendicant leaders (*ācārya*), (4) the mendicant teachers (*upādhyāya*), and (5) all the mendicants (*sādhu*) (Donaldson 2017; Jaini 2001/1979, 162–63).[35] Other acts of devotion include hymns of praise (*stava*) to the Jinas or the canon that transmits their teachings.

The preparatory restraints (*mūla-guṇa*) include eight restrictions regarding diet, namely refraining from eating meat, alcohol, honey, and five fruits in the fig family (ŚĀ 57–59). Although refraining from meat is an obvious restraint of *ahiṃsā*, the other food prohibitions are related to preventing harm to one-sensed *nigodas* considered prevalent in fermented, sweet, or seed-filled plants (GJK 186–91; Jaini 2001/1979, 166–68; see chapters 2 and 6). It is noteworthy that these preparatory restraints of the first *pratimā* are not a *result* of taking the five vows, but are *prerequisite* to the vows. In fact, Robert Williams states that for the Digambaras, the *mūla-guṇas* are "a category of interdictions which must be respected if even the first stage on the ladder of the *pratimās* is to be attained" (1963, 50; see also Kirde 2011, 9–10).[36]

*Pratimā* 2: The Vows *(Vrata)*. One who has appreciated the value of the fundamental devotions and preparatory restraints is ready for the next step in the *pratimā* path, called *vrata-pratimā*, or "the stage of taking the vows." There are twelve lay vows (*śrāvaka-vrata*), consisting of five minor vows (*aṇu-vrata*) and seven supplementary vows (see below). Each of the five minor vows represents a different restraint, to which we now turn.

*First Minor Vow: Nonviolence* (ahiṃsā)—The goal of nonviolence is rooted in two distinct, but overlapping, motivations. The first motivation, described above, is the recognition that all living beings are vulnerable to suffering and death, in accordance with which one should minimize all actions that could harm them. The second motivation is to restrain passions that inform the harmful activities of body, speech, and mind, and attract and bind karma ($TS^{Śv}$ 6.5–7;[37] Wiley 2006a, 438). In this latter understanding, violence "refers primarily to injuring oneself—to behavior which inhibits the soul's ability to attain *mokṣa*" (Jaini 2001/1979, 167). Jaini explains that "the killing of animals, for example, is reprehensible not only for the suffering produced in the victims, but even more so because it involves intense passions on the part of the killer, passions which bind him [*sic*] more firmly in the grip of saṃsāra" (167).

Because the minor vow of *ahiṃsā* is partial, it permits laypeople to commit some harms to beings with fewer senses in the activities of their daily lives (Jaini 2001/1979, 241–43). Williams explains how mendicants must avoid *sūkṣma-hiṃsā*, or "subtle violence," toward all life-forms, including one-sensed beings, while laypeople endeavor to avoid *sthūla-hiṃsā*, or "gross violence," toward beings with two or more senses (1963, 65–66; see also Balbir 2015, 91–92). This results in a functional hierarchy for those beings that mendicants must not harm (one- through five-sensed beings) and those that a layperson must avoid injuring (two- through five-sensed beings). Violating a being with more senses results in greater karma to the one causing injury.

*Second Minor Vow: Truthfulness* (satya)—The vow of truthfulness, which laity observe partially and mendicants fully, requires great care with the speech-related activities that might have destructive consequences. On one hand, this refers to utterances that are informed by the passions and, thus, injurious to the self that produces them. On the other, it also refers to the effects of speech acts that might be injurious to other living beings (Williams 1963, 71–78). In line with this, the vow of truthfulness prohibits speaking falsely; wrongly accusing another; insulting someone; causing embarrassment; encouraging another to perform injurious actions; wrong instruction; telling secrets; and so on. It is important to note that the considerations of the effects of actions that fall under this vow do not relate only to lying and deceit, but also to truthful utterances. Accordingly, the vow forbids speaking any truth that might lead to the destruction of embodied life-forms (77–78; Jaini 2001/1979, 174; SSi 7.14§689; YŚ 2.61). Jaini explains, for example, that a layperson may mislead a hunter who asks where a deer went in order to prevent harm, resulting in only a minimal intake of karma, while a mendicant's complete vow necessitates silence (174; see also Dundas 2002, 160). Nalini Balbir affirms that "lay Jains can knowingly utter a falsehood if this stops a greater wrong" (n.d.). The vow of truthfulness also involves positively directing speech toward worthwhile pursuits that serve self and others (Williams 1963, 77).

*Third Minor Vow: Nonstealing* (asteya)—Nonstealing involves a restraint against stealing (*steya*) or taking what is not given (*adatta-ādāna*). For mendicants, the vow refers primarily to alms and mendicant equipment (Balbir n.d.), whereas for laity, it relates to everything that has not been either inherited or obtained through legitimate means (Jaini 2001/1979, 175). In practice, this can refer to taking something belonging to another person; receiving stolen goods; using deceptive measurements; or cheating others with counterfeit goods, which also overlaps the previous vow of truthfulness. Many of these restrictions clearly apply to business transactions. Stealing is also highlighted as an expression of violence, since it robs people of possessions that are their source of consolation and, thus, "takes away" their lives (Williams 1963, 78–84).

*Fourth Minor Vow: Sexual Restraint* (brahmacarya)—Jainism recognizes three sexes, namely male, female, and "third sex," as well as three parallel sexual feelings or desires (SSi 2.52; $TS^{Dig}$ 8.9;[38] see chapter 5). While sexual restraint for mendicants means eschewing all sexual desires and activities, which represent damaging passions and attachments (Jaini 2001/1979, 176–77), laypeople are to content themselves in monogamous spousal relations with moderate sexual activity. Refraining from sexual relations for specific periods of time and for pleasure is seen as virtuous behavior. We will explore the topic of sexual restraint in more detail in chapter 5 in relation to reproductive birth control.

*Fifth Minor Vow: Nonpossession* (aparigraha)—Nonpossession is a restraint with two distinct aspects: forgoing *attachment* to internal and external possessions, and forgoing the *accumulation* of possessions (Balbir n.d.). Internal (*abhyantara*) possessions include attachments to beliefs, emotions, sexual urges, fears, and desires; external (*bahya*) possessions include attachments to assets such as land, homes, money, servants, and furniture (Jaini 2001/1979, 177; Williams 1963, 93–94). Being attached to such possessions can fuel passions that may injure self and others through the actions of body, speech, and mind (Williams 1963, 99). Nonpossession also includes forgoing the accumulation of possessions. While, for mendicants, who observe the vow fully, this means walking away from all social and material bonds (see below), laypeople, who observe the vow partially, fulfill it by setting limits to material, psychological, and relational possessions.

*The Seven Supplementary Vows*—Lay Jains can strengthen their five minor vows with seven additional supporting restraints (called *guṇa-vrata* and *śikṣā-vrata*). Laypeople may commit to these for the rest of their life, during holiday periods, or not at all.

Three *guṇa-vrata*s support the minor vows by placing additional limits on activity and contact with life-forms and objects through various restraints. The first supplementary vow (*dig-vrata*) addresses limiting the area in which one walks or travels in order to minimize harm (YŚ 3.2–3). A layperson can geographically demarcate the boundaries of movement by referencing specific locations, or commit to restrict movement to a certain radius. The second (*bhoga-upabhoga-parimāṇa-vrata*) requires refraining from pleasures or enjoyments that increase attachments and may result in harm. Hemacandra describes a variation of this vow as placing limits on items used once (*bhoga*), such as food or a decorative garland, or those used repeatedly (*upabhoga*) for pleasure, such as a lover, house, bed, or vehicle (YŚ 3.4–7). This vow includes the restriction of eating plants that contain infinite numbers of *nigodas* (*ananta-kāya*) and eating at night (*rātri-bhojana*), as well as drinking only filtered water. The restrictions of performing various occupations, which will be discussed in more detail below, likewise fall under this vow. The third supplementary vow (*anartha-daṇḍa-vrata*) requires one to avoid purposeless activities such as listening to stories that instigate violence, dwelling on dark thoughts, digging the earth or cutting trees, gambling, or providing a means of destruction for others (Jaini 2001/1979, 178–80; Williams 1963, 99–131).

Four *śikṣā-vratas* support the minor vows by introducing certain commitments that are to be observed on a regular basis, be it weekly, daily, monthly, and so on. These include (1) *deśa-avakāśika-vrata*, by which a layperson takes on an even more severe temporary restriction of travel than established with the *dig-vrata*, such as staying in a room, or limits communication, such as not speaking by phone or email, for a short term; (2) *sāmāyika-vrata*, by which one commits to regularly performing the meditative practice of equanimity (*sāmāyika*) for short periods; (3) undertaking a fast from eating and drinking, as well as refraining from performing household-related activities for a set period of time (*poṣadha-upavāsa-vrata*); (4) providing support to mendicants (*dāna-vrata*), such as preparing appropriate foods, as well as learning the acceptable modes of interaction and to recognize worthy recipients (Jaini 2001/1979, 180–81; Williams 1963, 131–72). Beyond these seven supplementary vows, lay Jains have the opportunity, though not the requirement, to take another supplementary vow of voluntary death toward the end of life, known as *sallekhanā* (also Śv. *saṃthāra*; detailed in chapter 7).

*Pratimās* 3–11. The remaining nine steps of the *pratimā* ladder require increased rigor in observing each of the twelve vows previously taken. An individual may or may not take these steps, demonstrating the wide range of advancement possible in this fifth *guṇa-sthāna*. Taking all nine of these remaining steps advances an individual to a state just short of the mendicant vows, which can be taken in the sixth *guṇa-sthāna*. These steps include (step 3) thrice-daily meditation (*sāmāyika*) akin to a mendicant's minimum requirement (*sāmāyika-pratimā*);[39] (step 4) fasting (*poṣadha*) from food and drink as well as refraining from social and business activities on four auspicious lunar days each month (*poṣadha-pratimā*); (step 5) giving up (*tyāga*) unboiled water,[40] green leaves, shoots, raw seeds and fruit, as well as root vegetables, and other foods that mendicants avoid (*sacitta-tyāga-pratimā*) (in

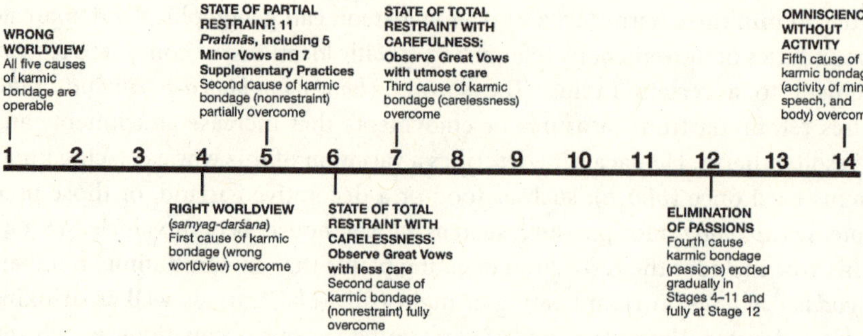


FIGURE 4. A diagram of the *guṇa-sthānas*, noting the particular causes of karmic bondage overcome at the respective stages. Credit: B. Donaldson.

addition to already eschewing meat);[41] (steps 6 and 7) increasing the vow of sexual restraint, including engaging in sex only at night (*rātri-bhakta-pratimā*) or possibly advancing to absolute abstinence (*brahmacarya-pratimā*); (step 8) withdrawal from all personal harmful activities, including abandoning one's occupation, though one's employees or agents may still engage in such efforts (*ārambha-tyāga-pratimā*); (step 9) releasing ties to possessions related to the lay life, including employees or agents, so that only one's family continues business activities, and so on (*parigraha-tyāga-pratimā*); and (steps 10 and 11) preparing for mendicant renunciation by total disengagement from household activities and, eventually, giving up all food and shelter prepared specially for oneself (*anumati-tyāga-pratimā, uddiṣṭa-tyāga-pratimā*). At the eleventh stage, one is considered "about to be a mendicant" (*śramaṇa-bhūta*) in the Śvetāmbara tradition. The layperson who has attained it emulates the mendicant lifestyle by carrying mendicant equipment, and possibly wearing mendicant clothes and shaving the head. The Digambara tradition divides this final step into two stages, that of a "junior/minor" (*kṣullaka*), who dons three pieces of clothing, and that of an *ailaka*, who wears only a single piece of clothing (Jaini 2001/1979, 182–84; Petit 2015, 106–8; Williams 1963, 175–81). One can get a sense of where the vows and *pratimās* fit within the larger ladder of karmic removal in figure 4 (noting where each of the five causes of bondage is overcome).

Jaini claims that historically these *pratimās* were intended to be practiced "for a period of months equal to the 'step number' of that *pratimā*"—that is, one month for the fundamentals, two months for the *vratas*, and so on, requiring five-and-a-half years of progress toward becoming mendicant-like (2001/1979, 185). "Thereafter," says Jaini, "the aspirant would usually (but not necessarily) decide to take the vows permanently," as a mendicant in the sixth *guṇa-sthāna*, though this timeline is no longer observed (185).

One who moves through all the *pratimās* succeeds in *partially* overcoming the second cause of bondage of nonrestraint (*avirati*), and is prepared for the next step of accepting the great vows.

### *Rungs 6 and 7: Mendicant Restraints: From Careless to Careful Practice of the Great Vows*

The sixth *guṇa-sthāna*, called "total restraint" (*sarva-virata*), signifies fully overcoming the second cause of bondage, that of nonrestraint (*avirati*) (AA 5; GJK 32). The *pratyākhyāna-āvaraṇa* passions, or "obstructors of complete renunciation," that prevented total restraint in the previous stage are now overcome, enabling one to take the five great vows (*mahā-vrata*) as part of a formal initiation (*dīkṣā*) or renunciation (*pravrajyā*) ceremony for entry into mendicant life. This ritual publicly signifies the rebirth of an aspiring monk or nun who has left their name, family, social status, occupation, possessions, and clothing (Jaini 2001/1979, 243–46).

In spite of one's having attained this significant milestone, Jaini points out that very subtle passions still operate at this level, known as "smoldering passions" (*saṃjvalana*, lit. "fuel") (120). While these passions "are not sufficiently strong to prevent one from entering the mendicant's path," he says, "they induce an insidious state of apathy or inertia (*pramāda*), a lack of drive with regard to the the actual purifactory practices entailed by that path" (120). Glasenapp refers to these as "flaming-up passions" that stoke the third cause of karmic bondage, carelessness (*pramāda*),[42] which undermines the newly achieved self-control (1942/1915, 82).[43] Wiley states that these smoldering passions "cause lapses or carelessness in observing the mendicant vows and an unconscious attachment to life" (2009, 121). Consequently, the sixth *guṇa-sthāna* is also known as the stage of "restraint with carelessness" (*pramatta-virata*).

In the seventh *guṇa-sthāna*, however, the third cause of bondage, carelessness, is overcome so that a mendicant can practice the great vows carefully. Hence, the seventh rung is called "restraint without carelessness" (*apramatta-virata*). Tatia describes this rung as "self-control with freedom from spiritual inertia (*apramatta-saṃyata*)" (1951, 277; see also GJK 45), while Glasenapp calls it "complete self-control without negligence" (1942/1915, 83).

As in previous stages, the movement between the sixth and seventh rungs is not linear. One may briefly suppress the "smoldering" passions that cause carelessness, and experience moments of careful practice, then slide back toward carelessness, repeating this advancement and regression many times (Glasenapp 1942/1915, 82). To aid in this transition as well as propel one to the further stages on the path of karmic removal, mendicants undertake several supporting practices, which will be discussed in the next section.

*Mendicant Supporting Practices.* In order to strengthen one's adherence to the five vows by continuing to reduce the frequency, duration, and space of one's actions, and thereby gradually stop the accrual of new karma (*saṃvara*), mendicants assume three additional restraints and five additional rules of conduct, known as the "eight matrices of doctrine" (*aṣṭa-pravacana-mātṛka*) (Jaini 2001/1979, 247; see also GJK 472). These eight supporting practices prepare one, as Jaini states, "for the advanced meditational states through which karmic matter is finally eliminated from the soul" (2001/1979, 247). The three restraints, or *guptis*, require one to further limit the activities of body (*kāya-gupti*), speech (*vāg-gupti*), and mind (*mano-gupti*), for instance by quieting the mind from thoughts and practicing silence and stillness (TS 9.4). The five supporting rules, or *samitis*, include using (1) extreme care in walking, to avoid injuring small living beings (*īryā-samiti*); (2) care in speaking infrequently and only when needed, to utter only truth or remain silent (*bhāṣā-samiti*); (3) care in accepting alms by making certain the food is appropriate, and eating it without excess pleasure (*eṣaṇā-samiti*); (4) care in picking up and setting down any object, such as a water pot or alms bowl, to avoid harming living beings (*ādāna-nikṣepaṇa-samiti*); and (5) care in executing excretory functions, by choosing a proper place, so as not to harm other beings (*utsarga-samiti*) (TS 9.5; Jaini 2001/1979, 247–48).

Mendicants also undertake twelve mental disciplines, called *anuprekṣās* (Dig.) or *bhāvanās* (Śv.), in which they reflect on impermanence (*anitya*), helplessness in the face of death (*aśaraṇa*), the cycle of rebirth (*saṃsāra*), the existential solitude of every individual's karmic path (*ekatva*), the distinction of body and *jīva* (*anyatva*), the karmic impurities that characterize a visually attractive body (*aśuci*), the reality of karmic inflow (*āsrava*), how to stop the inflow (*saṃvara*), how to erode existing karma (*nirjarā*), the nature of the cosmos (*loka*), the rarity of human birth alongside the greater rarity of true insight (*bodhi-durlabha*), and the absolute truth of the (Jina's) teachings (*dharma-svākhyātatva*) (TS 9.7; Jaini 2001/1979, 248; Sogani 2016, 155–58).[44] These twelve reflections are accompanied by cultivating the increasing perfection of ten moral virtues (*daśa-dharma*): patience (*kṣamā*), modesty (*mārdava*), honesty (*ārjava*), purity (*śauca*), truthfulness (*satya*), restraint (*saṃyama*), austerity (*tapas*), renunciation (*tyāga*), nonattachment (*ākiñcanya*), and sexual control (*brahmacarya*) (TS 9.6; Jaini 2001/1979, 248).

Additionally, mendicants assume six daily obligatory practices (*āvaśyaka*) that support discipline and provide a means of karmic expiation or austerities.[45] Some of these practices parallel those in the layperson *pratimās* of the fifth *guṇa-sthāna*, and they are themselves also recommended for laity. The six practices include (1) attaining a state of mental equanimity (*sāmāyika*), (2) venerating the twenty-four Jinas (*caturviṃśati-stava*), (3) honoring the mendicants (*guru-vandana*), (4) confessing one's daily harms (*pratikramaṇa*), (5) ascetic posture indicating the abandonment of the body (*kāya-utsarga*), and (6) fasting from certain foods or activities for a determined time (*pratyākhyāna*) (Balbir 1993; Williams 1963, 185).

By practicing these restraints and rules of conduct, mental reflections, moral virtues, and daily disciplines, mendicants prepare themselves to bear common "hardships" (*parīṣaha*) of mendicant life, which will help them stay on the spiritual path and remove karma (TS 9.8). The *Tattvārtha-sūtra*, for example, names twenty-two such hardships, ranging from hunger, thirst, cold, heat, and insect bites to injury and illness, among others (TS 9.9; see also US 2). These hardships gradually decrease as one progresses in the *guṇa-sthāna*s, as does one's reaction to them.[46]

Furthermore, in order to remove the karma that has already been accumulated, mendicants perform a wide range of voluntary ascetic practices (*tapas*). These are divided into twelve types, six external and six internal (US 30). The six external types are (1) fasting (*anaśana*); (2) reduced quantity of food (*avamaudarya*); (3) limitations relating to the gathering of alms (*vṛtti-parisaṃkhyāna*); (4) refusing tasty food (*rasa-parityāga*); (5) staying in isolated places (*vivikta-śayyāsana*); and (6) bodily mortifications (*kāya-kleśa*) (TS 9.19). The six internal types are (1) expiation of transgressions (*prāyaścitta*); (2) reverence (*vinaya*); (3) service to the teacher and other mendicants (*vaiyāvṛttya*); (4) study (*svādhyāya*); (5) renunciation of attachments (*vyutsarga*); and (6) meditation/concentration (*dhyāna*) (TS 9.20).

Finally, mendicants may also take the vow of *sallekhanā*, or the voluntary fast unto death, toward the end of their life (as detailed in chapter 7).

The sixth and seventh *guṇa-sthāna*s demonstrate that mendicants take the vows with varying degrees of carelessness and carefulness, or in Tatia's translation, "spiritual inertia" and "spiritual vigor" (1951, 275). He states that the *jīva* "fluctuates between the state of spiritual vigor and the state of spiritual inertia a hundred times before it reaches the state of steady progress" (275). Once a mendicant begins to increasingly overcome carelessness, the ability to rigorously practice meditation, particularly pure concentration (*śukla-dhyāna*), propels one to the next rung on the *guṇa-sthāna* ladder (Jaini 2001/1979, 253).

### *Rungs 8–12: Stages of Meditation to Suppress or Eliminate the Remaining Passions*

Having overcome three of the five causes of bondage at this point, individuals who reach the eighth *guṇa-sthāna*—called *apūrva-karaṇa*, or "unprecedented activity"—will proceed to diminish the remaining passions and karmas either through a path of suppression (*upaśama-śreṇi*), which is the less effective route, or a path of elimination (*kṣapaṇa-śreṇi/kṣapaka-śreṇi*), which is the more effective route.

The eighth rung is considered "unprecendented" because one can, in a relatively short period that one stays in the rung (one *antar-muhūrta*, or less than forty-eight minutes), begin to reduce the duration and intensity of previously bound karmas, as well as new karmas, more effectively than at any other point in their history (Tatia 1951, 271–72, 277). In this rung, the meditative practices of pure concentration (*śukla-dhyāna*) enable the mendicant to confront the remaining "smoldering" passions (*saṃjvalana-kaṣāya*), as well as a lingering group of subsidiary passions, called *no-kaṣāya*, including mundane emotions such as laughter, pleasure and displeasure in sense activity, sorrow, fear, disgust, and sexual feelings/desires (Jaini 2001/1979, 118–21; Wiley 2009, 158). Jaini explains: "The degree to which these *no-kaṣāya*s are manifest decreases with spiritual advancement; hence a monk is likely to laugh or weep or feel revulsion much less than ordinary people do, while for the *kevalin* [rungs 13 and 14] there are no such activities or feelings whatsoever" (120).

The emotional passions of *no-kaṣāya* are "rendered inoperative" in the eighth as well as the ninth rung, called *anivṛtti-karaṇa*, or "no return process" (Jaini 2001/1979, 257). Nearly all the smoldering passions are overcome in the tenth rung, called *sūkṣma-sāmparāya*, because only the most subtle (*sūkṣma*) passion of greed (*lobha*) is still operative (Glasenapp 1942/1915, 87). Tatia states that this form of greed "can be interpreted as the subconscious attachment to the body even in the souls which have achieved great spiritual advancement" (1951, 278).

What happens at the eleventh *guṇa-sthāna*—called *upaśānta-moha*, or "pacified delusion"—depends on whether one has taken the less effective path to suppress (*upaśama-śreṇi*) or the more effective path to eliminate (*kṣapaṇa-śreṇi/kṣapaka-śreṇi*) the remaining passions and karmas through the previous three rungs of meditation. Suppressing the karmas and passion is effective enough to enable an individual to reach the eleventh stage for a short delusion-free period, which is immediately followed by a fall to a lower rung (Glasenapp 1942/1915, 88). If one has taken the path to elimination, one "will pass over the eleventh guṇasthāna altogether" (Jaini 2001/1979, 257), and reach the twelfth *guṇa-sthāna*—called *kṣīṇa-moha*, or "destroyed delusion"—in which all of the subtle smoldering passions are totally eliminated, meaning that all the deluding (*mohanīya*) karmas are destroyed.

With this achievement, the fourth cause of karmic bondage—the passions, which have been operative for the entirety of embodied existence across innumerable rebirths—are finally overcome, and one gains a state of perfect conduct (*yathākhyāta-cāritra*) (Jaini 2001/1979, 258). One who reaches the twelfth rung of perfect conduct and obliterates passions will not fall below this stage again and guarantees the inevitable push toward liberation.

### *Rungs 13 and 14: Attaining Embodied Omniscience and Liberated Omniscience*

As the last passions are overcome, all the remaining *ghātiyā* karmas (karmas destructive of the *jīva*'s qualities; see chapter 2) are eliminated. The *jīva*'s qualities of perception, knowledge, energy, and bliss are fully realized in the thirteenth *guṇa-sthāna*. One who reaches this stage is a "supreme" (*parama*) self (AA 1, 7–8, trans. Petit) known as *arhat* or *kevalin*, the latter referring to the possession of omniscient, unobstructed cognition called *kevala-jñāna* (see chapter 2).[47] At this stage, the only remaining cause of karmic bondage is activity (*yoga*) of body, speech, and mind, which is why the practitioner who attains it is called *sayoga-kevalin*, or "omniscient with vibratory activity" (GJK 64, trans. Jaini). The only karmas still active are the nondestructive *aghātiyā* karmas related to body, longevity, status, and feeling (see chapter 2). As Glasenapp summarizes, "the Sayogi-kevalī [*kevalin* with activity] knows everything, sees everything, is capable of everything, yet he has a body and a certain activity which is conditioned by matter, and a number of [nondestructive] Karmas obtained earlier are produced in him" (1999/1925, 225). It should be pointed out that if one attained particular name-determining karmas associated with teaching in a previous lifetime, the Kevalin will become a Jina, a propagator of Jain teachings, in this rung ($TS^{Dig}$ 6.23[48]).

An individual remains in the thirteenth rung until the time of death. No karma is generated during this time. Digambara sources, in fact, say that a kevalin does not even eat or drink at this point, though Śvetāmbara sources dispute this, saying that food and drink are ingested as usual by the mendicant, just without karmic accrual (Jaini 2001/1979, 268). In the last stages of embodied life, one undertakes the final forms of meditation related to subtle movement (*sūkṣmakriyā-anivartin*), by which all gross bodily activities as well as gross and subtle mental and verbal activities cease, and absolute nonmotion (*vyuparatakriyā-anivartin*) (270), by which even subtle bodily activities are brought to a stop (Jaini 2001/1979, 269–70; Tatia 1951, 279–80).

This latter state of nonmotion is the fourteenth *guṇa-sthāna*, in which the practitioner is called *ayoga-kevalin*, or "omniscient without vibratory activity" (GJK 65, trans. Jaini). The *jīva* in this state is free of the last cause of karmic bondage of activities of body, speech, and mind. This immobile state is very brief,[49] and at the instant of death, longevity-determining karma expires and the *jīva* follows a natural movement upwards to the highest point in the cosmos, where it will remain as a disembodied liberated being (*siddha*) (see chapter 2).

## VALUE OF THE *GUṆA-STHĀNAS* FOR BIOETHICAL REFLECTIONS

It is important to remember that the *guṇa-sthāna* ladder is only a theoretical model; it is unclear to what degree modern lay Jains follow the technical details of these stages, especially when they cannot surpass the fifth level, nor can mendicants living in our time period surpass the sixth (Dundas 2002, 151–52). However, the framework is worth considering in a Jain approach to bioethics because all living beings are linked within it, including non-Jains as well as Jain laypeople and mendicants, in a continuum of right worldview, knowledge, and conduct (Petit 2015, 97). Although the state of liberation exceeds detailed description, it promises the possible culmination of immense efforts across lifetimes in which all beings can participate.

The logic of the *guṇa-sthāna*s in the overall framework of Jain ethics becomes clearer as we look backwards. The five causes of karmic bondage—wrong worldview; nonrestraint; carelessness; passions; and activities of body, speech, and mind—are overcome as one progresses along the ladder of karmic removal. The ordering of these five causes is also significant. The fifth cause of activity, for instance, is the last to be removed because activity itself is the most foundational cause of bondage for any living being (as discussed in chapter 2). Activities of body, speech, and mind condition passions, the next most persistent cause of bondage, of which the most subtle forms are operational until the twelfth rung. Activity and passions underlie carelessness, the third cause of bondage; these three together underlie nonrestraint, the second cause of bondage; and these four together underlie wrong worldview, the first cause of bondage. Tatia explains that "of these five [causes], the succeeding ones necessarily exist on the existence of the preceding ones, although it is not necessary that the preceding ones should exist on the existence of the succeeding ones" (1951, 147). Hence, the ladder of karmic removal is, in effect, the stripping away of symptoms generated by the subsequent cause of bondage, until even the primary cause of activity itself is neutralized.

However, lay Jains, who live and work in occupational and social settings where bioethical calculations are part of daily life, remain engaged in activity, as well as passions, carelessness, nonrestraint, and perhaps even wrong worldview if they have not yet reached the fourth rung of the ladder. Even a very disciplined layperson, who takes the minor vows and progresses through the eleven *pratimās*, can only attain the fifth *guṇa-sthāna* by virtue of having partially overcome the bondage of nonrestraint. Additionally, as is clear by the description of the mendicant path above, even mendicants who have taken the great vows may still be overcome by causes of bondage at the higher rungs.

Hence, the *guṇa-sthāna*s offer a perplexing framework. On one hand, Jain ethics is rooted in extremely rigorous disciplines directed at the effects of body, speech, and mind. On the other hand, these are not always practiced in a uniform way. A single person will advance and regress continuously. The overall aim is to persistently strive to overcome the causes of karmic bondage unique to one's path of existence, to cultivate right worldview, right knowledge, and increasingly right conduct. Jain ethics will not always look the same, but the *guṇa-sthāna*s provide a collection of concepts illuminating the highest ideals, strategies of practice, and the damaging reality of careless, passion-driven activities.

## VICES AND THE VIOLATIONS OF THE MINOR VOWS

The *guṇa-sthāna*s make clear that harm is inescapable for a layperson entangled in responsibilities of family, community, and work. As Jaini puts it, these efforts to systematize lay conduct "outlined a path of nonviolence that would allow a lay adherent to conduct his [*sic*] daily life with human dignity while permitting him to cope with the unavoidable reality of the world in which violence is all-pervasive" (2004, 60). The fact of harming, however, does not lead to apathy or an "anything goes" attitude toward injury. On the contrary, texts reflect efforts to circumscribe the limits of harm, and to distinguish violations of vows that fall outside those limits, as well as vices that fuel harmful actions. Since bioethical issues largely concern laity and since a substantive portion of part 2 of this book will analyze contemporary Jain medical professionals, it is important to explore these vices and violations of lay vows more closely, as well as specifically discuss the occupational restrictions for laity.

The *Tattvārtha-sūtra* lists five violations (*aticāra*) for each of the lay vows. Five violations of the minor vow of nonviolence (*ahiṃsā*) include "Tethering, beating, piercing the skin, overloading, and withholding food and drink" (TS$^{\text{Dig}}$ 7.25[50]). Five violations of the minor vow of truthfulness (*satya*) include providing wrong instruction, divulging secrets, forging documents, misusing entrusted funds, or sharing confidential thoughts of others (TS$^{\text{Dig}}$ 7.26[51]). Five violations of the minor vow of nonstealing (*asteya*) include "Abetting theft, dealing in stolen goods, transgressing the limits of a hostile country, using false weights and measures, and dealing in counterfeit goods" (TS$^{\text{Dig}}$ 7.27[52]). Five violations of the minor vow of sexual restraint (*brahmacarya*) include "Matchmaking, intercourse with a woman temporarily taken to wife, intercourse with an unmarried woman, unnatural sexual practices, and excessive sexual passion" (TS$^{\text{Dig}}$ 7.28[53]). Five violations of the minor vow of nonpossession (*aparigraha*) include "The failure to keep within the set limits of cultivable land and houses, silver and gold, livestock and grain, male and female servants, and of base metals, clothes/furniture" (TS$^{\text{Dig}}$ 7.29[54]). The text goes on to list five violations for each of the seven supplementary vows, as well as the vow of *sallekhanā* (TS 7.25–32), lists that are also included in the commentaries on this text.[55] Those violations that are particularly relevant for bioethical issues will be explored further in part 2.

Specific vices (*vyasana*) and sub-vices (*sodara*) unique to laypeople are also cited in medieval manuals of lay conduct written by authors of both main Jain sects. A list of seven vices is found in multiple Digambara texts, suggesting a common source. These include gambling, consuming alcohol, eating meat, engaging with prostitutes, hunting, stealing, and adultery (Williams 1963, 247). The *Śrāvaka-ācāra* of the Digambara teacher Amigati (eleventh century CE) considers these seven acts vices because they engender particularly strong passions or lead to other vices in the laity; eating meat, for instance, can encourage drunkenness, making religious progress impossible (248).

Śvetāmbara texts do not display the same uniformity regarding the vices, but many similar warnings are found therein; Hemacandra's *Yoga-śāstra*, for instance, explains the potent power of alcohol: "Judgment, (self-)control, knowledge, truth(fulness), purity [of conduct and] compassion, all are extinguished by liquor, just as a haystack is [extinguished] by a spark of fire" (YŚ 3.16, trans. Qvarnström). These vices reflect the social setting of Jain laypeople likely engaging in activities among non-Jains. In fact, the last two vices named by Amigati, stealing and adultery, were also punishable by civic law, making one susceptible not only to immense karmic bondage and personal torment, but also to legal punishments (Williams 1963, 249–50).

*Forbidden Occupations for Householders*

Jain texts also specify occupations that are forbidden to lay Jains. The canonical *Upāsaka-daśāḥ* (Pkt. *Uvāsaga-dasāo*)[56] lists fifteen forbidden occupations that are also cited by at least one Digambara author.[57] Several of these modes of employment (marked with an asterisk below) have direct bearing on medical professions and bioethical contexts, including pharmaceutical production, cultivating medicinal plants, animal research, and beyond, which we reference in the following chapters. Forbidden jobs include earning a livelihood from

(1.) making, buying, or selling charcoal or smelting other metals that kill multiple types of living beings*
(2) destroying plants, such as cutting trees, plants, or grinding grains or pulses*
(3) construction or sale of carts hauled by animals, which binds the animals and crushes living beings on the path
(4) transporting goods by vehicles or animals*
(5) excavating soil for agricultural purposes, wells, or rock quarries, which disturbs mobile and immobile beings*
(6) trade in animal byproducts such as shells, ivory, yak tails, bones, pets, or goose down, which instigates industries of killing*
(7) trade in chemicals or pigments used in poisons, dyes, or alcohol in which insects or minute living beings are destroyed in the cultivation or fermentation*
(8) trade in alcohol or forbidden foods such as meat, honey, butter, and other foods that torment animals or foment violent passions in those who ingest them*
(9) trade in men and animals, especially for profit, which restricts others' freedom and often involves hunger, thirst, beating, and being tied up*
(10) trade in weapons or tools that can kill plants, animals, and people, such as swords, guns, and farm implements*
(11) work in mills, such as crushing of sugarcane, seeds, or beans, which destroys plants and water-bodied beings
(12) work involving the mutilation of animals, such as castration, tail docking, nose piercing, or cutting of ears or other body parts
(13) burning to clear fields or for ritual purposes, which destroys many life-forms
(14) taking water from tanks, lakes, or ponds for irrigation or other purposes, which destroys aquatic lives
(15) breeding or rearing children for prostitution or as eunuchs, or breeding animals for use* (Williams 1963, 117–21)

Exceptions have been made to the above guidelines, especially in Digambara texts, for a member of a warrior caste required to bear arms or a member of an agricultural caste required to till the soil. Phyllis Granoff refers to these exceptions as "temporary lapses" (*chiṇḍikā*)—a term seemingly present only in medieval literature—in which a Jain could knowingly violate a precept to accommodate significant outside pressures (2000, 139–40). If one could maintain right worldview during these "lapses," the action would not be viewed as a karmic violation, nor would it prevent the ability to continue on a devout path.

Śvetāmbara and Digambara texts on lay conduct[58] offer short lists of permissible occupations (*upāya*) for laity. Digambara sources describe the merchant trade, clerical occupations, agriculture, artisanal crafts, and caste-related military occupations. Śvetāmbara texts forgo military occupations, but agree with the remaining list, adding practice of medicine, service to a political ruler, and begging (Williams 1963, 122).

## JAIN FOUNDATIONAL PRINCIPLES FOR ETHICS

Jain philosophy and textual history demonstrate a central and unparalleled concern with nonviolence to one- through five-sensed beings. However, neither the single concept of nonviolence nor its relation to the other four vows offers a sufficient summary of Jain ethics. Rather, the ethical outlook of Jainism includes a complex framework of disciplines that contains various principles, all of which are significant when considering a Jain engagement with contemporary bioethics. We have identified three key principles.

First, since its earliest texts, Jainism is characterized by a special attention to violence and nonviolence. The ancient concept of *parigraha*, for instance, identified attachments to objects, pleasures, and social relationships as leading to physical actions that cause inevitable violence, or *ārambha*. Additionally, early texts describe a triple harm in body, speech, and mind, committed in a triple manner of doing, causing others to do, or approving of what others do. Nonviolence, as the most central of the five main vows now synonymous with contemporary Jainism, is an evolving expression of these early concepts.

Second, Jainism offers distinct paths for non-Jains, Jain laity, and mendicants, and these paths are marked by progression and regression in the *guṇa-sthāṇa*s. All one- through five-sensed living beings, as well as Jains and non-Jains, are said to exist along this ladder of karmic removal. As a social discipline, bioethics primarily applies to laity up to the fifth stage of the ladder. Consequently, the context of modern bioethics, when seen through a Jain philosophical lens, is subject to high degrees of karmic bondage and should not be confused with the highest *guṇa-sthāṇa*s characterized by overcoming all karmic passions and, ultimately, activity itself.

Third, within the realm of lay ethics, there are numerous guidelines to help restrain the inevitable harms of one's professional, family, and social life. Although the highest stages of karmic removal are inaccessible to one who lives and works in the world, Jain ethics includes considerations and practices meant to decrease harm to one- through five-sensed beings, which could shape modern bioethical calculations, inform one's occupation, and demarcate lines of ethical compromise and ethical non-negotiables.

In summary, Jain ethical principles exist in a broad framework centered on nonviolence, but exceed any single concept. Jain ethics reveal an adaptive philosophy for an evolving community accounting for elements of action and inaction, intervention and withdrawal, compassion and isolation, and karmic injury and karmic benefit. While Jain ethics may be characterized by the goal of emulating the twenty-four Jinas, it must at the same time be understood as a gradual process of striving to overcome the causes of karmic bondage, namely wrong worldview, nonrestraint, carelessness, passions, and, ultimately, all activities of body, speech, and mind. This rich ethical framework also informs Jain attitudes toward medicine from antiquity to the present, to which we now turn.

4

# Jainism's Evolving View of Medicine

In this chapter, we explore how Jain texts view physical and mental illness, as well as the rules and exceptions they propose regarding medical treatment. After exploring a range of factors that Jain texts consider to either directly cause or contribute to the occurrence of illness, we examine the approaches to medicine in the early strata of the Śvetāmbara canon. We argue that these early canonical texts open up space for the later use of medicine with emerging accommodations and a "duty to care" for the sick, and we discuss several factors that influenced the changing attitudes. Then we examine the liberalization of medicine in the later canonical and postcanonical periods, followed by an overview of some important medieval Jain medical treatises. We conclude by summarizing five Jain principles for medicine and medical care that arise through our analysis. We focus here on the general principles of Jain medicine, and on the medical treatment of mendicants in selected canonical and postcanonical texts up to the medieval period; we mention laity mainly in relation to the treatment of mendicants. Lay and contemporary mendicant attitudes to medicine will be discussed in more detail in part 2 of this book.

It should be pointed out that the history of Jain medicine has scarcely been researched. While some valuable textual studies have been conducted on illnesses, medical treatises, and the mendicant attitudes to medical treatment, contemporary mendicant attitudes to medical treatment and the history of the lay approaches to medicine, to our knowledge, remain largely unexplored. The Digambara sources are likewise less researched. This means that much work still needs to be done in order to gain a comprehensive insight into Jain approaches to medicine, their relationship with other Indian medical traditions, and their potentially unique developments. Our present examination is one contribution to that ongoing effort.

Because Jain texts reflect accommodations for mendicants and laity at diverse points of karmic and spiritual development, and these, further, express various historical, cultural, and social contexts, there is no single unified "Jain view" of medicine. However, certain perspectives and values can be identified which may iluminate a Jain approach to medicine that informs an engagement with contemporary bioethical issues. As will be evident in this chapter and in part 2, several bioethical issues that arise for Jains today—despite bioethics being a relatively young discipline—are historically prefigured in the encounters between the Jain tradition and medicine.

## WHAT CAUSES AN ILLNESS?

As explained in chapter 2, Jains believe that the embodiment of living beings who are trapped in the cycle of rebirths is determined by karma they have accumulated throughout their lives. Accordingly, Jain texts often explain illness—as a particular condition of the embodied state—in terms of karma (BhS 16.2§701b), but as we will discuss in the following sections, karma is not understood to be the only factor that causes it. While mainly exploring the factors that generate illness, this section also touches on the methods of healing, with a particular focus on their effectiveness in relation to the various underlying causes of ailments.

### *Physical Illness*

In Jain cosmology, illness (*roga, vyādhi*)[1] affects only those human beings born in the "lands of action" (*karma-bhūmi*) of which our world is part. These humans are susceptible to aging and illness, unlike those born in the "lands of enjoyment" (*bhoga-bhūmi*) whose bodies do not age and who die naturally when their longevity-determining karma (*āyu-karman*) is exhausted.[2] While humans have several bodies, as discussed in chapter 2, illness affects only their principal body, which is the gross physical body (*audārika-śarīra*) (Wiley 2000a, 267).

More specifically, illness is considered an efficient or instrumental cause (*nimitta*) that harms the vitalities (*prāṇa*) of embodied beings. Among these, the principal one is the vitality of life (*āyu-prāṇa*), which is the product of longevity-determining karma. The others include the five sense vitalities, the vitality of respiration, and the vitalities of mind, speech, and body, all produced by name-determining karma (266–67).[3]

The efficient cause of illness itself is understood to be feeling-producing karma (*vedanīya-karman*), a nondestructive type of karma that is associated with the experience of pleasure and pain (*vedanā*), as explained in chapter 2. Śvetāmbaras and Digambaras both associate illness with the subtype of this karma that produces pain or unpleasant experience, called *asātā-vedanīya-karman* (TS 9.16; TVā 8.8.2; Wiley 2000a, 271).[4] Digambaras, further, maintain that the operation of certain other karmas makes the human body more prone to falling ill.

One such karma is the so-called *upaghāta-nāma-karman*, a type of name-determining karma that is thought to be always accompanied by pain-producing karma (Wiley 2000a, 271). As noted in chapter 2, Digambaras understand the *upaghāta-nāma-karman* to be a factor that causes self-annihilation (Glasenapp 1942/1915, 17; Wiley 2000a, 171–72).[5] Apart from playing a significant role in bringing about fatal injury, this karma is an important factor in the production of illnesses arising from the three humors (*tri-doṣa*) of wind (*vāta*), bile (*pitta*), and phlegm (*śleṣman/kapha*).[6] Drawing from Vīrasena's *Dhavalā* (ninth century), Wiley notes that without this specific kind of karma there would be no affliction arising from the three humors (2000a, 270).

Mari Jyväsjärvi Stuart points out that the presence of the doctrine of the three humors in Jain texts indicates that Jain authors were familiar with traditional Indian āyurvedic medicine, which posits a foundational theory of three humors whose imbalance causes illness (2014). In his commentary to the *Tattvārtha-sūtra*, J.L. Jaini lists wind, bile, and phlegm as secondary constituents of the body (*upadhātu*), along with tubular vessels (*śirā*), muscle (*snāyu*), skin (*carma*), and digestive fire of the stomach/gastric fluid (*udara-agni*); the primary constituents of the body (*dhātu*) include chyle (*rasa*),[7] blood (*rakta*), flesh (*māṃsa*), fat (*meda*), bone (*asthi*), marrow (*majjā*), and semen (*śukra*).[8] Two types of *nāma-karman* cause the proper and improper functioning and circulation of the primary and secondary bodily constituents, namely *sthira-nāma-karman* and *asthira-nāma-karman*, respectively (Jaini 1920, 168–69; see also Wiley 2000a, 170). As a cause of the imbalanced circulation of wind, bile, and phlegm, along with other bodily dysfunctions, *asthira-nāma-karman* can, then, also be understood as a factor that contributes to the arising of illnesses.

*Asthira-nāma-karman* weakens the body and exposes it to ailments in other ways as well. In his commentary to the *Tattvārtha-sūtra*, Akalaṅka follows his predecessor Pūjyapāda in stating that while *sthira-nāma-karman* causes a firm bodily constitution, which enables one to undergo austere ascetic practices without falling weak and ill, *asthira-nāma-karman* in combination with even the lightest austerities results in an exhausted body:

> From the rise of this [*sthira nāma*] *karma*, upon performing austerities such as severe fasts, etc., the limbs and minor limbs remain unchanged, in other words, the body remains robust and in good health. It does not become emaciated or weak. *Asthira nāma karma* causes unsteadiness and weakness and emaciation of the body from undertaking only one fast or from exposure to ordinary cold and heat. (TVā 8.11.34–35, trans. Wiley 2000a, 170)

Akalaṅka highlights that a person with a weak bodily constitution is not only prone to illness but also cannot perform rigorous austerities that Jain texts prescribe for mendicants, suggesting that a healthy body is necessary on the path of karmic purification, which we will return to later in this chapter.

Ugrāditya (c. ninth century) mentions blood as a cause of disease in addition to the three humors (KK 15.255–273),[9] but he sometimes also lists it as a humor (KK 3.67), or as something that can get corrupted by the humors (KK 9.15; KK 9.35)[10]

(Meulenbeld 2000, vol. IIA, 152; Meulenbeld 2000, vol. IIB, 175). As a primary bodily constituent, blood is also regulated by *sthira-nāma-karman* and *asthira-nāma-karman*, much like the three humors.[11]

The idea that ailments can be a result of bodily disturbances—specifically, the imbalances of the three humors of wind, bile, and phlegm—can be found already in the *Bhagavatī-sūtra* and the *Sthānāṅga-sūtra*. Each illness is named in accordance with the imbalance that causes it, be it wind (*vātika*), bile (*paittika*), phlegm (*śleṣmika*), or a combined imbalance of the three (*sānnipātika*) (BhS 18.10§758a; SthS 4.4.515).[12] Texts indicate that these imbalances can be caused by external factors. For example, the *Bhagavatī-sūtra* recounts a story of a mendicant called Jamālī who had been consuming improper foods (tasteless, leftover, too meager, dry, untimely, excessive, and so on) and consequently suffered from bilious fever (*pitta-jvara*), running a high temperature (BhS 9.33§484a).[13] J.C. Sikdar explains that in Jamālī's case "the normal function of the physical system was disturbed by the generation of more heat from the bile on account of unsuitable and untimely diet" (1964, 348). In accordance with this, Ugrāditya in his *Kalyāṇa-kāraka* pays great attention to the kinds of foods that should be consumed. However, it was not only food that was considered as being able to influence the condition of the humors. Apart from other changes in one's lifestyle, such as walking when one's humoral imbalance has been caused by excessive sitting (for more on lifestyle choices and illness, see below), Stuart also mentions the provision of massages, resting on or wrapping oneself in animal skins, and specific bed arrangements (2014, 78–79) as methods of treating illnesses arising from the humors. Sen, further, lists various treatments with powders and oils aimed at restoring the balance of the humors (1975, 185; see also Stuart 2014, 79).

The *Bhagavatī-sūtra* contains an account of an encounter between Mahāvīra and Makkhali Gosāla, where bilious fever is stated to be a result of a hot ray emanated from a powerful ascetic. Makhali Gosāla was the leader of the Ājīvikas, but according to the Śvetāmbaras, he was for six years also a student of Mahāvīra before the latter's attainment of omniscience. During this time, Mahāvīra taught Gosāla the power of emitting fiery heat (see chapter 2, note 57) after a particularly dangerous encounter with another ascetic. Their relationship, however, came to an end, when Gosāla left his teacher and proclaimed himself a Jina. Sixteen years later, when Mahāvīra had already attained omniscience, Gosāla tried using his yogic power of emitting heat on Mahāvīra himself in order to kill him, announcing that Mahāvīra would die of a bilious fever in the course of six months. The fiery ray, however, rebounded from Mahāvīra, striking Gosāla instead. Gosāla became delirious and died soon after the event as a consequence (BhS 15.C7§677b, 15.C9§682a). The *Bhagavatī-sūtra* states that Mahāvīra himself also got bilious fever soon after the attack, and the topic of how he recovered from it is quite controversial. The text states that he consumed meat of a cockerel that was killed by a cat and therafter regained his strength (BhS 15.C11§685b),[14] but commentators have offered alternative interpretations that are in accordance with the strict rules of the meatless Jain diet.[15] In any case, the narrative suggests that bilious fever was a direct result of overheating the body due to an external factor, similar to the case of Jamālī.

Jain texts—particularly medieval didactic stories and narrative literature—sometimes, further, assign illnesses to various divine and human curses. Especially prominent are narratives about leprosy as a result of malicious curses. Phyllis Granoff recounts a story of King Kumārapāla:

> The famous Jain king Kumārapāla is said to have suffered from leprosy . . . caused . . . by the curse of a goddess who felt slighted. He is cured by water consecrated by his preceptor, the Jain monk Hemacandra. This same Hemacandra is similarly said to have suffered from leprosy as the result of an ancient curse and to have cured himself through meditation. (1998a, 220; see also 230–34)

It seems that Jain religious rituals (recitations of hymns; use of consecrated water; meditation; worship of Jina images, deities, and texts; and so on) and contact with spiritually accomplished mendicants (through their bodily parts and bodily residue)[16] are particularly helpful in treating physical illnesses that are caused by malevolent deities and ascetics (224–25), where conventional medicines can perhaps be less effective.[17] However, religious healing is also used for illnesses caused by other factors, such as bodily imbalances (219, 239–41).[18]

More generally, Jain texts describe illness as being induced by certain lifestyles and behaviors, which include dietary choices and modes of eating. *Sthānāṅga-sūtra* lists nine reasons (*sthāna*) for illness: (1) sitting for prolonged periods or overeating (*atyāsana*), (2) sitting in a "harmful" posture or eating "harmful" foods (*ahita-aśana*),[19] (3) too much sleep (*atinidra*), (4) too little sleep or staying awake too long (*atijāgarana*), (5) restraining the urge to pass stool (*ucchāra-nirodha*), (6) restraining the urge to pass urine (*prasravaṇa-nirodha*), (7) excessive walking (*adhvagamana*), (8) unsuitable meals (*bhojana-pratikulata*), and (9) excessive sensuous pleasures (*indriyārtha-vikopana*)[20] (SthS 9.13). While the text provides only the list of reasons without any further explanation, N.L. Jain suggests that they result in the four kinds of disturbances of the humors mentioned above, which is aligned with the recommendation of walking and proper bed arrangements as ways of balancing the humors, discussed earlier (1996, 533).[21] Stuart notes that lists such as this one indicate that Jains were interested in etiology and possibly in preventing illness (2014, 71). Controlling the mind and body, she states, might deter illnesses or diminish the possibility of their occurrence (68). "The regime of moderation and simplicity that Jain mendicants are expected to follow," she writes, "represents the polar opposite of these deleterious habits. It is not unimaginable that this list may have provided a basis for a rudimentary conception of health maintenance among Jain mendicants" (71).[22]

Finally, a decline in bodily power (*bala-prāṇa*) and old age are also associated with physical illness (US 10.21–27). As explained in chapter 2, the age of fifty initiates the start of a gradual decline in a person's strength, which may lead to illness.

It is interesting to note that while some of the causes of illness that were discussed seem to be interrelated, certain texts strictly differentiate between them. Granoff points out that the story of Vimala in Maheśvarasūri's *Jñānapañcamī-kathā* (Pkt. *Nāṇapaṃcamī-kahāo*) emphasizes that illnesses arising from bad food or bad digestion can be treated, whereas those that arise due to karma cannot and can only be terminated upon death (1998a, 235). This differentiation suggests a fundamental distinction between illnesses generated by karmic causes and those stemming from more general lifestyle choices. The idea of karmically induced illnesses being resitant to cures seems to be based on the belief that every living being needs to work through the karma they have accumulated due to their own previous deeds (see chapter 2). Granoff observes that texts allow for exceptions, and she recounts a story of a young girl whose illness, which was caused by karma, is cured with a religious ritual (1998a, 234). However, she adds, some texts point out that even if illnesses resulting from karma are cured in the present, they will manifest again in the future until they are fully experienced (246–47). One's own past activities are, thus, understood as a deeper cause of the present ailments.[23] Granoff indicates that karmically caused illnesses can be properly healed only through the performance of austerities, which bring about the destruction of inauspicious karma (220, 248). This way, the cure for physical illness is also the means of progress on the religious path (249–50).

To summarize, physical illness afflicts the gross physical body of living beings that inhabit the "lands of action." Illness is described as being caused in several different ways, including karma associated with pain or unpleasant experiences, karma causing disfigurement or self-destruction, and karma causing a weak bodily constitution as well as improper functioning and circulation of the primary and secondary bodily constituents. Some of these are noted as being related to the imbalances in the bodily humors as causes of ailments. Other external instruments that can cause illness and are sometimes directly mentioned as being related to the imbalances in the bodily humors are unhealthy lifestyle habits and even malicious ascetic powers. Various curses are also described as triggering illnesses. A more general factor in bringing about illnesses is the decline in vitality due to old age. It is indicated, moreover, that a weak body and illness can hinder one's ascetic practice.

Jain texts do not seem to clearly explain how all of these different causes of illness are related. There are some indications of interrelation between them, but there are also passages that suggest certain fundamental differences among them. Karmically induced illnesses are specifically highlighted as those that are most difficult or even impossible to heal, with one's past activities being understood as the root cause of afflictions. The conventional types of medical treatment for physical illness that were mentioned in this section include changes in lifestyle choices, provision of massages, and treatments with powders and oils. Further kinds of conventional medical treatment will be mentioned in the later parts of this chapter. The unconventional types of medical treatment that were described are various types of religious healing. It was indicated that the most successful form of medical treatment is austerities, which eliminate inauspicious karmas.

*Mental Illness*

As with physical ailments, Stuart describes the imbalance of the humors as one cause of mental illness, which can be treated by providing food suitable to that condition (2014, 90). In the above-mentioned passage from the *Sthānāṅga-sūtra* that lists various lifestyles that can lead to the arising of illnesses, the commentator Abhayadevasūri interprets the last reason of excessive sensuous pleasures (*indriyārtha-vikopana*) as a cause of potentially fatal mental illness. He glosses it as "sexual excess" (*kāma-vikāra*), "for mental illness (*unmāda-roga*) arises because of affection for women, etc.; as it is said: first there may be affection, then pensiveness, then recollection, then praise of qualities, admiration, raving, mental illness [*unmāda*], then [physical] illness [*vyādhi*], apathy, and, finally, death" (trans. Bollée 2003–2004, 162, fn. 10, modified). As noted above, some have interpreted these lifestyle choices as disturbing the balance of the humors, which then leads to illness.

Many texts, however, seem to classify mental illnesses (*unmāda*) under a distinct category, reflected in their attribution to different causes from those that generate physical illness. The *Bhagavatī-sūtra*, for instance, lists two causes of mental illness: (1) being possessed by a demon (*yakṣa-āveśa*) and (2) the rising of deluding karma (*mohanīya-karman*). Similarly to physical illnesses, where karmically caused types are described as being resistant to cures, the text asserts that "it is easier to bear and get rid of the first kind [i.e., possession]. . . .[24] Beings contract the first kind when (they ingest) impure particles . . . (which) are sent off by a god (*deva*)" (BhS 14.2§634a, Deleu 1996/1970, 204).[25] The *Bṛhatkalpa-bhāṣya* explains that in the case of mental illness caused by deluding karma, "the inauspicious matter arises in one's own body.[26] In case of beings possessed by a *yakṣa*, it is necessarily coming from outside one's body" (BBh 6256; trans. Stuart 2014, 88).[27] Sikdar comments on these two kinds of mental illness: "The *Yakśāveśa*-insanity [*sic*] brings the state of happiness (*sukhavedanataraka*) and its cure is accompanied by happiness, while the *Mohanīyakarma*-insanity is full of suffering (*duḥkhavedanataraka*) and the cure or release from it is attained with pain (*duḥkhavimocanataraka*)" (Sikdar 1964, 349).

In his list of diseases in the canon, Jain mentions the following diseases that he describes as "demonal": *indra-graha, skanda-graha, kumāra-graha, bhūta-graha, yakṣa-graha*, and *nāga-graha* (1996, 536).[28] The word *graha* indicates that a person is "seized," and Bollée translates it as "possession" (2003–2004, 176). He interprets *indra-graha* and *skanda-graha* as astral possessions, and *bhūta-graha* as possession by a *bhūta* (malignant demon). Bollée additionally mentions possession by a *piśāca*, another demonic type of being (179).

An example of a mental illness caused by *yakṣa-graha* is described in the *Antakṛd-daśāḥ* (Pkt. *Aṃtagaḍa-dasāo*).[29] In this story, a garland-maker named Ajjuṇae gets possessed by a *yakṣa* called Moggarapāṇī whom he had worshipped as a protective deity. One day, as his wife Bandhumaī and he started their worship, a group of attackers tied him up and sexually assaulted Bandhumaī. Witnessing the violence, Ajjuṇae started to doubt the existence of the protective deity he had been worshipping, and as a response the *yakṣa* entered his body.

Possessed by the *yakṣa*, Ajjuṇae killed the attackers and his wife, and went on killing for days until he encountered a deeply religious Jain merchant, Sudaṃsaṇe, on his way to pay respects to a Jain ascetic who had just come to town. As Ajjuṇae advanced to attack and kill him, Sudaṃsaṇe stayed fearless and undisturbed. He raised his hands with joined palms, paid homage to the Jinas and the ascetic, and took the five great vows. Consequently, because of the power he attained, Ajjuṇae could not reach him, and so he stopped before Sudaṃsaṇe and stared at him for a long time. Finally, the *yakṣa* exited the body of Ajjuṇae and went away. Ajjuṇae himself went on to become a Jain monk and eventually attained liberation (AD 6.3).[30]

Perhaps the calm demeanor of Sudaṃsaṇe could be interpreted as the state of happiness that cures the *yakṣa*-induced type of mental illness, mentioned by Sikdar above. The emphasis on Sudaṃsaṇe's religiosity, however, seems to locate the healing power in the Jain religion itself (Aukland 2013, 117). Accordingly, Stuart states that mental illness caused by possession can be treated by mantras and similar esoteric techniques that overpower the *yakṣa* (see also Wiley 2000a, 268). This is in line with the previous section, where religious healing was found to be commonly used for treating physical ailments caused by ill-intentioned deities and ascetics.

Stuart explains that mental illness caused by deluding karma, on the other hand, is "essentially caused by weakness of one's mind and moral integrity, so that one gives into negative emotional states such as fear, passion, or arrogance" (2014, 88). One can become mentally unstable as a result of experiencing great fear or passion, not being treated well, or even being treated with excessive praise. Consequently, one might become overly fearful, arrogant, and so on, which points to an interesting link between emotions and karmically caused kinds of mental illness. Along with the four main passions (*kaṣāya*), emotions or subsidiary passions (*no-kaṣāya*) are considered products of conduct-deluding karma (Jaini 2001/1979, 118–21). Umāsvāti lists nine of them: laughter (*hāsya*), pleasure in sense activity (*rati*), displeasure in sense activity (*arati*), sorrow (*śoka*), fear (*bhaya*), disgust (*jugupsā*), and sexual desire or feeling toward women, men, and both women and men (*strī-puṃ-napuṃsaka-veda*) (TS$^{\text{Dig}}$ 8.9).[31] Based on the sources we have explored, it is unclear whether the difference between an excessive emotion and karmically induced mental illness is merely a matter of degree or whether there is a qualitative difference between the two. The case of sensuous pleasures mentioned above—which is not explicitly described as being tied to deluding karma—seems to identify excessive emotion as a *cause* of mental illness (see also Stuart 2014, 89). The sequence from admiration to raving and eventually mental illness indicates intensification of the same emotion, as does the case of extreme fearfulness, for example, as stemming from the experience of great fear. However, in the sequence, mental illness is followed by the effects of physical illness, apathy, and death, which indicates that the items on the list may also differ qualitatively.

This type of mental illness, Stuart states, can be treated in two ways: (1) a gentle approach that aims to induce the opposite emotions to the one that the patient is undergoing, and (2) an approach that she likens to a sort of shock therapy (88). The gentler approach might try to counter excessive fear by evoking reassurance in a person or humbling an excessively arrogant person, following a prior attempt to alleviate the patient's illness with religious instruction (89, 91). The latter approach might include bringing a tame lion to a patient who is afraid of them in order to pacify their fear. In the worst-case scenario, a mentally ill patient may be restrained in isolation by being tied up in a closed room or thrown into a well (92–93). "Such a shock therapy approach," notes Stuart, "is based on the assumption that the imbalanced state of mind is a temporary condition, and that the patient can be shaken out of it by having her undergo a shocking or otherwise powerful experience" (2014, 91).

However, drawing parallels with physical illnesses that result from karma, none of the conventional treatments for mental illnesses are able to reach the underlying cause of these ailments. At the karmic level, then, mental illnesses that result from deluding karma can be cured "by the destruction-cum-suppression (*kṣayopaśama*) of this *karma*" (Wiley 2002a, 268).

In the context of mental illnesses, Jain texts also open up a question of agency. Is a person who is mentally ill responsible for their actions? Colette Caillat cites postcanonical mendicant texts stating that a mendicant is not responsible for actions done while mentally ill, for such a person lacks freedom.

> The teacher affirms that if a religious is, for example, suffering from a mental illness, his [*sic*] conduct is predetermined. He does not accumulate any *karman* and has therefore nothing to expiate. . . . To illustrate his arguments, the teacher gives the example of the marionette whose many actions are in fact caused by someone else and bring it no benefit. (1975, 110; see also Deo 1954–55, 437)[32]

Although an individual suffering from mental illness may not be karmically responsible for their actions, such behavior does impact the immediate mendicant community, requiring some response. Caillat cites instructions for fellow mendicants to guard a mentally distressed mendicant closely, since they would be responsible for any injurious actions committed by that mendicant, and to use extreme care when seeking food or other articles of care for their treatment (110).

In sum, whereas some textual passages attribute mental illnesses to bodily imbalances that can be treated with changed lifestyle choices, they are usually categorized differently from physical illnesses. As we saw, they are caused by a different kind of karma or may even be brought about by an external force entering the body. As such, they sometimes also seem to require healing approaches that differ from those used for treating physical diseases. However, just as in the case of physical illnesses, religious healing may be used for mental illnesses induced by malevolent beings, and ascetic practices are highlighted as a way to eliminate the underlying cause of mental illnesses that result from karma. Mental illnesses, furthermore, open up discussions about human agency, responsibility, and karmic retribution.

## MENDICANTS AND MEDICAL TREATMENT IN THE EARLY ŚVETĀMBARA CANON

One central issue in the field of Jain medicine is whether mendicants can give and receive medical treatment. Does illness weaken or strengthen mendicant practice? Is it another physical hardship to be endured, just like extreme cold and scorching heat, or can/should it be treated? If the latter, who can provide treatment and what kinds of medicines may they use? Does a healthy body have a function in Jain mendicancy? The issue of the medical treatment of mendicants is significant because it raises ethical questions about proper conduct in the face of illness that are unique to Jain history and practice, establishing foundational guidance for other topics that relate to medicine. These considerations involve two parties: the ailing mendicant and the care provider. In this section we will discuss both perspectives.

As indicated in chapter 3, the practices of Jain mendicants today often do not entirely align with those described in the early textual sources, even though these sources—for Śvetāmbaras at least—are generally considered authoritative and are believed to contain the original teachings of the last Jina, Mahāvīra. This holds also in the case of medical treatment. For example, while the early texts encourage a mendicant to endure all pain—including illness—with calm and without seeking aid, some monks and nuns today consent to receiving medical care, ranging from plant-based curatives to full-scale surgery, as we will further explore in chapter 6. What explains this shift and when did it happen?

In his analysis of medicine in Buddhist monasticism, Kenneth Zysk states that "medicine generally played an insignificant role in Jaina monasticism" (1991, 8). He points out that mendicants clearly had knowledge of illness and medical treatments, but "because of the severity of their ascetic discipline, the cultivation and practice of techniques to remove and ease suffering operated essentially as a hindrance to spiritual progress. Hence Jainas did not codify medicine in their monastic tradition" (38; see also Stuart 2014, 64).

Some scholars have challenged the notion of a strict prohibition of medical treatment in Jain mendicant texts. While they have recognized mostly negative approaches to the medical treatment of mendicants in the early Jain canon, due to the strict adherence to performing austerities while accepting pain, discomfort, and illness, they have also highlighted a later shift to more lenient attitudes. Granoff mentions the canonical example of Mahāvīra taking medicine in the *Bhagavatī-sūtra* discussed above, but she, similarly to S.B. Deo and Stuart, locates a greater acceptance of medicine in the medieval texts (Granoff 1998a, 222, 254; Deo 1954–55, 29–33; Stuart 2014, 65–67).[33] We will return to these analyses later in the chapter.

Based on her study of the approaches to medicine in the Śvetāmbara canon, Stuart notes:

> On the basis of the canonical texts alone . . . it is not possible to conclusively determine to what degree early Jain mendicant communities resorted to the medical treatments of which they were clearly aware. However, the fact that exceptions to monastic rules for the sick are recorded even in these early texts suggests that Mahāvīra's example of perfect tolerance of discomfort very quickly turned out to be a difficult one for his followers to emulate. (2014, 72)

In line with this, we argue that the rare accommodations for ill mendicants that are permitted in the early canon in specific circumstances may have contributed—together with the emerging duty to care for the sick and the idea of a healthy body as the vital instrument of spiritual attainment—to the development of more lenient attitudes toward the medical treatment of mendicants later on. This means that the historical gap between the early and the later sources with regard to the care directed toward ill mendicants may not have been all that great.

In the next section, we explore the evolution of attitudes toward medicine in what are commonly understood to be four of the earliest canonical sources: *Ācārāṅga-sūtra* I, *Sūtrakṛtāṅga-sūtra* I,[34] *Uttarādhyayana-sūtra*, and *Daśavaikālika-sūtra*.

### *Medicine as Violence and the Illness of* Saṃsāra

As discussed in chapter 3, the *Ācārāṅga-sūtra* I is a manual of conduct that encourages individuals to cut off familial and community ties in order to pursue a path of strict mendicant practices that erode karma, ultimately freeing one from the cycle of rebirths. As a text that promotes the ideal of solitary mendicancy, the *Ācārāṅga-sūtra* I mainly provides guidance for individual mendicants who face illness, and only briefly discusses proper interactions when a mendicant falls ill. The text describes the body as something transitory and impure, to be overcome, even while that very body is the instrument with which one performs religious austerities. Since liberation is described as the only worthwhile aim, any activity that impedes liberation—which includes taking medication that causes harm to other life-forms and increases bodily attachment—should be avoided. Likewise, householders or doctors who provide harm-causing treatment are also denounced. At the same time, the text admits that the rigors of mendicant life require health and strength, and encourages individuals to take up austerities while their bodies are still able to perform them. We will discuss each of these unique features in turn.

The notion of karma in this text is not as extensively defined and theorized as it will be in later texts (see chapter 3). The view, simply stated, is that the varieties of embodied experience of living beings arise from karma (ĀS 1.3.1.4), including their birth state, bodily condition, and occurrences of illness (on which more shortly). Since one's karma is determined by actions, the text emphasizes that everyone is responsible for their own rebirths, meaning that the agent of an action not only reaps the fruit of that action, but is also the only one who can prevent the accrual of new karma. Mendicants manage their karma-causing actions in several ways, primarily by controlling their attachments (*parigraha*) and minimizing actions that cause harm (*ārambha*). As described in chapter 3, harm-causing activities can be performed directly, or one can cause or approve of another doing them.

One way in which wandering mendicants are instructed to observe these guidelines is by collecting alms from householders rather than preparing or purchasing their own food, all the while being extremely vigilant so as not to become attached to their donors. Mendicants are, further, encouraged to rigorously expose themselves to various bodily discomforts (ĀS 1.2.6.3). The causes of discomfort may be involuntary, such as calmly withstanding severe weather conditions and the mockery of householders, or voluntary, such as undergoing austerities like assuming an uncomfortable position for a long time or fasting. As described in the text, "Enduring cold and heat (*śitoṣṇa-saha*), pain and pleasure (*arati-rati-saha*), the unbound (*nirgrantha*) does not feel the hardship (*paruṣatā*)" (ĀS 1.3.1.2).

These strict practices are based on a sharp dualism between the *jīva* and the body, with the body being described as something that should be abandoned as ephemeral and impure (ĀS 1.2.5.5). However, even though mendicants are encouraged to transcend their bodies, it is precisely their bodies that function as instruments for the performance of austerities required for the liberation of the living self. After serving as a vehicle to liberation, upon reaching liberation, the body-as-instrument is discarded (ĀS 1.5.6.4). As noted in chapter 3, the *Ācārāṅga-sūtra* I presents liberation as a goal that is immediately attainable and the only worthwhile aim of spiritual practice.

The uncompromising approach to austerities and liberation is reflected in the attitude toward medicine evident in the text. The text lists sixteen illnesses or bodily conditions understood to be a result of one's own actions:[35]

> Now, look at those born in various kinds of families as a result of their own actions! [They undergo the ailments of] having goitre/boils (*gaṇḍin*) or leprosy (*kuṣṭhin*), consumption (*rājayakṣmin*), epilepsy (*apasmārika*), one-eyedness (*kāṇaka*) and stiffness/paralysis (*jāḍya*), lameness (*kuṇitva*) and hunch-backedness (*kubjita*) also. Having dropsy (*udarin*), look, and dumbness (*mūka*), inflammation/swelling (*śūnika*), excessive appetite/over-digestion (*grāsin*), trembling (*vepakin*) and immobility (*pīṭha-sarpin*), elephantiasis (*ślīpada*), [and] diabetes (*madhu-mehanin*). These sixteen illnesses have been enumerated in due order. (ĀS 1.6.1.3)

Seeking medicine for any of these conditions is discouraged in the text, since any curative would result in harm to other beings used in the treatment itself, and all just for the sake of maintaining one's frail body (ĀS 1.6.1.4):

> Knowing [that they are attacked by] diseases (*roga*) of various sorts, the afflicted ones (*ātura*) torment [other beings for the sake of treatment]. But mind you! [All these treatments] are not [competent] enough [to remedy the afflictions caused by karma]. Refrain from these [therapeutic measures that torment other living beings]. . . . One should not harm anything [even for the sake of treatment]. (ĀS 1.6.1.4)

The prohibition against harm means that not only animal-, but also plant-, earth-, water-, air-, and fire-based medical treatments are unacceptable, no matter what the medical condition. Moreover, it is indicated that such treatments would ultimately be ineffective. Illnesses are, after all, the result of one's own actions and, therefore, karma (as discussed above). The real illness that needs to be overcome through austerities, according to the *Ācārāṅga-sūtra* I, is thus not any one bodily condition, but *saṃsāra* itself.

In spite of the general aim toward liberation rather than curing bodily conditions brought on by karma, the *Ācārāṅga-sūtra* I invites mendicants to enter a mendicant path while still in good health, before falling ill. The text states that so long as hearing, sight, smell, taste, and touch remain strong, one should pursue liberation: "Seeing that strength (*vayas*) has not yet declined, wise man, recognize the moment!" (ĀS 1.2.1.5). Although this idea is not further developed in this text, the underlying suggestion seems to be that a strong body is necessary for performing austerities.

In addition to describing the medical conditions and treatment guidelines for an ailing mendicant, the *Ācārāṅga-sūtra* I addresses those who might provide care for the sick; the text primarily discusses householders as potential caregivers. In keeping with the negative picture of householders presented in this text, one scenario describes family members who abandon a sick person. Here, the *Ācārāṅga-sūtra* I emphasizes that family, just like medicine, cannot save and protect one from illnesses (that are karmically induced) (ĀS 1.2.1.4).

Doctors are also denounced in the text as those whom a mendicant should avoid. Not only do doctors blindly perform violent actions, their patients are also implicated in the violence:

> Proclaiming himself to be an expert in medicine (*cikitsā-paṇḍita*), [a doctor] kills, cuts, pierces, breaks, tears to pieces, and destroys [life] [for the purpose of medical care]. Thinking "I will do what has not been done yet," [he continues indulging in violence]. The one whom he treats is also [involved in the violence]. Enough of the company of this unwise person! Whoever receives [such a cure] is also unwise. This is not suitable for a houseless [mendicant]. (ĀS 1.2.5.6)

Commenting on this passage, Stuart notes that "early Indian medical prescriptions often included meat, honey and alcohol, substances whose production or extraction inevitably involved harming life-forms. . . . [T]he Āyurvedic use of these prohibited 'violent' ingredients likely contributed to their [i.e., the Jains'] misgivings about medicine" (2014, 70).

While assistance from laity is precluded, the *Ācārāṅga-sūtra* I does permit mendicants to help their sick fellow mendicants under very limited conditions. A passage toward the end of the text notes that in case of frailty, a mendicant should not accept food from a householder but may accept services of fellow mendicants when sick, should they offer it without being asked. Similarly, one may offer services to others when they are ill. However, these actions should be performed only if a mendicant had previously resolved to act in these specific ways. The rules of interaction regarding illness are thus established particularly with reference to the strict observance of one's own individual ascetic restraints and are not patient-oriented or framed as a duty to care for sick fellow mendicants. If one's prior resolution is not to accept or provide assistance in any situation, this decision should be upheld even in case of illness (ĀS 1.7.5.2–4).

When mendicants become so weak, due to factors such as disease, that they can no longer maintain their vows or austerities, the *Ācārāṅga-sūtra* I states that they may undertake a fast unto death (ĀS 1.7.5.1–1.7.8.25). This religious practice is described in more detail in chapter 7.

As a text for wandering mendicants, the *Ācārāṅga-sūtra* I details the ideal conduct required for liberation. In this context, medicine, as well as those who might provide it, not only results in violence to other living beings and damaging attachments to the body, but is ultimately considered ineffective in curing ailments brought about by karma. The text provides an option to accept and offer services in case of illness, but only if one's previous resolutions allow it. A religious solution that is presented as an option to deal with weakness and illness is the practice of fasting unto death. At the same time, the text encourages people to enter the spiritual path while their strength has not yet left them.

### *The Emerging Duty to Care*

Similarly to the *Ācārāṅga-sūtra* I, the *Sūtrakṛtāṅga-sūtra* I encourages mendicants to abandon the needs of the body. However, this goal is balanced by a growing duty to care for mendicants who have fallen ill. In the text, mendicants are instructed to endure every involuntary pain and, at the same time, voluntarily pursue austerities. The text suggests that one should view one's body as a corpse (SKS 1.13.17), though it warns against longing for death, which was probably an important caveat for novice mendicants: "A person who has left the householding life, free from desires (*niravakāṃkṣin*), should abandon his body. . . . He should desire neither life nor death" (SKS 1.10.24).

Like the *Ācārāṅga-sūtra* I, the *Sūtrakṛtāṅga-sūtra* I discusses situations in which fellow mendicants fall ill; however, unlike the former, it establishes a *duty* to care for them. In one passage, the text describes mendicants collecting alms-food for their sick brethren whose illness made them exempt from seeking their own alms. Although this practice is criticized by rival groups, the text defends mendicants seeking alms for a sick monk as much more preferable than a householder bringing food to the ailing mendicant. This preference, which was indicated already in the *Ācārāṅga-sūtra* I, seems to reflect a belief that mendicants should never accept food that householders prepared especially for them. Even though the passage demonstrates an awareness that such behavior might be seen as reflecting relationships of attachment, it nevertheless concludes that "a healthy mendicant should, steadfast, help a sick one" (SKS 1.3.3.8–11, 15, 20). This excerpt does not discuss medical treatment, yet it importantly establishes—perhaps for the first time—the *duty*, rather than merely an option, to provide care for a sick fellow mendicant. It also suggests, without reference to any previous individual resolutions like in the *Ācārāṅga-sūtra* I, that mendicants who have fallen ill are exempt from performing certain obligatory activities, such as collecting alms.

The duty to provide care opens space for a wide variety of interpretations of what exactly "care" consists of. Moreover, it is precisely within the domain of the duty to provide care for fellow mendicants that the lenient attitudes toward the medical treatment of mendicants in the postcanonical period, described by Granoff and Stuart, flourished.

Why did a duty to care emerge in the *Sūtrakṛtaṅga-sūtra* I? Taking care of sick fellow mendicants seems to be one aspect of a broader restructuring of the rules of proper conduct and its rewards in the text, which could be interpreted as reflecting the growth/stabilization of the Jain mendicant community, as well as a concern for its unity. As noted in chapter 3, the text recognizes that some mendicants may be too weak to emulate the solitary and rigorous lifestyle of Mahāvīra. It also encourages students to stay with and serve their teachers, another way in which service is underlined as important. Along with this, the text records the emergence of the idea of a good rebirth as a worthy goal of practice. Any or a combination of these developments could perhaps be the reason behind the (at least seemingly) novel idea that fellow mendicants are obliged to provide care to sick mendicants, who may be exempt from performing certain religious obligations.

### *The Body as an Instrument of Liberation*

The contents of the *Uttarādhyayana-sūtra* reflect the general avoidance of medicine found in the previous texts, while recognizing the body as a vital instrument for the performance of karma-destroying austerities. Aligned with the *Ācārāṅga-sūtra* I and the *Sūtrakṛtāṅga-sūtra* I, the *Uttarādhyayana-sūtra* urges mendicants to cultivate indifference to pleasant and unpleasant experiences toward the ultimate goal of leaving the impure body behind. Accordingly, a mendicant who falls ill "should not wish for medical treatment (*cikitsā*), but continue to explore the self. Thus, he will be a proper mendicant by neither acting himself nor causing others to act" (US 2.33). This view reflects the threefold notion of action described in chapter 3, namely that mendicants should not wish for medical treatment themselves, but also not cause others to provide care.[36]

The *Uttarādhyayana-sūtra*, further, discourages mendicants from lamenting their fellow mendicants' condition or participating in their medical treatment. The text cautions: "*Mantra*s, roots, various kinds of medical consideration (*vaidya-cintā*), emetics, purgatives, fumigation, eye [treatment], and bathing, [sharing in] the sick one's lamentation and his medical treatment, one who, understanding, renounces these is a [true] mendicant" (US 15.8). As in the previous texts, rather than paying attention to bodily illness, the ultimate goal of a "true mendicant" is to overcome the disease of *saṃsāra*. With this attainment, "one becomes free from all suffering that always afflicts humankind. Freed from the long illness (*dīrgha-āmaya*) and praiseworthy, he becomes infinitely happy, obtaining the [final] goal" (US 32.110). Similarly to the *Ācārāṅga-sūtra* I, the *Uttarādhyayana-sūtra* also presents the option of fasting unto death as one's end nears (US 5.32).

At the same time, the *Uttarādhyayana-sūtra* opens a space to consider a particular value of medical treatment, namely maintaining the body for the practice of austerities. While the idea that the body is a tool of spiritual progress is largely implicit in the other early canonical texts discussed in this section, the *Uttarādhyayana-sūtra* unambiguously explains that one should sustain one's body only in order to destroy previously accumulated karma (US 6.12). This perspective presents the body as a vital instrument for attaining spiritual goals, and, similarly to the *Ācārāṅga-sūtra* I, the text explicitly identifies illness (*roga*) as one of the factors that renders rigorous disciplines difficult (US 11.3). This is one avenue by which space opens up for a reconsideration of medical treatment as a means to sustain a healthy body capable of performing karma-destroying austerities to the extent that they are prescribed and, consequently, effective.

### *Moderate Accommodations for the Sick*

While instructing mendicants to bear bodily hardships, the *Daśavaikālika-sūtra* also demonstrates a clear concern for the sick and a developed duty to care for fellow mendicants. Like the previous texts, the *Daśavaikālika-sūtra* maintains the uncompromising ideal of a true mendicant who "is unperturbed in the face of hunger, thirst, and lying on uncomfortable ground, cold and heat, distress and fear, [for bearing the] suffering of the body [brings] great results" (DVS 8.27). The text continues: "A mendicant who is standing firm in the eternal good, should forever abandon the impure and impermanent body. Having cut off the bondage of birth and death, he reaches the state from where there is no return" (DVS 10.21).

The text, further, names several transgressive activities related specifically to medical treatment, such as "rubbing [the body] and cleaning teeth . . . medical treatment . . . application of enema and purgatives, rubbing the body with unguents. . . . None of this is undertaken," it states, "by the unbound (*nirgrantha*), the great sages, intent upon restraint, wandering like the wind" (DVS 3.3–10). This passage clarifies that any effort to clean, strengthen, and heal the body is a deviation from the religious path. In fact, even telling someone that a certain item has curative power is considered unacceptable, since a mendicant could be indirectly involved in violence should that person decide to use it. The text, thus, warns that the householder should not be told about what can be used as medicine (*bheṣaja*), since it may be something that contains life (DVS 8.50). Moreover, according to the *Daśavaikālika-sūtra*, the virtues should be observed equally "by the novices and the wise, [the healthy] and the sick, without a break and as a whole" (DVS 6.6).

Yet, amid these strict ideals, the *Daśavaikālika-sūtra* also makes accommodations for those afflicted with old age (*jarayā abhibhūta*), the sick (*vyādhita*), and those (weak after) practicing rigorous austerities (*tapasvin*); for example, individuals in these states are permitted to sit down while on an alms round, which was typically forbidden (DVS 6.60). However, even these individuals are allowed only minor transgressions. The verse immediately following discourages additional accommodations, stating that "a sick or healthy [mendicant] who wishes to bathe, transgresses proper conduct and abandons restraint" (DVS 6.60). A sick mendicant, then, can sit down while on an alms round, but something like washing would be too great a deviation from what is considered proper mendicant conduct.

### *Changing Approaches to Sick Mendicants*

These earliest strata of canonical texts generally discourage mendicants from seeking treatment for unpleasant and painful bodily conditions, such as illnesses, as scholars have noted. They present two main objections to medical care. First, the production and consumption of medicine—whether by a mendicant or a third party—requires violence toward other life-forms. Second, seeking medical care deviates from the practice of austerities through which a mendicant cultivates nonattachment and equanimity in the face of discomfort in order to eventually transcend bodily existence. However, as shown, these texts also contain accommodations for sick mendicants and the emerging duty to care that seem to have been mostly overlooked in scholarship.

These changing aspects possibly reflect a developing interpersonal code of conduct, perhaps as a result of a stabilizing mendicant community. Certain passages explicitly seem to be a result of specific situations where the community needed to consider how to deal with old, emaciated, and sick mendicants. While the *Ācārāṅga-sūtra* I discusses medicine mainly from the perspective of the solitary ailing mendicant, it nevertheless provides an option to accept and offer mendicant services in case of illness if such actions are aligned with one's previous resolutions. The other three texts address how a mendicant should behave when a fellow mendicant falls ill in more detail, suggestive of an increasingly communal orientation. The *Uttarādhyayana-sūtra* urges the mendicant not to participate in the lament and medical treatment of sick brethren. The *Daśavaikālika-sūtra*, however, expresses a concern for the sick, and the *Sūtrakṛtāṅga-sūtra* I develops a concept of the duty to provide care, for example, by collecting alms for them. Accordingly, these two latter texts permit minor transgressions of general rules by those who are ill, such as sitting down while on an alms round or, as indicated, being altogether exempt from going on alms rounds. In these contexts, ill mendicants seem to stay part of the community despite their illness.

As discussed in chapter 3, these early canonical strata gradually open the possibility of karmic merit and good rebirth in the heavenly realm for mendicants and householders who demonstrate proper conduct toward mendicants, and they soften the restrictions of interacting with the householders, a liberalization that will shape later medical exchanges. Still, in this early period, a mendicant remained the preferred choice as a caretaker for an ailing mendicant, over a householder.

Another important feature that emerges in these early portions of the canon is highlighting the role of the body in the attainment of liberation. The body is the tool for practicing austerities and, thereby, as some texts explicitly express, annihilating karma. In line with this, texts, further, point to the importance of a *healthy* body for the observance of rigorous asceticism, either by encouraging householders to enter the religious path while they are still healthy and strong or by indicating that illness can prevent one from performing difficult disciplines properly. There seems to be only a small step from recognizing that only those who are strong and healthy can fully observe religious practice, to promoting medical treatment for illnesses, in order to be able to get rid of as much karma as possible. As we will see later in this chapter, this is one of the directions in which the Jain approaches to the medical treatment of mendicants evolved.

## LIBERALIZATION OF MEDICINE IN LATER SOURCES

Later sources from both the Śvetāmbara and Digambara sects offer an increasingly detailed account of medicine. In this section, we shift from the early canonical texts examined above (sixth/fifth to fourth centuries BCE) to later canonical texts (third century BCE to fifth century CE)[37] and texts from the postcanonical period. These periods are not discrete, and certain ideas overlap within and between texts and periods. However, this division provides a useful, if conditional, guide to view the development of attitudes toward medicine within Jain texts over time.

Following the early canonical view, and with the above-mentioned factors of change in mind, we suggest that attitudes toward medicine in the later sources develop in several ways: (1) communal, rather than solitary, life among mendicants becomes the central concern; (2) the duty to care for a sick fellow mendicant shifts from an emerging idea in the earliest layers of the canon, to regulated practices in the later canon, to an expectation to provide care, including medical treatment, against the threat of penalty, in postcanonical texts; (3) medicine shifts from a karmic burden to a karma-destroying activity; (4) monks and nuns, and even householders, are permitted to act as medical providers; and (5) Jain mendicants compose elaborate medical treatises, contributing Jain values to the wider literary traditions of Indian medicine.

### *Later Canonical and Postcanonical Śvetāmbara Texts*

Under later canonical texts, we include strata of the sources analyzed in the previous section that were composed at later dates, as well as other later canonical texts. In this period, Jain authors clearly display familiarity with various aspects of medical treatment and with the wider Indian tradition of medicine known as *āyurveda*, as indicated in the first part of this chapter. In the Śvetāmbara canon, the *Sthānāṅga-sūtra*, for example, notes that medicine (*cikitsā*) is arranged around four components: (1) doctor (*vaidya*), medicine (*auṣadha*), patient (*ātura*), and nurse/medical assistant (*paricāraka*) (SthS 4.516).[38] Furthermore, experts on the body (*kāya-naipuṇika*), ash-thread therapists (*bhūtikarma-naipuṇika*),[39] and doctors (*cikitsā-naipuṇika*) are listed as three out of nine kinds of experts (*naipuṇika*). The *Sthānāṅga-sūtra* also lists eight branches of *āyurveda*, including (1) treatment of children (*kumāra-bhṛtya*); (2) diagnosis and treatment of bodily diseases/internal diseases (*kāya-cikitsā*); (3) minor surgery/treatment of eye, ear, nose, and throat (*śālākya*); (4) surgery/removal of substances that entered the body (*śalya*); (5) toxicology/science of antidotes (*jāṅgulā*); (6) treatment of mental illness (*bhūta-vidyā*); (7) science of aphrodisiacs (*kṣāra-tantra*); and (8) alchemy and science of elixirs (*rasāyana*) (SthS 8.26).

Later canonical texts additionally include various lists of illnesses, similar to the one mentioned in the previous section, as well as a wide range of healing methods. The *Vipāka-śruta* (Pkt. *Vivāga-suyaṃ*),[40] for example, enumerates the following types of āyurvedic medical treatment, some of which overlap with the treatments that are described (and prohibited) in the early canon:

> Oil massages, massages using powders, oily drinks, inducing vomiting, purgatives, burning, medicated baths, enemas, head treatments, dressing, opening of veins, scraping, piercing, oil-baths for the head, oblations, medical herbs cooked in a special way, bark, roots, bulbs, leaves, flowers, fruits, seeds, bitters, pills, drugs, and medications. (VŚ 1.1.9, trans. Stuart 2014, 71–72)[41]

At the same time, later canonical texts retain an aversion toward medicine that is typical of the early canonical strata. While the *Sthānāṅga-sūtra* clearly shows an understanding of the medical discipline, as shown above, it also describes medicine (*cikitsā*) as one of the eight types of false/inauspicious learning (*pāpa-śruta*) (SthS 9.27). Along with studying medicine, undergoing medical treatment is likewise disapproved of. The *Niśītha-sūtra*,[42] for example, reproaches mendicants for even cleaning out a wound:

> Whichever monk, for the sake of beautification, cleanses or washes out a wound on his body . . . massages or rubs it . . . smears or massages it with oil, ghee, fat, or butter

> . . . wipes or rubs it with clay or grass . . . cleanses or washes it with cold or hot water . . . blows on it or paints it . . . is [guilty of] enjoying himself. (NS 15.112–17, trans. Stuart 2014, 70)

Though associated with the "beautification of the body," several items on this list refer to methods of healing that are commonly censured in canonical texts. Since it does not refer to other medical providers, this passage particularly highlights the proscription of medical self-care.

However, similarly to the earliest canonical strata, mendicants are also warned against receiving medical care from another party (70). Following the early canonical approach, receiving care from householders remains supremely suspect during the later canonical period. The later strata of the *Ācārāṅga-sūtra*, for example, warn mendicants against seeking shelter with householders because they may unintentionally get involved in improper conduct. This is a particular danger if a mendicant who stays with householders suddenly falls ill. In order to help, the text states, the householders may smear the mendicant's body with various substances, such as oil, rub it, clean it, and so on, thereby violating rules of mendicancy (ĀS 2.2.1.8; see also Stuart 2014, 74–75). In line with this, the *Jñātṛdharma-kathā* offers a cautionary tale of an ascetic called Śailaka who fell ill due to a bad diet. When he came to pay respects to Śailaka, King Maṇḍuka noticed how unwell the ascetic was and offered to help him get medical treatment as well as provide a place for him and his students to stay. The ascetic accepted the help, and the doctors (*cikitsaka*) started to treat him, prescribing him alcohol (*madyapāna*) among other therapeutic methods.[43] The treatment was effective and Śailaka recovered. However, instead of returning to his mendicant way of life, he continued drinking alcohol and eating abundantly, and, thus, strayed from the path of ascetic discipline. It was only after a time that he found his way back to religious practice. The story emphasizes the dangers of medical care and the underlying attachments that lead to the perpetuation of one's stay in the cycle of rebirths (JK 5).

Yet, even as medicine remained marginal, the duty to care for fellow mendicants for the sake of communal solidarity and stability seems to have become more central and regulated. The *Sthānāṅga-sūtra* warns that an *ācārya* who does not take care of ailing mendicants can create disputes among the community (5.48), indicating that far from being only a private matter, illness can potentially fracture mendicant groups. Taking care of sick fellow mendicants is thus not placed only in the hands of individual mendicants, but is rather highlighted as a responsibility of the community leader, whose task is to ensure that the sick receive proper support.[44] In tandem with this concern about communal conflict and unity, the later strata of the *Uttarādhyayana-sūtra* reiterate the early canonical accommodations for mendicants in certain situations and conditions. The text states that a mendicant can forgo collecting alms for six reasons, one of them being illness (US 26.34–35).

Texts from this later canonical period reveal a more candid familiarity with medicine and medical treatments. Still, even though providing care and accommodations for sick mendicants seems to be an essential part of maintaining a strong community, efforts persist to regulate such concessions within the framework of stringent mendicant rules of conduct.

In the postcanonical period, the disinclination toward providing and accepting medical treatment remains especially prominent in medieval Jain didactic stories and narrative literature, discussed by Granoff and mentioned in the first section of this chapter (1998a). This literature is characterized by a persistent ambivalence toward healing, particularly when it comes to mendicants. Advanced mendicants who have healing powers are reluctant not only to heal others, whom they occasionally do heal, but also themselves—emphasizing the importance of abandoning the body for the purpose of exiting the cycle of rebirths. Importantly, mendicants who use their powers to heal others are sometimes praised, while texts remain suspicious of those mendicants who accept treatment. In this context, agreeing to medical treatment is portrayed as a temptation of sorts by which mendicants might deviate from the strict ascetic path (244–45). If they do decide to either receive treatment or heal themselves, their resolution is usually justified by a reason other than their own well-being, such as the reputation of the Jain religion or community. One such case is the story of Abhayadevasūri, who fears that his illness might shed a wrong light on the Jain teachings, if people interpreted it as arising from his commentarial misinterpretation of the doctrine (239–41).

The mendicant manuals in the postcanonical period that we will explore next reflect much more lenient approaches to the treatment of ailing mendicants than the canonical sources and medieval stories just discussed. While considerations of treating ill mendicants continue to be a struggle, the difficulties seem to be more practical and communal than soteriological. In this regard, it is interesting to compare the different genres of Jain literature, their purpose, and the related ideals of mendicancy they expound. Juan Wu notes:

> The somewhat divergent stances on medical healing in medieval Jaina narratives and legal commentaries [i.e., mendicant manuals] might be explained in view of the different genres of the two types of sources. While legal commentaries address pragmatic concerns of mendicants and thus tend to accommodate the needs of physical care, narrative literature functions as a medium instantiating religious ideals and values, thus laying more emphasis on the ascetic commitment to tolerating bodily suffering. (2017, 328)

In examining postcanonical mendicant manuals, it is, first of all, important to point out that discussions of the treatment of ailing mendicants are no longer marginal, as they are in the canonical texts. Based on her analysis of three Śvetāmbara commentaries (*bhāṣya*) composed around the sixth to seventh centuries CE—the *Niśītha-bhāṣya*, the *Vyavahāra-bhāṣya*, and the *Bṛhatkalpa-bhāṣya*—Stuart writes that they "reveal not only an interest in, but an urgent insistence on, practices of healing and how they might apply to Jain monks and nuns. These texts acknowledge that the ascetic body, weakened by years of arduous penances and fasts, can be subject to illness, and that this is a matter of collective concern for the monastic community" (2014, 72). A concern that was indicated in the early canonical strata through the emerging duty to care and minor nonmedical accommodations for ailing mendicants is now transformed into complex considerations of how to treat the sick and becomes one of the central preoccupations of mendicant authorities (66).

In these new contexts, the duty to provide care becomes a strict obligation. In his 1954 analysis of Jain monasticism, Deo asserts that caring for an ailing fellow mendicant is no longer optional in the postcanonical texts, but is a standard duty of all mendicants. He writes: "It was expected of every monk that he should wait upon the ill. Even if the ill belonged to his own or other gaccha [i.e., mendicant lineage], or was at a distant place, the monk had to go to him" (1954–55, 437; cf. Granoff 2017, 31–34). Granoff concurs that, in the postcanonical texts, "it is the duty of every monk to rush to the aid of sick brethren" (2017, 23; see also Stuart 2014, 75, 80), adding that the obligation to care was required even in the face of grave danger (36–37; see also Stuart 2014, 79).[45] An ideal that is celebrated in these texts is, therefore, not so much the endurance of illness and pain, but rather loyalty and service of mendicants or community leaders to the sick.

Beyond mere duty, Granoff explains that the *Bṛhatkalpa-bhāṣya*—a sixth-century CE commentary upon the earlier *Bṛhatkalpa-sūtra* (c. first century CE)—details penalties for the *ācārya* and mendicants who fail to provide such care (2017, 31–34).[46] The penalties for medical neglect are based on the degree of harm incurred by a sick mendicant. Granoff explains:

> The penalty grows in severity as the harm done to the patient increases; the penalty is lightest if the patient is simply inconvenienced, greater according to the degree of suffering he endures, even more severe if he falls unconscious and greater still if he is in danger of his life. If the patient dies, the *ācārya* is to receive the severest penalty possible; he is to be expelled from the monastic community. . . . [M]onks who have failed to help their sick member are also subject to penalties. (34)

Alongside these penalties, the same commentary notably defines caring for the sick as a way to *destroy* karma (Granoff 2014, 237). This is a significant change that associates the duty to care with karma-burning austerities rather than with accumulating nonmeritorious or even meritorious karma.[47] In relation to this, it is emphasized that mendicants should not have any ulterior motives, such as receiving good meals, in providing care to the sick, bringing attention to intention behind offering service (237–38).

In accordance with such a strictly prescribed duty to care, a later, twelfth-century Sanskrit commentary on the *Bṛhatkalpa-sūtra*, written by Malayagiri and

Kṣemakīrti, claims that Jain mendicant communities care for their ailing fellow mendicants much better than other mendicant groups, such as the Buddhists, do for theirs (Granoff 2017, 23, fn. 2). This is a bold statement, considering the renown of the Buddhist monastic medical tradition, and it demonstrates just how far the notion of care for fellow mendicants had developed since the early strata of the canon that allowed only minor nonmedical accommodations for the ill.

What motivated the Jain community to establish so rigorously regulated mandatory services to sick members? Granoff suggests that "compassion, a sense of responsibility, and obedience to the commands of the Jina,[48] which were said to include tending the sick, might well have been the primary impetus behind attentive care of the physical illness" (2017, 24). To this list, however, she adds another major motivating factor, that is, safeguarding the wider mendicant community (24). As Stuart observes:

> The Jain communities as reflected in the commentaries perceived themselves as belonging to a religious minority whose very existence and survival was constantly under potential threat from rival religious sects, a persecuting ruler, war, famine, or displeased lay communities. Their numbers were already small and their existence precarious, yet they were appointed with the sacred task of maintaining the Jina's teaching and practice of non-violence in the world. If Jain monks and nuns are not treated when ill, and become physically or mentally compromised or die, the Jain tradition too is weakened and its teaching lost. (2014, 95)

This is at least partly aligned with the justification of religious healing in medieval didactic stories and narratives.

Granoff notes that in relation to the efforts aimed at protecting the mendicant community, the need to keep a patient satisfied is called attention to (24). The possibility of a dissatisfied patient who might pose a threat to the community hearkens back to the earlier warning within the *Sthānāṅga-sūtra*, mentioned above, that an *ācārya* who fails to provide proper care for sick mendicants can trigger communal disputes. Based on the *Bṛhatkalpa-sūtra* and its commentaries, Granoff explains why a dissatisfied ailing mendicant might prove a threat to the mendicant community as a whole:

> Dissatisfied with what their fellow monks were doing for them . . . [t]hey might hightail it out of the monastic community and make for the nearest householder, whom they might pester for medicines. This ran the risk of alienating the householder, upon whom the monks all depended for their daily necessities. Disgruntled patients might even badmouth their fellow monks or in a final act of anger, they might even disrobe. . . . A dissatisfied monk who disrobed would mean one less monk, but more importantly an angry patient could weaken the essential support of the laity. (2017, 24)

Granoff emphasizes that care for ill fellow mendicants was, consequently, twofold. First of all, illness needed to be attended to properly, but at the same time, caretakers had to make sure that the patient was satisfied with the treatment and "felt that he was getting the best possible care" (2017, 24). In trying to address both of these demands—fulfilling the commitment to safeguard the reputation and unity of the community—the postcanonical commentaries show that mendicants occasionally broke their vows, such as the vow of nonpossession (e.g., by storing food and medications for the ill)[49] and truthfulness (e.g., by lying to patients or laypeople, sometimes even pretending that they were representatives of another tradition, such as Buddhism) (25–27; see also Granoff 2014, 238–39, 246; Stuart 2014, 82–83, 92). Stuart points out that the *Bṛhatkalpa-bhāṣya* even goes so far as to say that a seriously ill mendicant may consume any kind of food, be it Jain or not (BBh 1024–261; Stuart 2014, 77).[50] The texts show that these deviations are not reproached by the mendicant community, but are rather considered suitable behavior in specific circumstances.

Postcanonical mendicant texts also include complex discussions on who can treat a sick mendicant. In contrast to the strict prohibition of even such simple self-care as cleaning out a wound in the canonical sources, the postcanonical commentaries allow self-treatment when reasons for it are sufficient. Stuart cites the *Niśītha-bhāṣya* as an example of allowing a monk to clean and treat his own wound: "For the sake of the continuity [of scriptural learning]; for the sake of living beings; or so that he may die in *samādhi*, a monk conducts himself properly when washing etc., vigilantly" (NBh 1504; trans. Stuart 2014, 74). One reason behind this accommodation is the concern for the preservation of the Jain tradition and community, which was already discussed above. Stuart interprets the other two reasons as maintaining health in order to continue protecting living beings with one's religious practice, and in order to die "in a state of mental equipoise (*samādhi*) rather than aggravation" (2014, 74). In all cases, though, as emphasized in the text, a monk should remain vigilant in his conduct. In continuity with the canonical sources, the *Bṛhatkalpa-bhāṣya*, similarly, points out that "the religious life cannot be pursued without a body," highlighting the necessity of a relatively healthy body for the proper observance of religious practices, and thus justifying its medical treatment (BBh 2900, trans. Stuart 2014, 95–96).

Further, Deo asserts that if a monk or nun within the community was familiar with medicine, they were allowed to treat their fellow mendicants in times of illness (1954–55, 437; see also Stuart 2014, 75, 82). We can speculate that at least some mendicants were trained in medicine prior to their ordination, or they may have obtained medical knowledge in some other way (Granoff 2017, 26; Granoff 2014, 237–38). The *Vyavahāra-bhāṣya* encourages mendicant teachers to acquire medical training in order to be able to provide care to their students (VBh 2427–28; Stuart 2014, 76–77). Stuart points out that the monk who authored the *Bṛhatkalpa-bhāṣya*, for instance, "was both fascinated by and familiar with the world of medicine" (2014, 81). She notes that not only does his commentary reflect knowledge of specific medical treatments, *āyurveda*, and the doctrine of the three humors, but it also lists eight kinds of doctors, of whom two are Jain mendicants, that is, one that is spiritually mature and the other that is not (82). Moreover, the *Niśītha-bhāṣya* refers to hospitals (NBh 3649), suggesting mendicants' familiarity with institutionalized medicine, and even "sanctions the monks' use of certain sharp instruments for removing splinters, thorns, or the venom of a snake" (NBh 3437; Stuart 2014, 73; see also 82). This is in direct contrast to the canonical texts, in which cutting into flesh for any minor reason, as discussed above, was prohibited.

Ideally, mendicants would treat only mendicants of the same sex, but in extraordinary circumstances, mendicants of the opposite sex were also permitted to provide care (Stuart 2014, 75–76, cf. 80). Mendicants could also ordain a person of the "third sex" (*paṇḍaka*; see chapter 5)—who was previously prohibited from taking vows—if that person was a physician (Stuart 2014, 83). Importantly, even mendicants without any knowledge of medicine were urged to offer their services to the sick. "There is always something that a monk might do to help," Granoff notes. "He might massage the patient, grind the medicines, stay up at night and keep watch" (2014, 238).

Some postcanonical texts note that certain patients are not physically able to fulfill the requirements of treatment. Granoff specifically mentions the example of rigorous fasting as a remedy for some illnesses. In such cases, alternative medication, such as restorative tonics, may be provided (2017, 27). Granoff, further, points out that fasting unto death was recommended for mendicants who could no longer properly observe their religious duties; however, if they were not able to undergo such a fast, they were entrusted to the care of the mendicant community, with strict rules for how long specific members and groups at various communal levels should provide it (2017, 35; see also Deo 1954–55, 437).

If no mendicants were capable of medically attending to a sick mendicant, a doctor had to be found outside the community (Granoff 2017, 26; Granoff 2014, 239). Granoff describes the hierarchy of preferred caretakers enumerated in the *Bṛhatkalpa-bhāṣya* in the following way:

> The doctor of first choice would be a Jain monk; the least desirable choice would [be] a doctor who is not a Jain but an adherent of another faith. . . . [T]his means a Buddhist or another type of renunciant. The author also prefers a doctor who is not wealthy or famous; they are too much trouble. Ever practical, however, the text allows that if there is no competent Jain doctor, monk or layman, the monks should seek out the most competent person, regardless of his religious persuasion. (2014, 239)

Seeking medical care from a householder physician who was a relative of the ailing mendicant was considered an appealing option because this way the treatment did not have to be paid for. However, it was also considered a dangerous choice, as the ailing mendicants' families might try to reclaim them while they were seeking treatment (Granoff 2014, 241; Granoff 2017, 27–28; see also Stuart 2014, 75). In line with this, some texts emphasize that only mendicants who are very firm in their commitment to their renunciant life can seek such care (Granoff 2017, 28–29).

Regular householder physicians, on the other hand, required payment, which posed additional problems for the mendicant community, since Jain mendicants are not allowed to possess money. If they cannot convince the doctor to offer medical services for free, by appealing to having no possessions, the texts state that they may either use the possessions that have been renounced by a mendicant who had been wealthy as a layperson; find wealth buried in a secret place with the aid of mendicants with extraordinary cognitive abilities; go on alms rounds asking specifically for donations they can pay the doctor with; and offer various services and skills in exchange for money (Granoff 2014, 244–45; Stuart 2014, 86).[51] Another concern that emerges is how mendicants without possessions may offer a comfortable stay and other proper services to the doctor who is visiting in order to provide medical care to a mendicant patient. The texts offer a broad range of accommodations, including being allowed to bathe and massage the doctor, as well as arrange for a special meal, prepared either by householders or, in certain circumstances, even by the mendicants themselves (Granoff 2014, 243, 245–46; Stuart 2014, 83–87). One solution to these medical challenges was reliance on the help of former mendicants who had returned to lay life, called *paścātkṛta*s (Granoff 2014, 229, 232). Although early texts were extremely critical of monks who left the fold, by the postcanonical period, *paścātkṛta*s were essential intermediaries between mendicants and householders, and they were particularly helpful in the case of providing medical care for sick mendicants, for example by assisting in interactions with physicians (229, 235, 237).

In seeking the most proper physicians and care providers for ailing mendicants, the postcanonical texts suggest, as Stuart points out, that the "concern is not medical care itself, but simply the potential for association and physical intimacy with members of the opposite sex—or monastics' association with heretics and householders" (2014, 75). The continuous underlying worry is that such associations may bring mendicants to renounce their vows and leave their mendicant life (Granoff 2017, 28).

While the postcanonical texts and the early canonical sources seem to be divided by a large gap at first sight, we can see several lines of continuity between them. It seems that the early emergence of the duty to care and the idea of the body as an instrument of spiritual progress may have set the precedent for the later developments. The open recognition that mendicants do get ill generated a whole new set of concerns rooted in the desire to keep the community stable as well as ensure the mendicants' ability to properly perform their religious practices. With this, care for the sick became an obligation and a sign of a compassionate, loyal, and dedicated mendicant. Medieval didactic stories and narrative literature, on the other hand, retain a stronger tension between the treatment of illnesses and the ultimate goal of liberation, reminiscent of the early portions of the canon.

### *Digambara Sources*

Digambara sources are much less explored than those of the Śvetāmbara tradition in relation to medicine and the medical treatment of mendicants. We know of no study in English that overviews the Digambara medical textual sources, and only one text, the *Kalyāṇa-kāraka* (on which more shortly), is slightly better researched. Since the Digambaras consider their canon to be lost, the sources that describe medicine are all postcanonical (see chapter 3). In light of this, we will here offer only a few remarks on these sources based on a small number of selected texts, paying particular attention to the continuities and discontinuities with the Śvetāmbara sources that have been discussed so far.

There is an indication in some texts that Digambara attitudes toward the medical treatment of mendicants may have undergone a development that parallels the Śvetāmbara sources. For example, we see the tension between the emphasis on abandoning the body, on one hand, and maintaining the body for religious practices as well as offering services to the sick, on the other, exemplified in Pūjyapāda's sixth-century *Sarvārtha-siddhi*, a Digambara commentary to the *Tattvārtha-sūtra*. The root-text and the commentary stress the importance of enduring twenty-two hardships (*parīṣaha*) (TS 9.9), including illness (*roga*) and injury (*vadha*) (see chapter 3). Here, Pūjyapāda attempts to reconcile the importance of the body as a vehicle on the path of purification with a detached attitude toward the body. He describes the body as "the repository of everything impure (*sarva-aśuci-nidhāna*), impermanent (*anitya*), and defenseless (*aparitrāṇa*)" (SSi 9.9§830). In line with this, an ascetic is neither to think of the body nor adorn it. At the same time, Pūjyapāda likens the body to an essential tool in need of maintenance, drawing an analogy between an ascetic eating food and taking care of an axle or applying ointment to a wound. It is interesting that he uses the example of the wound (*vraṇa*), the treatment of which was, as discussed above, prohibited in the Śvetāmbara canon.

Should ascetics fall ill due to unsuitable food or drink, they are supposed to endure the illness. Pūjyapāda notes that an ascetic may have, through the practice of various austerities, attained extraordinary powers, such as *jallauṣadhi*. Wiley explains that "*jalla* means impurities (*mala*) originating from the ears, mouth, nose, eyes, tongue, and the body. By this attainment these impurities become pleasant smelling and cure all diseases" (2012, 160).[52] Pūjyapāda stresses that despite possessing healing abilities, ascetics should not use them to cure themselves, paralleling the reluctance to cure oneself through religious healing in medieval didactic stories and narrative literature discussed above.[53]

However, both the root-text and the commentary also describe an internal austerity of service (*vaiyāvṛttya*) to the sick (*glāna*) (TS and SSi 9.20, 9.24; see chapter 3). Pūjyapāda defines "service" as "attending to" (*upāsana*) with bodily activity (*kāya-ceṣṭā*) and other things (*dravya-antara*) (SSi 9.20§862). He further notes that service is done for the purpose of effecting *samādhi* (*samādhi-ādhāna*), dispelling of doubt (*vicikitsā-abhāva*), and expression of affection (*pravacana-vātsalya*), among others (SSi 9.24§866). Medical treatment is not explicitly mentioned, and it seems that *service* here refers primarily to nonmedical help. Service is, additionally, considered as being aligned with the spiritual path, even leading to spiritual attainments. In this regard, the commentary resembles the late Śvetāmbara canonical sources better than the postcanonical mendicant manuals. This again highlights the function of different literary genres, noted above.

However, the absence of an explicit reference to medical treatment does not mean that Digambara sources rejected the use of medicine entirely. On the contrary, it seems that Digambara texts view not only service but also medical gifts in a positive light. The *Trilokaprajñapti* (Pkt. *Tiloyapaṇṇatī*), composed by Yativṛṣabha around the sixth to seventh centuries CE (roughly the same period as the Śvetāmbara commentaries explored above), suggests that people who give the gift of medicines (*auṣadhi-dāna*) may earn auspicious rebirth in the *subhoga-bhūmi* lands of the cosmos (Wiley 2000a, 59), linking medical provision with auspicious karma.[54] The possibility of beneficial rebirth suggests that medical care was, at least to a certain extent, also promoted.

These few textual examples indicate that Digambara sources contain similar themes and considerations to Śvetāmbara sources when it comes to medicine and medical treatment. Further research in Digambara sources is needed in order to more precisely identify similarities and differences.

### *Jain Medical Treatises*

According to the Jain tradition, the earliest canonical scriptures contained knowledge about illnesses and their treatment. *Prāṇa-vāda* (Pkt. *Pāṇā-vāya*), the twelfth Pūrva, is supposed to have discussed medical topics and contained an account of eight kinds of medical science. Wiley identifies these as "the eight *aṅga*s of *āyurveda*" (2000a, 268). As the twelfth Pūrva is lost, it can, however, only be speculated what the version of medicine imparted by this text was and in what ways it reflected specifically Jain ethical values.

Much research still needs to be done on the history of Jain medical treatises. Gerrit Jan Meulenbeld's extensive, five-volume *History of Indian Medical Literature* and R.P. Bhatnagar's *Jaina Āyurveda kā Itihāsa* are rich resources for future scholarship in this area. In part 2 of this book, we will mainly refer to two medical treatises that have already received some, albeit limited, scholarly attention: the Śvetāmbara *Taṇḍula-vaicārika* (Pkt. *Tandula-veyāliya*), written in Prākrit (post-seventh century CE) and the Sanskrit *Kalyāṇa-kāraka* (c. ninth century CE), written by the Digambara monk Ugrāditya. The *Kalyāṇa-kāraka* is presently available only in Hindi translation. The *Taṇḍula-vaicārika* was translated into French as a two-part analysis by Jain studies scholar Colette Caillat; Brianne Donaldson has recently published English translations of Caillat's work (Caillat 2018, 2019).

The *Taṇḍula-vaicārika* is a short treatise belonging to a collection of the Prakīrṇaka-sūtras or "Mixture" texts that exist on the margin of the Śvetāmbara canonical corpus. The title refers to the total "grains of rice" that a male individual consumes over the course of a hundred-year life span. The text includes descriptions of embryology, gynecology, anatomy, the duration of life, and the inevitability of disease and death (Caillat 2018, 2019). In her analysis of the treatise, Caillat claims that "the teaching [that the *Taṇḍula-vaicārika*] dispenses recalls, without being identical to, elements of classical Indian medicine" (2018, 4).

The Digambara *Kalyāṇa-kāraka* of Ugrāditya seems to be the most detailed and comprehensive extant manual on Jain medicine, consisting of twenty-five, and two additional, chapters, and roughly eight thousand verses and some prose. The text proclaims medicine as something innate to the Jain tradition, claiming that āyurvedic knowledge originated with the first Jina Ṛṣabha, who passed it on to the first universal emperor (*cakravartin*) Bharata, from whom it was passed to each subsequent Jina, teacher, and student (Meulenbeld 2002, vol. IIA, 151).[55]

Ugrāditya claims to have consulted earlier Jain medical texts, but unfortunately none of these seem to be extant (Ghatnekar and Nanal 1979, 94). He describes the *Kalyāṇa-kāraka* as an abbreviated version of an extensive text on the eight limbs of *āyurveda* by Samantabhadra (KK 20.86), while claiming the ultimate source of all medical works to be the *Prāṇā-vāda* mentioned above (KK 21.3, 25.54). Meulenbeld explains that Ugrāditya belonged to the mendicant lineage of the eminent Digambara philosopher-monk Kundakunda (2002, vol. IIA, 155), a pedigree suggesting that medicine was fully accepted in Digambara circles by the ninth century.

Like the *Taṇḍula-vaicārika*, the *Kalyāṇa-kāraka* is in conversation with the classical āyurvedic treatises of the time, but also adds its own Jain twist by removing three forbidden foods (*vikṛti*) of honey, alcohol, and meat from the accepted lists of medicines. Rao suggests that the removal of meat and alcohol from medical treatments "assumes a position against even *Caraka* in this regard" (1985, 64). He continues:

> Diseases (*āmaya*) and meat (*māṃsa*) are both alike caused by sin (*pāpajatvāt*), by the three *doṣa*s, and by the involvement of bodily constituents (*mala-dhātu-nibandhanāt*), and, therefore meat cannot be employed to cure a disease (*na pratīkārakam*). . . . The work recommends only the medicines derived from the vegetable kingdom, and that too in little quantity (*svalpam*) and taken in an agreeable manner (*sukham pathyatamam*). (64)

The *Kalyāṇa-kāraka* also prohibits honey as a medical treatment since it is a substance that consists of infinite minute beings. Other substances of animal origin can be used, however, such as hair, nails, bones, or excrement (Meulenbeld 2002, vol. IIA, 152). The text addresses many topics, such as prognostics, embryology, anatomy, obstetrics, and various modes of treatment, including sixty kinds of therapeutic procedures, directions for taking drugs, bloodletting with leeches, and alchemy.[56]

## JAIN FOUNDATIONAL PRINCIPLES IN MEDICINE

There is little scholarship addressing Jain views on medicine and medical practices in the canon. However, the canonical texts reveal a period of dynamic change within the Jain community that led to accommodations and duty to care for sick mendicants within circumscribed regulations, and these adaptive practices possibly opened space for the later liberalization of medicine within the postcanonical period. The examination of the development of the Jain approaches to medicine and medical treatment highlights several foundational principles that must be considered within any contemporary engagement between Jainism and bioethics. These principles establish fundamental attitudes toward the understanding of illness and the body, the relation of illness and the body to mendicant practice, the karmic costs and/or benefits of medicine, and the social dimensions of medical treatment.

First, the body is an essential instrument upon the path to liberation. Each individual body is the product of past karma, and each body is also the medium through which one strives toward karmic advancement in one's present existence. Jain texts encourage mendicants to overcome—often through rigorous physical austerities—attachments to the body itself, to its beauty, comfort, or longevity. One who can practice equanimity in the face of bodily illness or discomfort, can attain immense spiritual gains. Nevertheless, Jain texts also recognize that ascetic disciplines require a body healthy enough to withstand the efforts, and that illness can impede that progress.

Second, physical illnesses are said to affect the gross physical body of those beings living in the "lands of action" and to have diverse causes. Physical illness is produced through karma associated with pain or unpleasant experiences, karma causing disfigurement or self-destruction, disturbances in the three bodily humors, damaging lifestyle habits, ascetic powers, human and divine curses, or the decline in vitality due to old age. Mental illness may be caused by delusion-producing karma, possession by a *yakṣa*, or an imbalance of the humors. Depending on the cause, illnesses of various types can be more or less responsive to treatment, modification, and improvement. For instance, adjusting lifestyle habits is said to alleviate many health issues. Conditions affiliated with karma, however, may require an entire lifetime to influence through severe austerities.

Third, Jain approaches to medical treatment vary. In the earliest texts, disciplined, individual mendicants were expected to forgo medicine, medical treatment, and using their own skills to heal others or themselves. Receiving and providing medical treatment was deemed a source of attachment (*parigraha*) and violence (*ārambha*). However, these costs could eventually be accepted for ill mendicants for the sake of communal health and stability, so long as they were regulated with additional rules. The texts record a gradual emergence of a duty to care, first by mendicants collecting alms for sick fellow mendicants and circumscribing specific situations when sick mendicants could violate communal rules, and eventually providing and/or procuring medicines or treatment that would keep the community stable and patients satisfied. In order to provide care for the sick, Jain mendicants could even violate certain vows such as storing food or medications for the sick. Nevertheless, some texts, especially didactic stories and narrative literature, express a persistent unease in encounters with healing.

Fourth, the understanding of the effects of caring for the sick is likewise not uniform. In the texts, caring for ailing mendicants transforms from a karma-accumulating activity to a karma-destroying practice that aids one on the path of purification.

Fifth, and finally, the notion of an acceptable medical provider expanded from the early canon through the postcanonical period. Doctors and other householders were decried as violent and deluded in the earliest texts. However, the need to safeguard community health meant that mendicants could eventually provide care for themselves and their fellows. The view of householders also gradually softened as the dependence of the mendicant community on householders deepened, and if no mendicants were available to provide medical care, doctors were regarded as suitable to offer medical services. In the postcanonical period, a formal hierarchy of healthcare providers begins with Jain mendicants themselves (who may have been physicians prior to ordination), to Jain former mendicants, to Jain householder physicians, and finally to non-Jain providers. Jains also developed their own medical treatises and contributed to the wider medical literature of the time.

In part 2, we will explore contemporary views of medicine that draw upon insights from the canon and from postcanonical texts, as well as from individual Jains' personal and clinical experience. Drawing upon the foundational principles we have identified in part 1, we attempt to distinguish principles of application that can inform a Jain engagement with modern bioethics.

PART TWO

# Principles of Application

5

# Potentials of (Re)Birth

In part 2 of this book, we aim to identify Jain perspectives on the bioethical dilemmas of birth, life, and death. Since Jain primary texts rarely address any of these dilemmas specifically, we draw upon four sources to identify various insights, competing values, and provisional principles of application for engaging with contemporary bioethical issues. First, we examine Jain canonical and postcanonical texts, varying from mendicant and lay manuals to narratives and medical treatises. Second, we look to modern lay Jains and Jain studies scholars who interpret traditional sources for new ethical situations, and to modern scholars of Indian medicine whose work provides comparative and historical context for the Jain view. Third, we utilize data gathered from a survey we conducted in 2017–18 of international Jain medical professionals, described in the next section. Fourth, where available, we examine the views of contemporary Jain mendicants through their personal writing, interviews, and academic anthropological accounts.

Throughout part 2, we also engage aspects of Western bioethics to provide a frame for understanding contemporary issues in their evolving contexts. This variously includes definitions, key terms, legal precedents, philosophical commitments of other religious communities, and, to a lesser extent, Western normative ethical theories that feature in bioethics debates such as deontology and utilitarianism, among others. Our aim is not to equate Jainism with any term, precedent, or ethical theory. On the contrary, Jain foundational principles or perspectives rarely align easily with any singular view. For that reason, we identify a plurality of positions and concepts to illuminate what is at stake in current debates and where Jainism may resonate, diverge, or raise alternate questions. Although there is no single Jain view on any of the ethical challenges herein, we identify five provisional Jain principles of application for reproductive ethics at the end of the chapter.

## SURVEY OF JAIN MEDICAL PROFESSIONALS, 2017–2018: DESIGN AND METHODOLOGY

Today, Jains are firmly entrenched in modern medicine. Although they constitute less than 1 percent of the Indian population, the National Health Portal of India lists over two hundred Jain-sponsored hospitals and clinics in India.[1] There are at least twenty-five Jain medical colleges, and the Jain Medical Doctors Association of India has a partial directory of some 23,400 Jain physicians.[2] Jain medical professionals are also a visible part of the global diaspora. Many Jains came to the United States through the 1965 Immigration Act, which favored those with advanced training in science, engineering, and medicine. Consequently, the estimated one hundred thousand Jains living in the United States[3] have high representation in medical fields. As of 2017, the Federation of Jain Associations in North America (JAINA) reported a directory of about six hundred Jain medical professionals.[4]

Given the high number of Jains who work in medical fields, we designed an online survey titled "Foundations for Bioethics in the Jain Tradition." We vetted this survey with two Jain physicians to clarify language and modify any question for accuracy. During spring 2017, after ethics review, we solicited the help of Jain medical professionals involved with JAINA, several medical associations in India, and Jain physicians and researchers in the private sector in order to disseminate the survey through email, along with a two-minute introductory video.[5] The survey included 130 multiple-choice and open-ended questions related to demographics (17 questions), professional and religious identity (32 questions), ethical reflection (69 questions), and Jain religious education (12 questions). The survey was open from mid-July through mid-September 2017 on the Qualtrics platform of Rice University in Houston, Texas.

Our data include survey answers from a total of 48 respondents. Of these, 35 completed the entire survey, and 13 answered at least 10 percent or more of the survey, meaning that 35–48 participants interacted with each question. The gender ratio was 19 female to 29 male. The ages, places of birth, and countries of residence for participants were as follows:[6]

**Age** (*n* = 48)
18–23 (8%)
24–29 (8%)
30–39 (8%)
40–49 (21%)
50–59 (15%)
60–69 (19%)
70–79 (17%)
80–89 (4%)

**Birth country** (*n* = 48)
India (58%)
United States (19%)

Kenya (13%)
United Kingdom (4%)
Tanzania (4%)
Canada (2%)

**Country of residence** (*n* = 48)
United States (67%)
United Kingdom (8%)
India (8%)
Kenya (8%)
Canada (6%)
Australia (2%)

Most of the respondents selected a sect affiliation, with the majority identifying as Śvetāmbara (73%, *n* = 48), with the subsects Mūrtipūjaka/Mandir Mārgī (51%, *n* = 35), Sthānakavāsī (29%), Bāīs Sampradāya (3%), and Śvetāmbara Terāpanthī (6%). A smaller minority identified as Digambara (25%, *n* = 48), with the subsects Bīsapanthī (25%, *n* = 12) and Digambara Terāpanthī (17%). Additional respondents identified themselves with two different sect identities (6%, *n* = 48) or as followers of Śrīmad Rājacandra (6%). Respondents reported their education levels as MD (56%, *n* = 48), PhD (4%), master's degree (13%), four-year college (17%), high school (4%), or other (6%).[7]

The majority of participants had attended Jain temple education (*pāṭhaśālā*) (75%, *n* = 36) in the United States, India, or their birth country, for 0–1 year (21%, *n* = 28), 1–3 years (11%), 3–5 years (36%), 5–7 years (14%), or 7 years or more (18%).[8] A considerable percentage of respondents had also taught in *pāṭhaśālā* (39%, *n* = 36), and a significant number were currently attending adult *pāṭhaśālā* classes (17%, *n* = 36) or teaching classes (22%, *n* = 36). In addition to their involvement with Jain temple education, many respondents had served in a leadership position with a Jain-related organization such as JAINA, Young Jains of America, Young Jains of Nairobi, Young Jain Professionals, Jain Vegans, their own temple board, or similar groups (42%, *n* = 36), demonstrating both exposure to Jain values and investment in the community's continuity. We have integrated these survey responses throughout this and the next two chapters to deepen our analysis of what constitutes a Jain response to bioethical dilemmas.

## BIRTH AS REBIRTH

As detailed in chapter 2, in Jain philosophy an individual birth (*janman*) is always a *rebirth* (*punar-bhava*), one of many transformations that an individual *jīva* will undergo on its karmic path.[9] Rebirth signifies the start of life in a new bodily form, but not the beginning of life itself. As Christopher Chapple suggests: "The question for Jainism is not who created life; life has always been present and can never be destroyed. The question for Jainism is how to advance the *jiva* toward a state of liberation through the gradual release of all karmas" (2013, 83). Consequently, the moment of birth is one significant event in a much longer trajectory. Furthermore, as discussed in chapter 2, a particular embodiment is not determined at birth but rather at the moment when longevity-determining karma (*āyu-karman*) binds in the previous life, establishing the forthcoming life span and the birth state to come (Wiley 2000a, 41–47). Past, present, and future lives are thus intricately connected.

Jain texts locate human beings in the viviparous-with-placenta (*jarāyu*) class of living beings born in a womb (*garbhaja*) (see chapter 2). Being born as an embryo (*garbha*) in a womb had spiritual and biological significance throughout Indian religious and medical traditions. In addition to being addressed in classical āyurvedic texts such as the *Caraka-saṃhitā* and *Suśruta-saṃhitā*, specific treatises such as the Vedic *Garbha-upaniṣad* and the Buddhist *Garbhāvakrānti-sūtra* focus on conception, gestation, and embryology (Kritzer 2009). The Jain medical texts *Taṇḍula-vaicārika* and *Kalyāṇa-kāraka*, introduced in chapter 4, include sections on embryology and conception. Jain embryology reflects wider trends within traditional Indian medicine, which, according to Zwilling and Sweet, "combines philosophical and metaphysical speculation with empirical observation" (1993, 592). The Jain medical treatises, for instance, offer a biological account of the embryo that often depends upon particular notions of karma, cosmology, purity, and well-being. Conversely, Jain texts that are more concerned with philosophy, karma, and cosmology also include references to biological knowledge and physiological processes of conception and birth.

## CONCEPTION, EMBRYOLOGY, AND FETAL LIFE IN THE JAIN TRADITION

As detailed in chapter 2, Jain texts describe the births of various living beings as occurring either through agglutination, through the womb, or "by descent" ($TS^{Dig}$ 2.31–35[10]). Whatever the mode, birth is understood as leading to inevitable suffering, death, and possible rebirth in an even more detrimental existence. Intercourse is believed to harm living beings, as we will discuss below, and requires damaging attachments to women who enable birth (YŚ 2.87), and to sexuality that undermines the mendicant path of vigilance over the passions. As stated in chapter 3, passions are one of the five primary causes of karmic bondage, and a prerequisite for the three causes of carelessness, nonrestraint, and wrong worldview. Conceiving a child thus contributes to the persistence of passions that generate violence, guaranteeing more rounds of rebirth. At the same time, the Jain tradition has viewed birth as a positive occasion for women, families, and society—especially the birth of a Jina. Conception and birth represent two of the five auspicious events (*kalyāṇaka*) in the life of a Jina, the other three being renunciation, achieving omniscience, and liberation. These events are sometimes reenacted by Jains during festivals and temple consecrations.[11]

### *Conception in the Womb*

Contrary to certain Buddhist[12] or Hindu notions of an intermediate period between life and death, Jain texts insist that the *jīva* starts a new embodied existence almost immediately after the death of its previous form. Umāsvāti explains this transition as lasting a minimum of one moment (*samaya*)[13] to a maximum of four moments, propelled by karma in a straight line or with up to three turns (TS$^{Dig}$ 2.25–29;[14] also BhS 1.7§85b). Juxtapose this with a Hindu view expressed in the *Chāndogya-upaniṣad*, in which potential life, after an indeterminate waiting period in the "realm of the fathers" (*pitṛ-loka*) and beyond, due to karma, becomes mist, then cloud, and then rain, before being absorbed in plant life; only after these plants are eaten by a male individual and later emitted as semen can a life be reborn (ChU 5.10.3–6). Padmanabh Jaini clarifies how this Upaniṣadic view clashes with Jain cosmology, which does not accept other life-forms as mere instruments: "For the Jainas . . . it is possible for a soul to be *reborn* as a 'water body' (*āp-kāyika*) or as a plant (*vanaspati-kāyika*), but not for these latter entities to function simply as insentient props in the life of a soul on its way to a human existence" (2010b, 125).

As noted in chapter 2, it is unclear how the embryo enters the body of the mother-to-be (Jaini 2010b, 124), but Jain texts typically depict human births as being a result of real sex acts, (*maithuna, maithuna-vṛttika*) (BhS 2.5§133b; SthS 3.1.10).[15] Jain medical manuals share the wider Indian medical view that a child is conceived when fluid from the father, commonly understood to be semen (*śukra, bīja*), mixes with the mother's fluid (*rasa, śoṇita*), variously described as blood, menstrual fluid, or another undefined procreative substance.[16] Classical Indian medical texts, as well as Jain mendicant and medical texts, describe these two fluids uniting with a third vital element—that of *jīva*—to form the living embryo at the moment of conception (KK 2.47; TV 11–15, p. 5,1–3, p. 5,6–12; cf. Das 2003, 4, fn. 6).[17] The semen present in the uterus retains the potential to form an embryo from a time range of less than one *muhūrta* (forty-eight minutes) to a maximum of twelve *muhūrta*s, or approximately ten hours (BhS 2.5§133a).[18]

The chances of conception are further limited by the potentiality of the female fluid and the fertility of the couple.[19] Following the *Taṇḍula-vaicārika* 9–15, Colette Caillat describes the female anatomy and its mechanism of releasing "drops of blood" through menstruation, and addresses male and female fertility:

> All the drops that reach the uterus, mixed with sperm, are able to be born in the form of "lives": up to 900,000;[20] but they are sterile after twelve *muhuttas* [Skt. *muhūrtas*]. Man's sperm remains active for the same period of twelve *muhuttas*; and a child can have up to ninety fathers. On our continent, a woman is no longer fertile after fifty-five years, a man after seventy-five years. (Caillat 2019, 4–5)

A child's temperament, health, and sex are also determined during conception. The condition of a child is said to be determined by the karma it has accumulated throughout its previous lives (BhS 1.7§86b). The *Kalyāṇa-kāraka* states that whichever one of the three "humors"—wind, bile, or phlegm—is dominant at the time of conception informs a child's character disposition and general health (KK 3.18–27; see chapter 4). The sex (*liṅga*) of the child is determined, in part, by the quantities of the parental fluids at conception. More of the father's fluid leads to a male (*puṃ-liṅga*) child; more maternal fluid leads to a female (*strī-liṅga*) child; equal portions result in a child that is neither male nor female, sometimes referred to as "third sex" (*napuṃsaka-liṅga*) (TV 22–23; Das 2003, 3–4; Jaini 1991a, 11–12; Sethi 2012, 71–74; Zwilling and Sweet 1996, 362–63, fn. 16).[21] The sex of the child is also influenced by the karma of the embryo, as noted in chapter 2, and is related to the womb position: a male embryo is on the right side of the uterus, a female on the left, and a third-sex embryo in the middle (Schubring 2000/1962, 142; TV 16).

The *Kalyāṇa-kāraka* describes disciplines for menstruation and intercourse that the mother should follow to ensure conception—what to wear, where to sleep, and rules for not speaking or committing violence (KK 2.42). Sex is permitted and prohibited on certain days, and the text also describes an accompanying ritual to ensure conception (*garbha-ādhāna*) (KK 2.43–47). For example, the fourth day of menstruation is proper for intercourse after bathing and eating certain foods or medicinal substances to increase virility (*vājī-karaṇa*). In keeping with prevailing Indian medical wisdom of that period, after intercourse the mother is to lie on her left side for a female child or on her right side for a male. This reflects the positions of the different sexes in the womb mentioned above.

The embryo's first food within the womb is the fluid of the mother, the fluid of the father, or a combination of the two (SKS 2.3.21).[22] These substances are considered impure (*kaluṣa*) and offensive (*kilbiṣa*) (Wiley 2000a, 191; TV p. 5,1–3). At the same time, early nourishment enables the growth of structures and limbs (*piṇḍa*), with matter transformed from the mother's fluid contributing flesh, blood, and brain, and matter transformed from the father's fluid contributing bones, marrow, hair, and nails. These parental contributions are said to stay with the child's body until its death (BhS 1.7§86b).[23]

### *Embryonic Development and Maternal Connection*

Jain texts understand a nine-month gestation period for human beings born in a womb (TV p. 6,31),[24] and they mostly agree on the details regarding human bodily development (Wiley 2000a, 190). The *Taṇḍula-vaicārika* and the *Kalyāṇa-kāraka* describe a child's growth as proceeding from a thick liquid form (*kalala*; seven days after conception) to a long round mass (*arbuda*; seven days after *kalala*), then to flesh-like and solid forms (*peśin* and *ghana*) until becoming a fully developed fetus (KK 2.53–57; TV 17, p. 5,6–12; Sikdar 1974, 240; Wiley 2000a, 192). During this developmental period, the texts describe how the *jīva* begins to attract various material particles to construct its body, sense organs, and respiratory organs, as well as the organs of speech and mind. Some human beings possess the ability to fulfill this process of bodily development (*paryāpta*), whereas others lack this ability (*aparyāpta*) and die soon after rebirth, a distinction to which we will return below in relation to genomic editing (Babb 1996, 200, fn. 36; Wiley 2000a, 128–30) (see also chapter 2).

In relation to the bioethical issues we will examine, it is important to note that a nascent human embryo possesses all five sense faculties (*bhāva-indriya*) that precede and correlate with the sense organs (*dravya-indriya*) that develop with the principal body (BhS 1.7§86b; see chapter 2).[25] The first sense organ to develop is that of touch, perhaps because it takes the longest to develop, followed by organs of taste, smell, hearing, and sight (Wiley 2000a, 178).

After the embryo's initial diet of fluids from both parents, when it is said to absorb food with its entire body, bodily construction takes place by taking nutrients from whatever food the mother ingests (BhS 1.7§86b; TV p. 5,27–29). The *Kalyāṇa-kāraka* prescribes the mother's diet for different stages of pregnancy, including fruit, milk, vegetables, grains, butter with rice, as well as certain medicinal drinks (*kaṣāya*) made from plants and bark, mixed with ghee, curd, and milk (KK 23.22–24). Since the embryo has no excretion during this time, food helps grow the body and the physical sense organs (BhS 1.7§86b; TV p. 5,11–14).

Jains share the view called "double-heartedness" (*dvai-hṛdaya*), according to which nutrients are transferred to the fetus by way of the "two threads"—possibly akin to umbilical connections—that develop around the third month of gestation. One of these threads leads from mother to fetus (*mātṛ-jīva-rasa-haraṇi*; lit. "liquid vessel of the mother's *jīva*") and another from fetus to mother (*putra-jīva-rasa-haraṇi*; lit. "liquid vessel of the child's *jīva*") (BhS 1.7§86b; Caillat 2018, 7–10; Kritzer 2008, 75; Schubring 2000/1962, 141). Through these two threads, the pregnant woman (*garbhiṇī*) influences her child's bodily development through what she eats. The *Taṇḍula-vaicārika* also states that the two threads permit the fetus to feel and influence its mother's cravings in the third month and cause the mother's body to swell in the fourth month (TV p. 5,7). Such pregnancy cravings (*dohada*)[26] can be positive or harmful, often appearing in Jain narratives to teach about karma, to explain seemingly unjust suffering, and to reflect relational concerns between women, maternal roles, husbands, family, and society, as is evident in the Jain narrative on abortion below (Bauer 1998, 256–57).

### *Auspicious Embryos* in Utero

Jain narratives depict an especially strong connection between a mother and the embryo of an important figure such as a Jina or a universal emperor (*cakravartin*). These stories are found in Śvetāmbara canonical texts such as the *Ācārāṅga-*, *Bhagavatī-*, and *Kalpa-sūtra*, among others. Later, postcanonical biographies in the Jain genre of "universal history" embellish the stories further, detailing the lives of one or all of the sixty-three great persons (*śalākā-puruṣa*) born in each progressive and regressive half-cycle of time (see chapter 2). Purāṇic texts, for example, pay special attention to their last incarnation and the unexpected ways that past karma ripens over numerous lives (Cort 1993, 188–89). This includes animated accounts of Jain heroes in the womb.

The life of Mahāvīra, the twenty-fourth Jina, begins with an especially lively gestation. In the Śvetāmbara canon, Mahāvīra descends from the heavenly world, taking the form of an embryo in the womb of Devānandā, the wife of a Brahmin, while she is asleep (KS 2.2). The account avoids any mention of the impurities of conception described elsewhere. Like all mothers of Jinas, Devānandā experiences fourteen auspicious dreams.[27] During Devānandā's pregnancy, Indra, the king of one of the heavens in the Jain cosmos, realizes that Mahāvīra—who was destined to be a great spiritual hero—had incorrectly descended into the womb of a Brahmin woman when warriors, including Jinas as "spiritual warriors," could only be born from the Kṣatriya stratum of society.[28] Indra calls upon Hariṇegamesī,[29] a leader of Indra's heavenly army, to gently transfer the embryo of Mahāvīra by hand from Devānandā, exchanging it with an embryo in the womb of a Kṣatriya woman named Triśalā.[30] The extreme care of this embryo transfer, recorded in the *Kalpa-*, *Bhagavatī-*, and *Ācārāṅga-sūtra*, is complete on the eighty-third day of gestation when Triśalā has the same fourteen dreams (KS 2.30, 3.32–46; BhS 5.4§218a).[31]

In these stories, the Mahāvīra-to-be-embryo has special knowledge of entering the wombs of both Devānandā and Triśalā (KS 2.3, 2.29; ĀS 2.15.3–5). He causes his mother no pain, increases her beauty, and is sensitive to her feelings, quivering when she fears he may be dead, and, according to Śvetāmbaras, takes his first vow within the womb not to become a monk until after his parents' deaths (KS 4.92–94). Beyond these insights, the fetus brings wealth to his family (Mahāvīra's birth name is Vardhamāna, meaning "increase/prosperity") and inspires his father, the king, to set prisoners free, cancel debts, lighten taxes, clean the city, forgo arrests, and invite all artists, musicians, and marginalized citizens to a ten-day celebration (ĀS 2.15.10–12; KS 4.90–91, 5.102–9).

In her analysis of Jain heroes *in utero* in the Purāṇas,[32] Eva De Clercq describes these events as the "Jina life blueprint," including dreams, the transformation of the mother (though the father is also affected, as noted above), and a series of supernatural events that reflect the status of the hero (2009, 51–52). She highlights elements of these stories that distance the conception, gestation, and birth from sexuality, as well as the embryo transfer. She discusses instances of pregnancy cravings, mentioned above, but also argues that despite the "double-hearted" threads between the mother and the child,[33] the mother is primarily an expression of her child's Jina-hood and a passive recipient of his one-directional influence (44–45). Other scholars, however, assert that the mothers of Jinas are counted as Jain heroes in their own right (Sethi 2009, 47–48).[34]

The Digambara tradition does not accept the embryo transfer as valid and understands Triśalā to be Mahāvīra's only mother. Digambaras also reject the first vow being made in the womb, asserting that Mahāvīra committed to mendicancy as an adult and renounced the worldly life while his parents were still alive, only after seeking their approval. Such variations notwithstanding, these epic stories of auspicious embryos add another layer to the diverse Jain sources of conception and fetal life by which we might approach modern issues in reproductive ethics—especially taking, facilitating, and altering nascent life—to which we now turn.

## TAKING AND PREVENTING NASCENT LIFE: JAIN VIEWS ON ABORTION, POPULATION CONTROL, AND CONTRACEPTION

We begin with the question of taking and preventing life through abortion, population control, and contraception. Jain texts either do not address these questions specifically or address them in no great detail. The death of nascent human life is described as a particular kind of death called *avyakta-bāla-maraṇa*—or "death of the undeveloped" (Settar 2017/1990, 10). Certain stories attempt to account for the difficult experience of pregnancy not coming to term. The *Bhagavatī-sūtra* asserts that the right posture for the fetus to emerge from the womb is by the head or feet, but if it is born side-first, it will die (BhS 1.7§86b; TV p. 7,1–2). The *Kalyāṇa-kāraka* acknowledges the possibility of miscarriage if a woman does not follow prescribed preparations for pregnancy (KK 2.46–47; Patil et al. 2015, 147). The *Taṇḍula-vaicārika* states that if maternal fluid (*ojas*) condenses, a mass (*biṃba*) is born (TV 23, p. 6,33–34), which Walther Schubring interprets as a result of a miscarriage (2000/1962, 142). Jain narratives sometimes depict mothers beseeching guardian deities to protect against miscarriage (Bauer 1998, 58), and, as mentioned above, the *Kalpa-sūtra* states that Mahāvīra quivered in the womb to assuage his mother's fear that he had died (KS 4.92–93). However, all these occurrences are unintentional; and we will discuss the intentional termination of nascent life shortly.

It is important to highlight that Jain texts warn about the processes and motivations of producing new life. As noted in chapter 2, sex (*maithuna*) is deemed one of the four instincts (*saṃjñā*) that define embodied life, fuel the passions, and thus maintain karmic bondage (Jaini 2010e, 284). In the male mendicant context, women are also seen as a perpetual source of delusion and karmic attachment because of their erotic allure (Sethi 2012, 51–86; YŚ 2.82–102). Consequently, celibacy, or *brahmacarya*, as one of the five great vows, allows monks and nuns to assiduously avoid the attachments that lead to the desire for procreation in the first place.

Even in the textual guidelines for laity that accommodate social norms of childbearing, procreation is not neutral. The Digambara mendicant Amṛtacandrasūri (c. tenth century) describes multiple living beings killed in the vagina[35] due to the friction of intercourse, comparing it to a hot iron rod being inserted into a tube filled with sesame seeds, which it burns up (PSU 107–9; Wiley 2000a, 140–41); and, as indicated earlier, texts suggest that sex can "create" and "destroy" up to nine hundred thousand progeny (TV 12; cf. Wiley 2000a, 139–40).[36] The minor vow of *brahmacarya* for lay Jains requires sexual restraint, often interpreted as monogamy, or as celibacy for particular durations. The *Kalyāṇa-kāraka*, for example, prescribes celibacy for lay Jains on certain days depending on hot and cold weather, during menstruation, and the eighth and fourteenth days of the lunar fortnight, when other ritual fasts are also prescribed (Patil et al. 2015, 143–44).

### *Abortion*

Jain texts describe rare examples of abortion utilizing various methods. The canonical *Vipāka-sūtra* tells the story of the wicked governor Ikkāi, who is reborn as the fetus Miyāputta in the womb of queen Miyādevī. Afflicted with great pain during the pregnancy, which also repels her husband, the queen tries unsuccessfully to abort the fetus by means of ingesting several salty, bitter, and astringent substances; Miyāputta is later born with severe physical and mental defects and nearly killed by infanticide before being rescued by his father (Bauer 1998, 245–48; Bollée 2003–2004, 182–83).[37]

The canonical *Nirayāvalī* (Pkt. *Nirayāvaliyāo*)[38] describes the attempted abortion of Kūṇika by his mother Celanā, a co-wife of King Śreṇika. During the third month of pregnancy, Celanā experiences pregnancy cravings (*dohada*) to eat her husband's flesh of the belly, baked, fried, and roasted. Unable to fulfill this craving, Celanā grows emaciated until her husband, with the aid of another son, devises a plan to pass off flesh and blood from the slaughterhouse as those of the king (NS 1.1.22–29). After eating them, Celanā is overcome with disgust that her unborn child had indirectly ingested his father's flesh and tries unsuccessfully to abort Kūṇika "by various means of ejecting, abortion, dropping and destroying" (NS 1.1.30, trans. Gopani and Chokshi). When Kūṇika is born, Celanā tries to leave him in a solitary place to die, but his father rescues him. Although—unlike Miyāputta—Kūṇika was born with a beautiful form, he later imprisoned his father, King Śreṇika, and took over the throne, which resulted in King Śreṇika's suicide (NS 1.1.31–39).

These two narratives illuminate various methods of abortion, including manual procedures and eating or drinking different medicinal tonics (Jain 1996, 549). They also offer distinct explanations for the attempted abortion and later results. In the first story, Ikkāi's karma is fulfilled as Miyāputta's embryo, including the painful pregnancy, attempted abortion, and subsequent deformity. In the second story, the inauspicious pregnancy cravings of Celanā, though deceptively fulfilled, seem to impact the character of Kūṇika (543–44). Before turning to current Jain views on abortion, it is important to have a greater understanding of the topic within contemporary medical and bioethical contexts.

*Contemporary Bioethical Debates on Abortion.* To understand the contemporary issue of abortion, one must consider the various reasons why a woman may seek abortion, appreciate the stages of pregnancy in which different forms of abortion can occur, and consider the bioethical arguments for and against abortion.

Ethicists explore several reasons why a woman may seek an abortion. In extreme cases, carrying a fetus to term may result in the mother's own death. At the other extreme, carrying a fetus to term may obstruct a woman's personal, relational, or vocational satisfaction. In between these poles, a woman might seek abortion because pregnancy may threaten her own mental or physical well-being, produce a child with severe impairments, subject her to social stigma due to being unmarried, or cause an undue financial burden for her or her family; a woman may also seek abortion if the pregnancy is the result of rape or incest (DeGrazia et al. 2010, 456).

Abortions can be performed at different stages and by different means. For example, nonsurgical medical abortion, first available in France and China in the 1980s, utilizes a pill taken in the first ten weeks of pregnancy.[39] These pills are now widely available in certain countries through clinics and online sources (Aiken et al. 2017).[40] Surgical abortions depend on the stage of development. Vacuum aspiration involves removing the contents of the uterus with a vacuum syringe or suction tube and can be performed from six to sixteen weeks. Dilation and evacuation (D&E) is performed after sixteen weeks of gestation; a surgical curette and forceps are used to scrape out the lining of the uterus and remove any larger fetal remains, followed by suction. Abortion can also be performed by inducing labor.

Modern debates over abortion typically involve disputes over (1) at what point in reproduction an individual life begins or attains "personhood"; and (2) at what point in fetal development, if any, and for what reasons, an abortion can be considered morally or ethically justified.

Regarding the beginning of life, there is no scientific consensus. Current biological perspectives place the start of life at various stages from fertilization of the egg, to gastrulation (when the blastocyst begins to establish distinct cell lineages), to birth, and even later. Philosophical bioethics typically consider the following possible stages:

*conception/fertilization* (when sperm joins egg)
*implantation* (when zygote implants into uterine wall)
*quickening* (when fetus starts to move)
*viability* (when fetus can live outside womb independently or with life-sustaining treatments/technologies)

Several religious bioethical views identify origin of life and/or personhood as significant markers that impact the morality of abortion. Pope John Paul II, for example, in a 1995 encyclical titled "Evangelium Vitae" (The Gospel of Life), stated the Catholic Church's formal position that individual existence begins at conception (John Paul II 1995). Jewish law diversely assigns "humanness" to a fetus at or after birth, though a pre-birth embryo/fetus still has great value as a "potential" human (Schenker 2008, 273). In his comparative analysis of Jewish and Catholic bioethics, Aaron Mackler helpfully explains how formal positions in each tradition coexist with diverse interpretations and applications by ethicists and practitioners (2003).

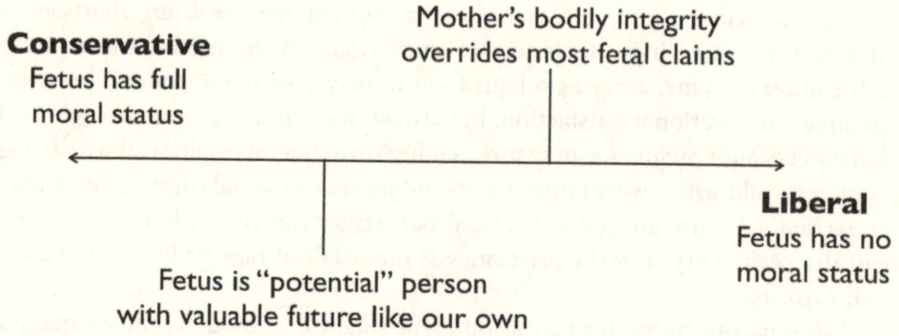


FIGURE 5. Basic continuum of contemporary abortion debates with two examples of intermediary positions. Credit: B. Donaldson (adapted from DeGrazia et al. 2010).

Likewise, the Islamic view is varied, ranging from ensoulment of the fetus at 120 days to divine involvement at every stage of development (Brockopp 2003, 24).

Regarding the point of whether abortion may ever be justified and for what reason, DeGrazia et al. present two corners of the debate. On one end, the oft-called "conservative" view assigns full moral status (or "personhood") to the embryo/fetus and demands ethical consideration equal to that of a fully developed adult (2010, 458). This is the formal position of the Catholic Church, articulated by Pope John Paul II, declaring abortion to be an "unspeakable crime . . . [of] deliberate and direct killing" of an absolutely innocent human person (1995). On the other end is the "liberal"-labeled view, which denies any moral status to an embryo/fetus. Feminist ethicist Mary Anne Warren defends this position by claiming that a fetus can only be considered "human" in the *biological* sense of species; to be a human person in the *moral* sense requires that a being possess *at least one* of the following traits: consciousness of objects and pain, reasoning, self-motivated activity, capacity to communicate, and self-awareness (2010, 469–70). There are a variety of intermediate positions, including affirming a fetus as a "potential person" with a valuable future or privileging a mother's right to bodily integrity over most fetal claims (Marquis 2010, 477; Jarvis Thomson 2010, 480–83). We map this continuum in figure 5.

*Current Jain Perspectives on Abortion.* Jain approaches to abortion do not easily map onto this sort of continuum. Few statements exist from contemporary mendicants on the topic of abortion. In a rare video interview, the current Bhaṭṭāraka Cārukīrti in Mūḍbidrī, Karnataka, who holds one of ten Digambara mendicant seats of authority in south India, engaged with several bioethical issues, including abortion, from a Jain perspective (Sarma 2013). The orthodox position he describes is fairly simple: abortion forces a *jīva* to be reborn when the goal is to break out of the cycle of rebirths. At its base, the Bhaṭṭāraka's view reflects the vow of nonviolence: do not kill a *jīva*, whether in the form of an embryo/fetus or any other embodied state. Yet his response quickly unfolds in multiple directions.

First, akin to the three activities of body, speech, and mind described in chapter 3, he explains that thinking about killing brings negative karma, but acting toward abortion and actually doing it invites the worst karmic cost, even if the aim is to save the mother (Sarma 2013). This point suggests that one who seeks an abortion and one who provides it, even with a positive purpose in mind, will still incur karma, indicative of the three methods by which one can harm directly, cause another to harm, or approve of another's harm.

Second, the Bhaṭṭāraka does not condemn abortion specifically, nor does he describe any social or institutional consequences for those involved. Like all actions in a karmic-based system, if a woman seeks an abortion for any reason, she will take the "penalty of karma," which suggests that abortion is a serious karmic harm against a five-sensed being, but it is one among many kinds of karmic harm (Sarma 2013). Notably, there is no reference to the origin of life, fetal personhood, or the phase of pregnancy, as characterizes many contemporary secular and religious bioethical views.

Third, he maintains an important distinction between the Jain mendicant ideal—which makes no provision for killing anything—and the lay practice of that ideal, saying, "The question [of abortion] is a social question, not a religion question" (Sarma 2013). This distinction reveals a persistent feature in Jain ethics—described in chapters 3 and 4—that one can uphold a "religious" ideal of absolute nonviolence as a functional aim, even while recognizing the "social" contexts and limits in which lay Jains, and even some monks and nuns, will lack the capacity to pursue the ideal in every moment or to the fullest degree.

Fourth, the Bhaṭṭāraka directs attention to activities that transpire *prior to* the ethical question of abortion, by practicing restraints of body, speech, and mind. *Brahmacarya*, or sexual restraint, he asserts, is "the best gift" of self-control that reduces one's karmic impact by freeing an individual from the potential of pregnancy, the need for abortion, and other related procreative dilemmas (Sarma 2013).

It should be noted that there are cultural examples of Jains taking a very strong position against abortion. For instance, some lay Jains in India have organized rare protests against the liberalization of the nation's abortion laws ("Jains Hold Rally," 2008), and there is at least one online proclamation by a Jain mendicant against abortion, intercaste marriage, and premarital sex ("No Abortion" 2018). At the same time, in a 2018 *Young Minds* article titled "Ahimsa in a Pro-Choice World," Jain youth Ayush Bhansali presses the Jain engagement with abortion beyond *ahiṃsā* and karma. Bhansali contends that "the debate around abortion often exists as a proxy for broad opposition to patriarchy, misogyny, sexual assault, and other types of systemic violence which affect women daily . . . [and] which under the complex of Ahimsa, Jains should be very much against" (2018). Bhansali argues that being a "responsible Jain" means examining nonviolence as it applies to personal choices as well as to wider social structures and conditions (2018).

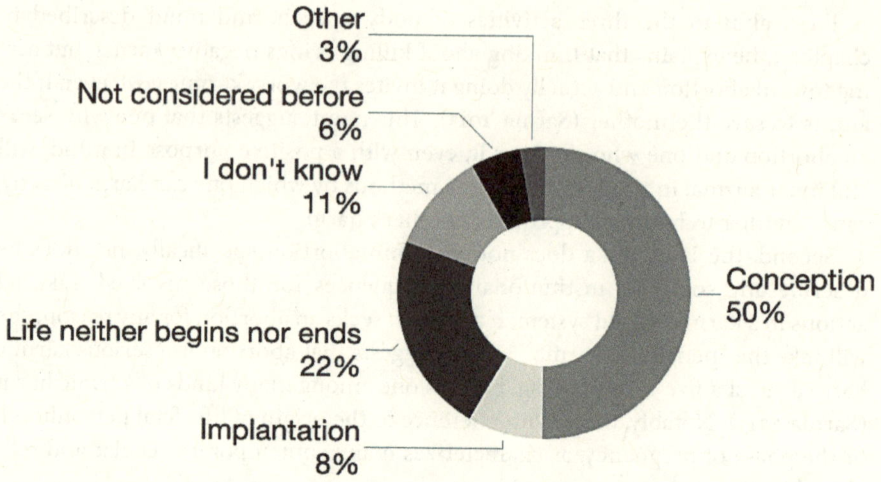


FIGURE 6. Responses of Jain medical professionals to the question of when life begins ($n = 36$).

Our survey of Jain medical professionals reveals diverse considerations in relation to the theory and practice of abortion, as well as the starting point of life. In keeping with the Jain concept of rebirth, a significant minority of respondents felt that life does not begin or end (22%, $n = 36$). Others privileged positions of philosophical bioethics, placing the beginning of life at conception (50%) or implantation (8%) (figure 6). No participants selected *quickening* (fetal movement) or *viability*, when the fetus can survive outside the womb with support. There was also a degree of ambivalence (17%), suggesting that notions of beginning may not be critical to ethical action in Jainism.

The majority of Jain medical professionals (64%, $n = 36$) considered abortion a form of violence. Yet over a third of respondents either disagreed, were unsure, or selected "Other," offering the following remarks:

> "[It] depends on strong medical reason [such as the] mother's health and her life."
>
> "[D]epends upon why abortion has to be done."
>
> "It is [a form of violence], but it needs to be taken on a case by case basis."
>
> "[I]f you are saving the life of the mother it should be okay. I would rather discourage the need for abortion."

When asked about providing abortion services, only a small minority had done so (6%, $n = 36$) while most had not provided such services (78%), with the following additional comments:

> "No, but [I] have referred patients."
>
> "I dispensed emergency contraceptives which I wish I never had to be part of; I worked for somebody and had no choice."

> "Only when it was medically indicated."
>
> "I do not even refer the patient to another doctor who might perform abortion."

Participants provided greater insight into their various perspectives when asked to review a series of statements related to abortion and choose all that apply. Those statements selected by the highest percentage of respondents were as follows: (1) abortion can be justified only when needed to save the life of the mother (58%, $n = 36$); (2) abortion can be justified when the child may have genetic or physical anomalies that could lead to a life of suffering or early death for the child (56%); and (3) the Jain tradition has influenced my attitude regarding abortion (44%) (figure 7). A significant minority felt that "abortion can be justified when a woman feels that she cannot emotionally or financially take the burden of another child" (28%). Only a few respondents believed that viability is a significant marker (8%), whereas no respondents felt that abortion can be justified when the child is an undesired gender (0%).

At opposite ends, a very small minority affirmed a more permissive position that "abortion can be justified at any stage prior to birth" (5%, $n = 36$), while a slightly larger minority felt that "abortion can never be justified" (11%). No respondents felt that "abortion can be justified by the mother for any reason whatsoever" (0%).

At the same time, a number of respondents felt that "providing abortion services and counseling is an important healthcare service for women and families" (28%, $n = 36$), and that "greater education regarding abortion and abortion laws among medical/healthcare professionals is needed to reduce stigma and increase safety and accessibility to abortive services" (22%). A similar percentage felt that there are too many obstacles for women seeking abortion (20%), while a very small minority believed "there should be additional regulations on women seeking abortion" (3%).

These responses make clear that abortion, although considered a form of violence by the majority of respondents, may be an accepted course of action in the face of other costs. As shown above, over half of Jain medical professionals calculate the costs to a mother's health, as well as a child's future suffering due to impairments, against the karmic cost of terminating fetal development *in utero*.

It is precisely this principled plurality of views that makes Jainism difficult to map onto bioethical continuums, or to compare with Western normative ethics. For example, one might see in the Jain vow of *ahiṃsā* certain overlaps with deontological duties that offer a more or less universal injunction against killing innocent persons. At the same time, in the Jain concern for the well-being of the mother, the suffering of the child, as well as social and economic hardships, one may see overlap with a utilitarian view in which the most ethical choice is determined not by following a set duty, but by maximizing pleasure and minimizing pain for the greatest number of those involved. Jain views that emphasize the importance of karmic responsibility within a specific context may look more like a virtue ethics

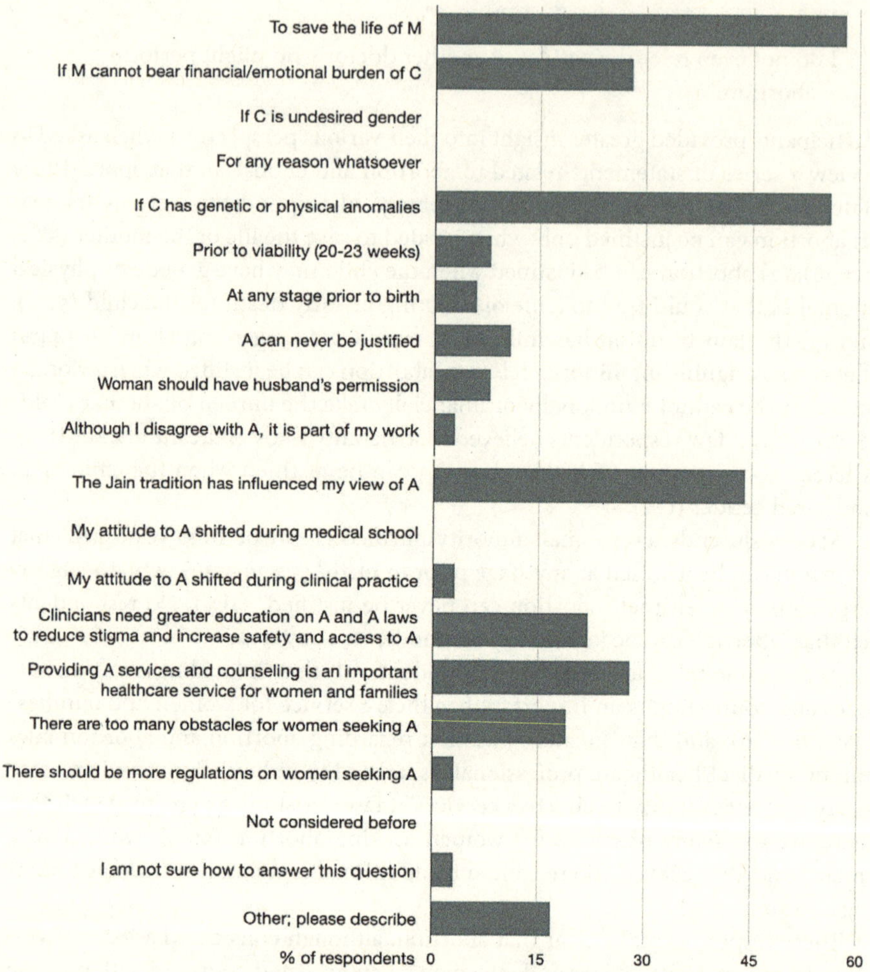


FIGURE 7. Responses of Jain medical professionals to the question "Which of the following statements [regarding abortion] is/are most true for you? Choose all that apply" ($n = 36$). Key: M = mother, C = child, A = abortion.

approach that explores what kind of person *to be* rather than what action to do. Jain principles and views that stress care and compassion might seem more akin to a feminist "ethics of care," which illuminates coexisting obligations, diverse relationship roles, and the historical subordination of certain members of society.

Jain medical professionals in our survey certainly do not reflect a strong public stance against abortion. Though the majority agreed it is a form of violence, only a small minority believed that additional abortion regulations are needed (3%, $n = 36$) or felt that abortion cannot be justified for any reason (11%). Even the

Bhaṭṭāraka Cārukīrti, whose view on abortion we described above, makes it clear that taking nascent life must be examined at various levels. He states: "The Jain answer is not about killing, dying, birth, [or] abortion. It is about understanding the karmic consequences of one's actions. If you want to [harm] someone and you ask someone else to do it, you are still responsible for the [harm]" (Sarma 2013). He inquires further: If our desire for sex leads us to consider killing a nascent life, or having someone else kill for us, might a different desire lead us to kill a person or an animal? These questions, along with the plurality of views from individual Jains, reveal that a Jain ethics of abortion exceeds any single issue of life's beginning, fetal personhood, or stage of pregnancy, and complicates a flat application of the vow of nonviolence. Jains who grapple with the issue of abortion offer responses that seem to reflect Jain principles within the constraints of specific contexts—for example, in India or abroad, in the medical field or not, as a mendicant or lay Jain, as a male or female, or as a young person striving to hold together Jain values with an emergent social and political consciousness.

### *Population Control*

The 2018 global population of 7.6 billion people is expected to near 10 billion by 2050, according to the United Nations. Bioethical debates regarding population control typically include concerns over maintaining reproductive freedom contrasted with managing the ecological effects of a fast-growing global population. Sixty-one percent of Jain medical professionals felt that humans have an obligation to address overpopulation through restrained reproduction (61%, $n = 36$).

In the Jain tradition, the presence of human beings in the world does not pose a challenge in and of itself. As noted in chapter 2, the attainment of human form is understood to be rare and valuable.[41] Further, within Jain cosmology, the total number of living beings is said to remain constant, though populations of individual groups may fluctuate over time (BhS 5.8§244a). The Jain time cycle of progress and regress, described in chapter 2, may also challenge any innate resistance to the damaging impacts of overpopulation, though lay Jains frequently understand this cosmology metaphorically, rather than literally (Donaldson 2020). Paul Dundas writes:

> Jain tradition is clear that, as we enter the final stages of each particular movement of the wheel of time, it is necessary and inevitable that both humankind and the natural worlds socially and ecologically decay. The world will be destroyed and human beings will degenerate intellectually and culturally, to be renewed subsequently with the next motion of time. (2002b, 97)[42]

Nevertheless, many global Jains—both mendicant and lay—have increasingly vocalized a strong commitment to environmental flourishing over the past three decades, which is often linked to the detrimental effects of overpopulation and its associated economic, health, and political impacts.[43] L.M. Singhvi's "The

Jain Declaration on Nature"—presented to Prince Philip at Buckingham Palace in 1990—marked a distinct entry of Jainism into the global conversation on religion and the environment. In that document, Singhvi stresses the role of self-restraint and the avoidance of waste in Jainism, stating that Jain laity "must not procreate indiscriminately lest they overburden the universe or its resources" (2002, 223–24).

In terms of their own population, Jains constitute a very small community. As noted in chapter 1, Jains make up approximately 0.42 percent of the Indian population, while around 285,000 Jains live abroad. The 2011 Census of India analysis shows that the Indian Jain community has increased by only 5.37 percent between 2001 and 2011; this phase of slowed growth, beginning in 1981, is less than other minority communities in the country (Bajaj 2016, 1–2). This stalled growth is attributed to several factors, including high urban habitation and high levels of female literacy (see chapter 1). Jains also have fewer children. Per hundred of the population, Jains have 8.9 children compared to 13.2 for Hindus (5). Some Jains have been prompted to question the survival of the tradition, both in India and abroad, due to issues such as intercultural marriage,[44] the disenfranchisement of young Jains, exposure to other religions, female feticide (on which more below), dowry obligations, and geographic assimilation (Jain and Malaiya 2011).

Contemporary Jainism hinges between a perceived need among some members of the community to bolster their own numbers while others see value in restraining wider trends in overpopulation. Yet it is unclear whether a Jain approach to population control would be socially prescriptive or an expression of personal restraint. As one survey respondent commented regarding population control, "My responsibility begins and ends with me. What someone [else] has to do or not is his or her responsibility."

### *Contraception and Sexuality*

The use of contraceptives has a double effect of preventing conception and protecting oneself from sexually transmitted infections. Modern debates often include questions of whether one should interfere with the natural process of fertility and whether contraception is a form of early abortion. Broader questions emerge from these concerns as to how contraception may redefine (a) the role of sex, (b) the family as a formative social structure, and (c) characteristics of responsible parenthood.

Classical Indian medical treatises say little about contraception beyond strategies of interrupting natural processes and establishing times of abstinence. Bhagwan Dash and R.N. Basu (1968) offer a fascinating account of antifertility measures in ancient and medieval India. Mira Roy (1966) explores methods of sterilization and sex-determination in the Vedas, while A.C. Kar Galib et al. describe the development of female contraceptive methods ingested orally or applied to the vagina that appear peripherally in medieval āyurvedic manuals (2008, 82–83).

The orthodox view of contraception in Jainism is the vow of *brahmacarya*, mentioned above and detailed in chapter 3. As already stated, *brahmacarya* is expressed as celibacy for mendicants and self-imposed sexual restraints for lay Jains. Bhaṭṭāraka Cārukīrti, in the above-mentioned interview, agrees that limiting the population is important but asserts that family planning methods, such as condoms, also kill sperm, which are living *jīvas* (Sarma 2013). From this view—between burdening planetary life through over-procreation on one hand and killing millions of sperm on the other—one can see why the Bhaṭṭāraka's preferred resolution is *brahmacarya*. However, the belief that semen contains life is not uniform in the Jain tradition. Pūjyapāda, for example, asserts that semen is nonliving, which presents a different karmic calculation to that of the Bhaṭṭāraka (SSi 2.32§324; 2000a, 136; see also note 17 in this chapter, and chapter 2 on the violence of sex acts). In any case, the Bhaṭṭāraka insists that the question of contraception is a response to social conventions and should not be confused with the more comprehensive aim of Jain celibacy. As in his discussion of abortion, he states, not that all Jains must practice *brahmacarya* in a uniform way, or at all, but that one should not dilute the Jain ideal to accommodate social norms.

Ācārya Tulsī presents an alternate mendicant view in his book *The Vision of a New Society* (1998), emphasizing the important role of self-restraint for lay Jains. He discusses the ways in which entertainment commodifies sexuality (28), describing popular media as selling the obscenity of "uninhibited sex" (24). He accepts the evolution of the tradition in light of changing social norms but simultaneously implores young people to explore a "new vision" of self-imposed limits for themselves (24–30).

Among lay Jains who interpret the vow of *brahmacarya* within the context of intimate relationships or marriage, attitudes on contraception are unclear. M. Whitney Kelting's research on Jain wifehood among Jains in Maharashtra offers anecdotal evidence that persistent social pressure to have children means that birth control is out of the question until a child, and ideally a son, is born (2009, 70). Conversely, in an editorial in *Young Minds*, a public online forum run by Young Jains of America (YJA), Shardule Shah asserts that *brahmacarya* has unique value in the US context, even though it is difficult to interpret (2009). Celibacy is not merely a prohibition, asserts Shah, but an invitation to "develop who you are as a person without the pressure of marriage, family, [and a] full-time job" (2009). Shah speaks candidly about complications that accompany sex, including STDs and emotional distraction, even with the use of condoms or birth control. This perspective seems to offer a hybrid view wherein strategic celibacy in certain life stages permits a layperson to retain the freedom of self-development prior to the expectations of adulthood. Given the high rate of education and literacy among Jains—which likely reflects historical periods of economic security among the community as a whole—a question emerges as to what role the value of *brahmacarya* might play, even for the period of adolescence and young adulthood, in facilitating educational opportunities and personal growth outside marriage among young Jains, especially women.[45]

The majority of Jain medical professionals we surveyed did not see a conflict between Jain principles and contraception (64%; $n$ = 36). A small minority believed that birth control violates Jain principles (6%), while others did not know (14%) or had never considered the issue before (11%). In the survey, we did not differentiate between preventative contraception, such as condoms, pills, devices, or implants, and emergency contraception administered in the short-term window after sex, which could raise different ethical considerations. Consequently, we can only cautiously infer that the attitude of Jain medical professionals toward contraception suggests that most of them may not see semen as comprising living beings, and/or that they may accept the loss of such living beings for the sake of other benefits related to nonprocreation.

## FACILITATING NASCENT LIFE: IVF, CLONING, AND STEM CELL RESEARCH

We now turn to practices and procedures that facilitate the production of life in special circumstances, including IVF, cloning, and stem cell research.

### *IVF*

In vitro fertilization (IVF) is an assisted reproductive technology (ART) introduced in the 1970s[46] to treat infertility in women with damaged fallopian tubes. Women who seek IVF may also be past the ideal reproductive age, have infertile male partners, or lack the ability to produce eggs, in which case a sperm or egg donor is needed. In most IVF procedures, a woman undertakes a regimen of hormone injections to overproduce eggs that are then removed and fertilized with sperm *in vitro*, or "in glass." The fertilized eggs develop to the blastocyst stage (at five to seven days), whereupon the nascent embryos are evaluated for quality, before one or more are transferred into the mother's uterus in hopes of implantation.

IVF is a basic process involved in many other reproductive technologies, multiplying its ethical significance, which we discuss throughout this section. Because IVF aims to enable procreation without sexual intercourse, bioethical debates often include the personal and social impacts of separating genetic, gestational, and traditional parent-child relations while also enabling single and same-gender parents. The production of excess embryos in IVF raises ethical questions about their storage, their use in research or for other purposes, and their destruction, as well as about the ethics of preimplantation genetic screening, and concerns over donors and donated embryos, eggs, or sperm.

The 2004 President's Commission on Bioethics also warned against unintentional harms to children born using ART, such as increased rate of prenatal death, premature birth, developmental abnormalities, multi-fetal pregnancies, and the disposal of unused embryos ("Assisted Reproduction" 2004). According to the US Centers for Disease Control, only 25 percent of all ART cycles completed in 2016 resulted in live births, meaning that numerous fertilized embryos were terminated in the IVF process ("ART Success Rate" 2016). In addition to failed pregnancies, excess embryos produced during IVF pose persistent questions of whether to destroy them, freeze them, or use them for embryonic stem cell research, which we will discuss shortly.

Multi-fetal pregnancies are also more common with IVF. Countries such as Canada, the United Kingdom, Australia, and New Zealand permit only two embryos to be transferred during IVF, in an effort to limit multiple births. However, the United States has no transfer limit; consequently, the incidence of triplet and high-number births increased by a factor of 6.7 from 1971 to 1998, including high-profile pregnancies with six to eight surviving infants (Kulkarni et al. 2013). While the US rate of multiple pregnancies decreased by 29 percent from 1998 to 2011—coinciding with a 70 percent reduction in the transfer of three or more embryos due to medical association recommendations—multi-fetal pregnancies remain more common for IVF patients, as does the practice of "selective fetal reduction" surgeries to remove excess or diseased fetuses (Kulkarni et al. 2013).

In the orthodox Jain view, the decision to produce life, regardless of the means, equates to taking on greater karmic attachments, as described previously. In his brief summary of Jain bioethics, Jain physician Dilip Bobra states that Jainism is indifferent to the method of procreation, but more concerned with the fact that "children are the cause of attachments and aversions leading to [the] influx of karmas" (2008). He goes on:

> [A] follower should be satisfied if they can have children by natural means. If not, then they have to accept it as a result of their past karmas [whereby a] childless experience provides them a chance to accumulate less karmas to improve future births. As we see, [the] life of a monk or a [nun] is one of renunciation of family and children for spiritual progress. (2008)

Childlessness, as Bobra suggests, is frequently attributed to karma within Jain texts and described as a malady that cannot be cured by medicine or ritual. Phyllis Granoff explains that Jain and Buddhist texts rejected the ritual treatment of infertility, in part, as a response to Hindu stories that depicted sages and gods granting a child to a devotee (1998a, 252, fn. 60). Yet we do find instances in Jain literature when laypeople—especially kings and queens whose social duty involves producing an heir—benefit from reproductive assistance. In addition to the transfer of Mahāvīra's embryo, described above, the third chapter of the *Antakṛd-daśāḥ* describes the reproductive failures and miracles experienced by Queen Devakī and Lady Sulasā, including the transfer of six embryos by Hariṇegamesī and an extraordinary conception earned through the austerity of fasting (AD 3.8; Bauer 1998, 67; Kelting n.d. [a]).[47] However, it should be pointed out that these royal birth stories, including those of the Jinas, tend to result in a child forgoing the bonds of marriage and parenthood in order to pursue the path to liberation.

As indicated above, Jain medical manuals also suggest practices to assist one in conceiving. These include selecting the optimal time for sex (daily during cold weather or approximately weekly during warm weather; neither morning nor evening, nor during particular auspicious days), eating foods that will enhance virility (milk and related products, sugarcane and jaggery substances, and cold beverages), and womb ceremonies to ensure conception (Patil et al. 2015, 143–44).

Bobra further illuminates collateral costs within IVF that invite reflection on the social harms of the practice, beyond Jain-only concerns, including the exploitation of low-income egg donors or surrogate mothers who risk their bodies for financial stability, as well as sperm donors who may produce children they never know (2008).

Yet many Jain women still feel that childbearing is crucial to their identity. Kelting found that, among Jain women in Maharashtra, many feared infertility; children offer their mother emotional support, social status, and economic security in their later years (2009, 69–70). Within the context of Indian marriage, when wives may struggle to integrate into their husband's family home, a woman's first child—especially a son—"mark[s] their full participation in their husband's lineage" (70). Conversely, Manisha Sethi's research on Jain nuns revealed that many female renouncers valued their freedom from maternal roles (*vairāgya*) as "superior to and more fulfilling than anything that [lay]women were capable of achieving in marriage and family" (2012, 38–39).[48]

This tension of freedom-versus-family between Jain nuns and laywomen is unexpectedly illuminated by feminist ethicist Susan Sherwin when she challenges the supposition that IVF expands women's reproductive independence. Sherwin draws attention to social arrangements and cultural values that drive women to take on the burden and risks of IVF, including women's lack of access to meaningful jobs; a dearth of close friendships with men and women, which might necessitate intimacy with "one's own" child; and persistent views that childbearing is a woman's greatest purpose (2010, 548–49). Akin to the lay Jain view stated earlier—that the sexual restraint of *brahmacarya* may enable greater personal development—Sherwin emphasizes the ability of women to redefine their roles in society without dependence on expensive technologies and the norms of marriage, while opening other possibilities for personal growth and social satisfaction (551).

The majority of Jain medical professionals in our survey supported IVF and other ART. When asked, "Do you feel that individuals or couples who cannot conceive naturally can ethically use reproductive technologies such as in vitro fertilization (IVF), egg/sperm donation, or surrogate mothers? Choose all that apply," a majority of respondents replied "Yes" to IVF (69%, $n = 36$), egg donation (58%), sperm donation (58%), and surrogate mothers (53%). A minority believed that "none of the above" treatments is acceptable (17%), while others felt that adoption is a preferable option (22%) or had not considered it before (3%) (figure 8).

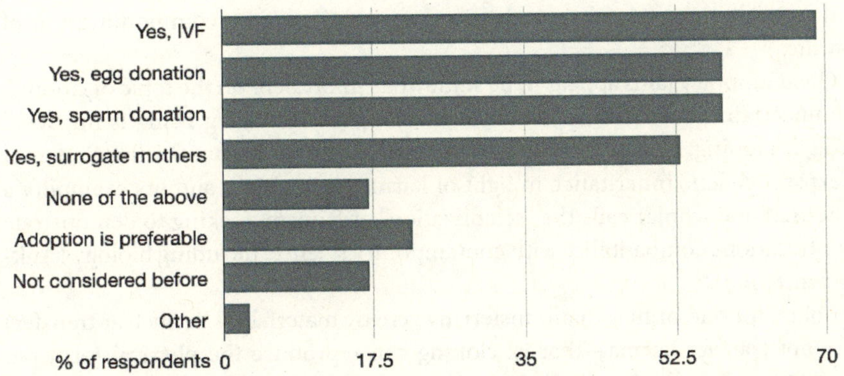


FIGURE 8. Responses of Jain medical professionals to the question "Do you feel that individuals or couples who cannot conceive naturally can ethically use reproductive technologies such as in vitro fertilization (IVF), egg/sperm donation, or surrogate mothers? Choose all that apply" ($n = 36$). Key: M = mother, C = child, A = abortion.

A relatively small number of respondents affirmed that the Jain tradition informed their view of ART, which suggests that this contemporary bioethical issue remains underexplored through a Jain lens (17%, $n = 36$).

### *Cloning*

After the 1996 cloning of a sheep named Dolly in Scotland, public fears erupted over the science-fiction potential of cloning human beings. Reproductive cloning of an entire organism requires transferring a DNA-containing nucleus from one cell into a second denucleated egg cell. This new cellular combination is then blasted with electricity so that it multiplies to become a blastocyst that is implanted into a surrogate's womb. The first cloning actually took place a century prior to Dolly when German biologist Hans Adolf Eduard Driesch successfully separated two-celled sea urchin embryos. Each cell grew into a complete sea urchin, demonstrating that embryonic cells contain full genetic instructions. Various cloning procedures advanced through the twentieth century with frogs, rabbits, and cows, among others. Dolly was the first animal to be successfully cloned from adult, rather than embryonic, cells.

Fears of cloning a human being have not been realized, and cloning animals is still a laborious and limited task. Researchers now say that Dolly's greatest contribution to science was the advancement of therapeutic cloning of DNA and cells, rather than organisms. For example, cloning is essential in embryonic stem cell research and in utilizing adult cells to generate "pluripotent" stem cells that can potentially produce any cell or tissue the body needs to repair itself (Weintraub 2016). Bioethical debates must differentiate between reproductive cloning of a whole organism and therapeutic cloning of DNA, cells, and embryos. Major topics of debate include creating embryos to be destroyed in research, health risks to mothers (whether human or nonhuman animals), the high rate of embryo and fetal loss, altering natural reproductive processes, and the commodification of new life.

Contemporary Jains appear to be somewhat ambivalent on the topic of cloning. The uncertainty seems to derive from what aspect of a living being is impacted through cloning, and/or how nuclear transfer impacts karma. In their attempt to explain genetic inheritance in light of karma, several Jain authors exemplify a trend that one scholar calls the "scientization" of Jainism, seeking to demonstrate their tradition's compatibility with contemporary science, including biology (Aukland 2016, 199).[49]

Bobra, for one, argues that transferring genetic material (as in nuclear transfer) does not transfer karma—that is, cloning can reproduce the physical form but cannot reproduce the karmic or luminous body that carries a *jīva*'s karmic history between rebirths (2008; see also chapter 2).[50] "A duplicate body does not make a duplicate person," he writes, maintaining that only the entrance of a *jīva* after fertilization can create a fully living being.

Conversely, Narayan Kachhara, a Jain mechanical engineer who has written extensively on Jainism and science, asserts that information from the karmic body may be transferred into a new life as part of DNA (2014, 39). Likewise, Sohan Raj Tater, in his book *The Jaina Doctrine of Karma and the Science of Genetics*, affirms that "karmas are [the] cause and genes are their effects," suggesting that transferring genetic material results in a karmic transfer as well (2009, 303). It is notable that Tater's book is prefaced with blessings from three Jain monks, each lauding the comparative study of karma and genetics (2009, viii–ix).

Survey responses among Jain medical professionals were split as to whether cloning represents a violation of Jain principles. A greater number of participants agreed that cloning living humans (44%, $n = 36$) and animals (46%, $n = 35$) constitutes a violation than agreed that cloning human and animal embryos (37%, $n = 35$) or cells (23%) does. Some respondents either did not know whether cloning is a violation of Jain principles (14–20%) or had not considered the issue before (9–14%), which suggests that cloning is an underexplored issue in Jain medical ethics. When participants were asked what Jain principles were violated in cloning, no uniquely Jain concepts were listed. However, we have cautiously inferred three different concerns, dividing the answers accordingly:

> "If a soul can enter into a cloned being, it is a different being."
> "A cloned embryo has a soul in it."

(1) The above answers suggest that the *theoretical* ability to reproduce a genetic copy is not inherently violent because a "copied" being remains a unique living being with a *jīva* of its own.

> "A 'live' adult cell is not a cell with a soul."
> ". . . cell [cloning is different] than cloning a person or animal life."

(2) These responses suggest that the genetic duplication of cells is either not a form of violence at all, or exacts less violence than reproducing a genetic copy of a living animal or human.

> "The embryo itself will have life and it is experimented on without that embryo having a choice."
>
> "The intention to make the copy is unethical."
>
> "[Cloning is] against the process of nature [and] can easily be used and abused."

(3) These comments suggest that the *practical* application of cloning constitutes a form of violence. This violence can occur at the level of intention, at the level of direct physical action that infringes upon the freedom of another being, or at the level of indirect violence caused by technology that overreaches the bounds of human activity, creating opportunities for injurious application.

### *Stem Cell Research*

Stem cells are the foundation for every organ and tissue in our bodies. The most common include embryonic stem cells that exist only during fetal development, and adult (or tissue) stem cells that emerge during fetal development and persist throughout our lifetime. Adult stem cells, such as skin cells, are tissue specific. Embryonic stem cells are considered "pluripotent" because they can potentially produce any cell or tissue the body needs to repair itself. These cells were first isolated in mice in 1981 and in primates in 1995; human embryonic stem cells were isolated in 1998 at the University of Wisconsin.

This advancement was controversial, however, because research teams derived their stem cells from the tissue of aborted fetuses and from embryos left over from IVF treatments. US stem cell research, then, has been closely related both to the legalization of abortion (in the 1973 *Roe v. Wade* decision) and to the development of IVF technology. Since 1998, more than a thousand different "lines" of self-renewing embryonic stem cells have been created and shared by researchers worldwide. These cells can be used to repair damaged tissue, replace cells associated with chronic diseases, and generate cells for bone and tissue transplants (Löser et al. 2010).

The debate over embryonic stem cell use centers on disagreements regarding the moral value of a human embryo. Many countries have enacted legislation prohibiting the creation of embryos for research while allowing use of already-existing embryos discarded from fertility treatments. In 2001, President George W. Bush affirmed earlier US legislative efforts to protect embryos by prohibiting federal funding of research utilizing embryonic stem cells derived after August of that year. Although this law did not affect private or state-funded programs, it did inhibit overall US research. In 2008, President Barack Obama expanded federal funding for embryonic cells so long as they were derived from IVF with consent from the donor families. Today, the countries with the most active embryonic stem cell programs include Japan, Singapore, China, South Korea, Australia, South Africa, the United Kingdom, Switzerland, Brazil, Mexico, and the United States (Dhar and Ho 2009).

Beyond the connection to abortion and IVF, embryonic stem cell advances are indebted to genetic cloning research. In the 1960s, John Gurdon's work on nucleus transfer showed that already-specialized tadpole cells inserted into the nucleus of an egg cell could still produce a complete living frog (Maayan and Cohmer 2012). These cells had been "reprogrammed" from specialized cells to pluripotent cells. Building on Gurdon's work and the successful cloning of Dolly the sheep in 1996, Japanese scientist Shinya Yamanaka published papers in 2006 and 2007 identifying four genetic factors in transforming specialized cells into an embryonic stem cell-like state, called "induced pluripotent stem cells," first in mice, then in humans (Philbrick 2011). Induced pluripotent stem cells are one of the most significant contributions derived from cloning research because the process creates embryonic cells without destroying embryos, thus sidestepping many of the earlier moral concerns.

A Jain approach to stem cell research appears to be conflicted. On one hand, embryos are considered living five-sensed human beings; injuring them interrupts their path of existence and brings negative karma to oneself. On the other hand, many lay Jains accept that certain forms of social progress may require some harm. In his sociological analysis of the Jain community, Vilas Sangave explains this tension succinctly: "Though [violence] is unavoidable in the sustenance of life, Jainism . . . tries to limit it for essential purposes only" (1997, 168). It bears restating here that "essential" activities for a mendicant are quite different from those for a lay Jain. Padmanabh Jaini highlights that any efforts "to improve the quality of life of one segment of society must be weighed against its negative impact on other humans, as well as on animals, plants, earth, water, and air" (2002, 151). In his brief examination of engineered biology in the Jain tradition, Chapple draws particular attention to the suffering of animals who are produced, often through cloning-related procedures, to carry disease and endure painful tests and death for research purposes, which most Jains would see as high-level karmic violations of five-sensed beings (2013, 86; see chapter 6).

Respondents in our survey felt that induced pluripotent embryonic stem cells pose a slightly lesser violation of Jain principles than cells sourced from embryos. Although the status of stem cells is unclear in Jainism (as discussed above), most respondents did not see a violation (figure 9).

Those who elaborated on the Jain principles violated in stem cell research described altering the formation of life "for a few selfish reasons," that "cloning a higher order organism is violence," and that cells should be used from dead embryos only. Another candidly states, "I'm not sure if [the] Jain tradition has

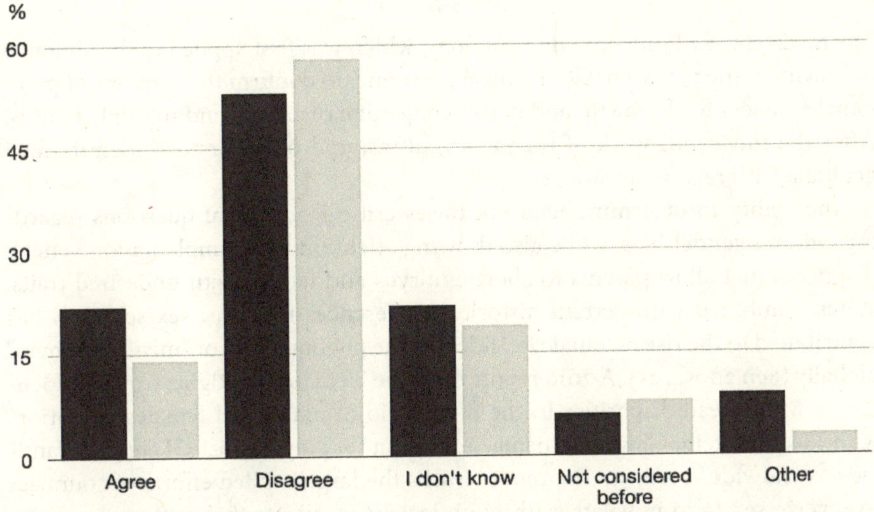


FIGURE 9. Responses of Jain medical professionals ($n = 36$) to the statements "Pluripotent stem cells can develop into a variety of adult cells such as tissue or organs. I consider research on pluripotent stem cells derived from embryos a violation of Jain principles" (black bars); and "Some adult cells can be 'reprogrammed' to be pluripotent stem cells. A normal skin cell, for example, can be 'reprogrammed' into a pluripotent cell. I consider research on 'reprogrammed' pluripotent stem cells to be a violation of Jain principles" (gray bars).

a position on this issue." In an online forum, Jain physician Mitul Mehta, who describes himself as "an imperfect follower" of the tradition, acknowledges that Jain mendicants would likely not support embryonic stem cell research but that the Jain doctrine of *anekānta-vāda* compels him to consider "millions of people's lives that can be saved/improved by deriving a single immortal cell line" (2015). Even though Mehta himself does not personally conduct research on stem cells—and implies he would not be comfortable doing so—he offers support for those who do. In this distinction, Mehta implicitly acknowledges his indirect approval of, though not an active participation in, stem cell research that would have significant health benefits for higher-sensed beings. He also stresses the utilization of *one* stem cell line—rather than proliferating multiple lines—to seek the proposed benefit.

## ALTERING NASCENT LIFE: JAIN VIEWS ON SEX SELECTION AND GENOME EDITING

In the realm of facilitating nascent life, what alterations, if any, are ethically viable from a Jain perspective? In this section, we examine practices and preferences that influence fetal characteristics, including sex selection and genome editing.

### *Sex Selection*

The medical use of ultrasound technology, which was first applied to the abdominal cavity in the 1950s, enables medical personnel to confirm the progress of pregnancies, assess fetal growth, and detect congenital disorders and multiple fetuses. After the thirteenth week of pregnancy, ultrasound operators can identify fetal genitalia with relative accuracy.

The ability to determine fetal sex raises critical bioethical questions regarding cultural gender bias, while also drawing attention to preimplantation genetic diagnoses that allow parents to abort embryos and fetuses with undesired traits. When combined with certain historical preferences for sons, sex-selection has contributed to the rise of female feticide and the phenomenon of "missing women" globally (Sen 2005, 225). A 2016 report from the UN Human Rights Council documents widespread disparities in the birth ratio of males and females by nation, with Liechtenstein, China, Armenia, and India topping the list ("Female Infanticide Worldwide" 2016, 3). The report tracks the largely failed efforts of countries to reverse sex ratio imbalances through legislative efforts that outlaw sex detection and/or incentivize female birth. It also tracks the rise of "reproductive tourism" in countries where sex detection is legal, such as Thailand. There, parents can utilize IVF technologies along with related preimplantation genetic diagnosis, preimplantation genetic screening, and sperm sorting for the additional purpose of sex selection.

In India, preference for male children has a long history. A well-known Vedic wedding blessing exhorts the new bride to "be the mother of a hundred sons" (Iyer 2002, 41). The classical Hindu law book *Manu-smṛti* offers mixed views of a woman's role in society (*strī-dharma*), but concludes that she can never live independently of the control of her father, husband, or son (MS 5.147–50).

Various cultural practices also value gender differently. The continued practice of dowry (*yautaka*), or the price families pay for their daughters to marry, though outlawed in India in 1961, makes females a financial liability.[51] Sons, on the other hand, may improve their mother's social and home-life status and increase parents' financial security in their later years. One study suggests that women's stated son preference is primarily due to financial concerns (Robitaille 2013).[52]

The Indian census has shown a significant gap between male and female children (0–6 years old) for the past hundred years, in spite of contemporary legislative efforts to outlaw sex-selective abortion or feticide ("Sex Ratio of India and Madhya Pradesh 1901–2011" 2011). Although the Indian government enacted the Pre-Conception and Pre-Natal Diagnostic Techniques Act of 1994, which regulates the sale and use of ultrasound machines, it later had to pass additional amendments to enforce this law as birth ratios continued to decline (Tabaie 2017).

The 2011 Census of India shows 940 females per 1,000 males nationwide; these differentials vary throughout the country, with the north having a greater absence of females and parts of south India having a largely equal gender ratio

(Diamond-Smith et al. 2008, 697; Klaus and Tipandjan 2015). The International Center for Research on Women (ICRW) concluded in their 2006 report on India that preference for sons was widespread but not universal. Among several findings, the ICRW concluded that wealth did not reduce son preference, but education level and access to media did result in a meaningful reduction in male child bias (Pande and Malhotra 2006, 5–6). In recent headlines, the 2017–18 Economic Survey published by the government of India reports twenty-one million "unwanted" females 0–25 years old, referring not only to sex-selective abortions, but also to girls who, according to the National Family Health Survey, "disappear" because of disease, neglect, or inadequate nutrition (Ministry of Finance 2018, 112).

Indian diaspora communities are not immune to this gender gap. Abrevaya (2008) shows that, even in the United States, Chinese and Indian girls are more likely than others to be sex-selectively aborted; the author estimates 2,000 missing girls in the United States between 1991 and 2004.

*Gender Disparity in Jainism.* Jain communities also show an imbalance in their gender ratios, with an average of 954 females per 1,000 males compared to 939 per 1,000 among Hindus, as reported in the 2011 Census of India (Bajaj 2016, 4). In states with large Jain populations, Jains have better ratios of females than neighboring Hindu communities—Gujarat (966 Jain/916 Hindu), Maharashtra (964/928), and Delhi (942/865)—with the exception of Chhattisgarh (947/990) and Karnataka (952/972). Jains have a significant disparity in Haryana, with only 895 females per 1,000 males. The reality of sex preference among Jains confronts us with a tradition that has, since its earliest texts, affirmed a fourfold community of monks, nuns, laymen, and laywomen, in which nuns have continuously outnumbered monks (Sethi 2012, 4; KS 5.132–45). Historically, women could marry, enter ascetic life, or remain single, pursuing education through any of these avenues (Sangave 2001, 147–50).

Yet gender disparity also exists in the textual sources and in modern practice. N. Shāntā's comprehensive treatise on Jain nuns, titled *The Unknown Pilgrims* (1997), and Padmanabh Jaini's landmark text *Gender and Salvation* (1991a) both detail historical debates over the ability of female nuns to achieve liberation. The Digambara position rejects the possibility of women's liberation, given bodily limitations such as menstruation, physical frailty that prevents austerities, psychological instability, and the prohibition of female nudity in society that is required for ultimate detachment from material goods (Balbir 1994b; Jaini 1991a; Shāntā 1997, 640–53). While Śvetāmbara mendicants disputed these assertions at length within historical debates, being born female was still considered inauspicious, and they concurred with their Digambara counterparts that once one has achieved the right worldview (see chapter 3), one will never again be born female (Jaini 2010c, 178–79). The Śvetāmbaras also assert that the nineteenth Jina, Mallī, was female—which the Digambaras deny—but her being born female is understood to be an extraordinary event (*āścarya*), and Mallī's rebirth as a woman is attributed to deceit, as the tradition holds for all women and "third sex" individuals (Jaini 2010c, 179–80; Zwilling and Sweet 1996).

Jain medical literature aligns with other Indian medical treatises on the various causes of a child's sex, such as the relative ratio of maternal and paternal fluids, the embryo's karma, and the position in the womb, as noted above. Rahul Peter Das describes cultural rituals to reverse the sex of a child in the womb (*vivartana*), especially the *puṃsavana* rite to ensure the birth of a son (2003, 4, fn. 7).[53] Although Jain texts do not mention this specific ritual, the *Kalyāṇa-kāraka* advises the mother to lie on her right side for a male baby and on her left side for a female, as already mentioned (KK 2.43).

Contemporary Jain practices regarding gender remain complex. Several Jain studies scholars, perplexed by the prevalence of Jain nuns within a tradition that privileges male asceticism, have conducted studies of nuns who persist in finding creative outlets for personal growth, higher education, and community leadership (Fohr 2006; Sethi 2012; Shāntā 1997; Vallely 2002a). Laywomen are seen as indispensable transmitters of the tradition—perpetuating recitations, songs, mantras (Kelting 2001), Jain education of children, and family fasts (Kelting 2009). Nevertheless, Digambara women are prevented from performing *pūjā* on the temple statues of Jinas, and menstruating women of all sects are often discouraged from entering the temple.[54]

Simultaneously, there are efforts to resist gender bias from within the Jain community. Three examples follow. In the first, Pravin Shah, the long-standing chair of the JAINA Educational Committee, released a 2017 summary of temple education in the United States. He named several unique features of the diaspora context, such as gender parity, that require alterations in Jain teachings. He stated that "Jain children have grown up in American culture where . . . [b]oth men and women are treated equally. Jain religious principles are not and should not be male dominated . . . [although] [s]everal of our [current] rituals are male dominated rituals" (2017).

The second example comes from Ācārya Candanā, a contemporary Jain Sthānakavāsī nun and *ācārya* who cofounded the nonprofit organization Veerayatan in 1973 to make the Jain tradition accessible for global Jains by emphasizing service, education, and personal development. Veerayatan now has programs in the United Kingdom, Kenya, Dubai, Nepal, and the United States. In an imaginative book titled *Walk with Me* (2009), Ācārya Candanā recreates canonical dialogues between Mahāvīra and his chief disciple Indrabhūti Gautama, with her own voice substituting for Gautama's. In the chapter concerning women's liberation, Gautama is disturbed that Mahāvīra has ordained a female mendicant by the name of Candanā.[55] After reflecting on the resiliency with which Candanā has met the obstacles of her life, Gautama concludes:

> [T]here was a time when I too was a strong believer in the superiority of men, but the bold step taken by Mahāvīra to ordain women like [Candanā] made me believe that our mothers, sisters, and daughters are no less! In the future, whenever men,

> in their ignorance and arrogance, try to oppress women, I am sure that [Candanā] will inspire women of the world to assert and trust themselves. (Chandanaji and Parikh 2009, 48)

The final example comes from Ācārya Mahāprajña (1920–2010), the tenth mendicant leader of the Śvetāmbara Terāpanthīs, who strongly condemns the practice of dowry in his book *The Happy and Harmonious Family* (2008). Ācārya Mahāprajña connects violence toward women and girls to an unchecked desire for wealth and status through dowry. "The notion that all these [material desires] will be fulfilled by dowry . . . has raised the value of commodities and has devalued women" (Mahāprajña 2008, 232). He suggests a "revolution" by exhorting Jains to consider new vows that reestablish marriage as a dowry-free institution (235).

In our survey of Jain medical professionals, the overwhelming majority believed that prenatal testing for the purpose of sex selection violates Jain principles (83%, $n = 36$). Among the participants who chose "Other," one explained, "I do not agree with sex-selective abortion, but [that disagreement] has nothing to do with my Jain principles." Two others described the Jain principles they felt were violated, stating: (1) "Of course it is against the Jain principles to kill a life no matter what the reason" and (2) "Any abortion is a violation of Jain principles." Recall from our survey analysis on abortion that no respondents felt that abortion can be justified when a child is an undesired gender (0%).

Although this response makes a strong statement against sex-selective abortion, modern gender selection often transpires through indirect means such as preimplantation diagnoses and IVF "selection," as well as gamete/zygote intrafallopian transfer. As Vibhuti Patel argues in his study of sex determination methods in India, these reproductive technologies enable some couples, including Jains, to ensure a male child, seemingly without direct abortion; rather, embryos are "selectively transferred" (2014, 243). Similarly, Sulekh Jain, an influential Jain layman in the United States, recently discussed the practice of sex selection among Jains in his book *An Ahimsa Crisis: You Decide* (2016). Intended as an invitation for the global Jain lay community to reassess cultural attitudes that have tempered the full impact of the Jain doctrine of nonviolence, the book draws special attention to Jain physicians who provide sex-selective services, lamenting that the community has remained largely silent on these practices (188–89).

Although there is evidence of gender bias against females in Jainism—within the textual tradition, in mendicant practice, and in the population disparities of certain Indian states—there is also strong resistance to sex screening among the Jain medical professionals we surveyed, and significant social statements directed against the discrimination of women and in favor of gender equality.

### *Genome Editing*

Genome editing emerged, in part, from developments in IVF and cloning technologies, and it shares many of the same bioethical concerns. In IVF, when an embryo reaches the blastocyst stages around day five, researchers can make a preimplantation genetic diagnosis of up to two thousand gene disorders—including cystic fibrosis and sickle cell anemia, among others—to ensure the implantation of a disease-free embryo, and preimplantation genetic screening to ensure that the embryo contains the standard forty-six chromosomes. After genetic anomalies have been identified, gene editing technology permits scientists to delete, modify, or replace a damaged portion of an organism's genome. The term *genome* refers to a complete set of an organism's genetic sequence. In humans, a copy of the entire genome is contained in the nucleus of each cell.

Early gene editing in the 1970s through 1990s involved isolating individual genes to evaluate how a change in that particular section of DNA (genotype) resulted in a change within the organism (phenotype). For example, scientists replaced the normal genotype of a white-fur mouse with a mutated gene that resulted in a creature being born with the phenotype of black fur. This process helped determine gene function in mammals, and also established a reliable way to model human diseases in mice. The ability to target genes to change the color of a mouse's fur, however, makes it clear that genome editing can be used for *therapeutic* purposes, that is, to target genes associated with illness and disease; and for *nontherapeutic* purposes, targeting genes associated with fur color or other desirable physical traits. During this early period of research, two additional gene editing tools emerged using enzymes called nucleases to cut the bonds between the nucleotides that make up strands of DNA and RNA. These tools, called zinc finger proteins (ZnFs) and transcription activator-like effector nucleases (TALENs), expanded gene editing beyond mice embryonic stem cells to rats, fruit flies, zebrafish, butterflies, and livestock, among others.

Recently a new gene editing technique has harnessed bacteria and enzymes to achieve the goals of ZnFs and TALENs faster, cheaper, and more accurately. CRISPR (clustered regularly interspaced short palindromic repeats)—also called Cas (CRISPR-associated) proteins—uses the immune system of bacteria to remember DNA segments from viruses. These bacteria then create an RNA "guide" that activates the next time the virus appears, directing an enzyme to cut the DNA at a precise location, which deactivates the virus. Throughout 2017, CRISPR/Cas technology was used in animal models to remove HIV and target the "master" genes in cancer that cause tumor growth; it was also used to limit fertility in disease-carrying mosquitos and to engineer fast-growing algae for biofuel production (Dean 2017).

Chinese teams have already begun using CRISPR/Cas techniques to alter disease-causing genes in human embryos, and work is under way in the United Kingdom and Sweden to study early embryonic development and miscarriage (Ledford 2017). In December 2018, Chinese scientist He Jiankui shocked the global research community by announcing he had successfully created the world's first "CRISPR babies," twin girls born through IVF. Jiankui claimed to have altered the genomes related to HIV transmission using CRISPR methods, and was subsequently fined and sentenced to three years in prison by the Chinese government; two of his collaborators were likewise fined and given lesser sentences (Normile 2019).

Many in the scientific community urge caution with CRISPR application, especially to germline, or reproductive, cells such as egg or sperm that will be incorporated into the DNA of every cell in the offspring's body in perpetuity (Kang et al. 2016). Even the scientist who pioneered CRISPR gene editing, Jennifer Doudna, has called for a pause in editing heritable genes until scientists, doctors, and the public have a better understanding of the ramifications of altering an entire line of descendants, and she has urged the development of standardized guidelines for what is ethically acceptable in genome research (2015). One of the persistent concerns with CRISPR technology is that the same methods currently in use for disease intervention can also be used for nontherapeutic embryonic enhancements related to an offspring's physical stature, memory, athleticism, sex, or hair/eye color, potentially creating, according to ethicist Michael J. Sandel, a socially sanctioned form of "liberal eugenics" (2012, 101).

While Jain texts propose various factors as causes of illnesses, as explained in chapter 4 and mentioned with regard to the health of the embryo above, the underlying cause of one's present bodily condition is karma. Karma affects the longevity of living beings as well as their specific birth forms with various disabilities and dysfunctions (see chapter 2). As discussed in chapters 4 and 6, the earliest Jain canonical texts implored mendicants to accept their afflictions without seeking treatment in order to exhaust their karmic debt, with an understanding that physical maladies are part of the suffering of *saṃsāra* that must be worked through to release karma. At the same time, the practice of curing illness gradually developed within the Jain mendicant community and became prevalent by the medieval period, as detailed in chapter 4. As noted there, Granoff explored Jain healing practices and identified a shift from seeing disease as a "natural" karmic effect that one had to live out, to mendicants seeking physicians' services and even themselves providing medical care for fellow monks and nuns (1998b, 286–87). Although these examples of medicinal therapies are not aimed at the genetic level, they offer a precedent for resisting disease with compassion, knowledge, and skill.

Consequently, we are left with an ambiguous relation between the roles of karma and biological genetics in understanding human health. If, as Tater asserts above in relation to cloning, "karmas are [the] cause and genes are their effect" (2009, 303), what happens when genes are deleted, modified, or replaced through editing techniques? Gene editing also challenges the Jain concept of *paryāpta/aparyāpta* (described in relation to fetal development above and in chapter 2). Are geneticists interrupting the karma of an *aparyāpta* being by removing a dysfunctional gene to permit its successful development?

Some contemporary Jains attempt to address the ambiguous relation between genes and karma in creative ways. In a recent analysis, Kachhara and colleagues correlate genetic inheritance with nondestructive karma responsible for embodiment, rather than destructive karma that affects the *jīva* (Kachhara et al. 2017, 133–34). Specifically, the authors state that genes—and, thus, gene editing—impact name-determining karma (*nāma-karman*) and status-determining karma (*gotra-karman*) (133–34).[56] It is not clear whether this version of gene editing—as only affecting embodiment—would be acceptable to other Jains.

Further, there are many strong statements regarding preventative health among contemporary Jains. Ācārya Tulsī, for instance, describes three aspects of protecting health, namely: (1) following lifestyle choices to aid in disease prevention; (2) trying to regain health with the help of natural means if an illness does come, due to negligence or certain conditions; and (3) taking the help of an experienced physician if the need arises (1998, 134). These three suggestions are geared toward healthcare after birth, rather than altering the genome before implantation. Although this view affirms various paths to health, Ācārya Tulsī privileges self-administered efforts in wellness, both preventative and therapeutic, seeking the help of a physician only if needed. Ācārya Mahāprajña also emphasizes the continual responsibility one has to maintain their own health, beyond inherited genes. In his book *Lord Mahavira's Scripture of Health* (2001), Ācārya Mahāprajña describes the various *paryāptis*—calling them "bio-potentials"—as *ongoing* foundations for life and health (2001, 42–52). "*[P]aryaptis* are our vitalities," he writes. "Health is very closely related to them . . . [O]nly when the power of resistance against diseases is linked not only with just one system but with all the [*paryāptis*], would it be possible to maintain health" (Mahāprajña 2001, 45). Since these "bio-potentials" require attentive upkeep beyond the womb, could one infer that gene editing may be permitted so long as it is accompanied by responsible care of one's body after birth? Or is preventative care the preferred mode to deal with inherited health ailments?

Without providing clear guidance as to a Jain lay view of genome editing, Bobra maintains that beneficial medicine, including gene editing, must be balanced with personal restraint. He says that "Jainism believes in preserving health of [the] physical and mental body in order to pursue spiritual progress while keeping the principle of nonviolence in the forefront" (2008). In other words, karmic advancement requires a healthy body, but achieving that health through harming of others ultimately undermines spiritual progress. Bobra seems to tentatively accept gene editing *if* its effects enable one to more effectively pursue the Jain path, and *if* the harm to other beings is negligible. He also sees gene editing as possibly a technology that could reduce current levels of medical research conducted upon humans and animals. Still, he warns against the possible abuse of gene editing technology for financial gain, and rejects genomic editing for the purpose of enhancement, which "could become an exclusive right of the rich" (2008).

Only a small percentage of the Jain medical professionals in our survey felt that gene editing for therapeutic purposes constitutes a violation of Jain principles when done to an animal's genome (11%, $n = 36$) or a human genome (8%, $n = 36$), meaning that most did not see a violation (figure 10). In fact, a greater number

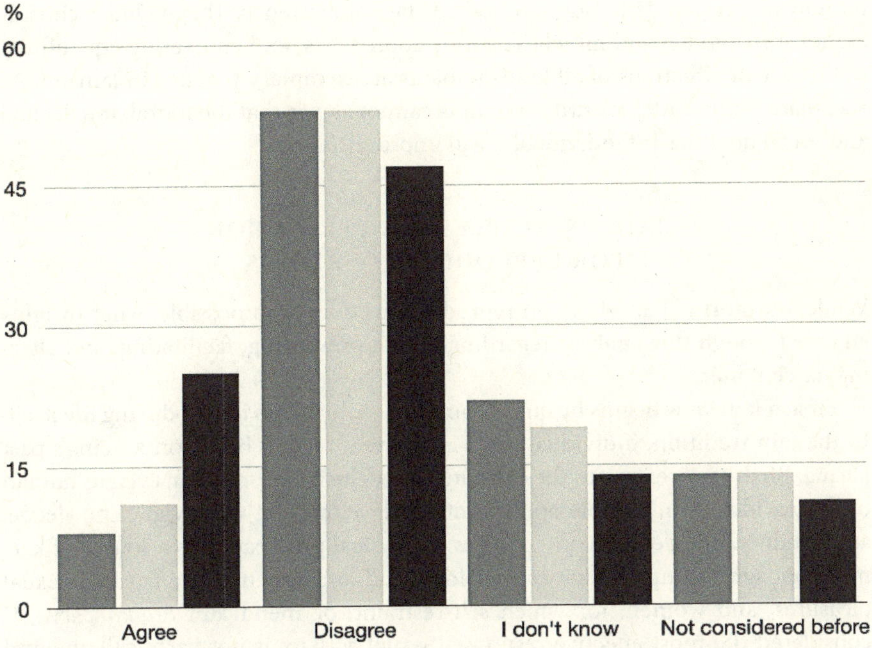


FIGURE 10. Responses of Jain medical professionals ($n = 36$) to the statements "I consider gene therapy (the ability to identify and change the *human* genome for therapeutic purposes, rather than desired traits) a violation of Jain principles" (dark gray bars); "I consider gene therapy (the ability to identify and change the *animal* genome for therapeutic purposes, rather than desired traits) a violation of Jain principles" (light gray bars); and "I consider genetically modified foods a violation of Jain principles" (black bars).

of participants felt that genetically modifying food violated Jain principles (24%, $n = 37$).

These survey responses suggest that Jain medical professionals might accept the benefits of gene editing technologies that target genes responsible for disease. When viewed in concert with the above views, however, we see a more complex network of issues, including the value of self-administered care rather than external intervention, a recognition that health (and, thus, gene editing) is primarily to enable one's karmic advancement, and the possible benefits of gene editing for humans and animals as well as its potential to be abused.

While Bobra points out that gene editing could relieve unnecessary medical testing on vulnerable populations, current genomic research requires the ubiquitous use of animal models, which necessitates the institutionalization of animal breeding, injury, and death, which many Jains reject (see chapter 6). Additionally, gene editing is already being used to alter animal and plant genes for industrial food production as well as transgenic applications for organ or cell transplants. It is likely that Jain attitudes to gene editing may change depending on the application. Regardless of one's genes, contemporary Jains place a great deal of emphasis on how one responds to one's embodied state of existence. This includes considerations that go beyond merely scientific approaches, and cultivating equanimity in the face of afflictions of all kinds remains an exemplary practice in Jainism. As Kachhara points out, "scientific attempts cannot assure that the moral, intellectual and social qualities [of individuals] will improve" (2005).

## JAIN PRINCIPLES OF APPLICATION FOR REPRODUCTIVE ETHICS

While a uniform "Jain view" on reproductive ethics is impossible, what insights emerge through this analysis regarding taking/preventing, facilitating, and altering nascent life?

First, a Jain view begins by questioning the motivations for producing life itself. In the Jain tradition, individual birth is always a *re*birth based on a being's past karma. Birth exposes one to the suffering and delusion of *saṃsāra*, even as human birth provides an invaluable opportunity to develop right worldview, knowledge, and conduct. The decision and process of physical procreation is a source of karmic bondage through activities, passions, and attachments to offspring, sexual pleasures, and women, for which self-restraint, or mendicant *brahmacarya*, is considered the most effective response. Sexual activity is not karmically neutral in the Jain view, insofar as living beings may be injured through intercourse and many possible progeny may fail to implant. Even lay Jains recognize that sex, marriage, and family can inhibit an individual's development, which suggests that the restraint of *brahmacarya* may offer a strategic, if temporary, abstention from sexual relations that supports personal and spiritual growth. In the face of infertility, for example, some Jains may pursue ART options, such as IVF, while others see infertility as a valuable limit that provides opportunities to adopt existing children, or to remain childless and increase one's karmic advancement.

At the same time, the period of gestation can produce a powerful bond between mother and fetus capable of nurturing an inclination toward spiritual advancement, and can satisfy social norms of lay life, norms that most lay Jains do not seriously challenge. Although all individuals are reborn due to their own varieties of karma—ideally into a mother's womb, family, and environment that are conducive to karmic progress—the ultimate goal in Jainism is to not be reborn at all.

Second, injuring nascent life is considered a serious act of violence comprising various components of body, speech, and mind and resulting in inauspicious forms of karmic bondage. Modern Jains, including surveyed medical professionals, frequently describe killing nascent life—whether through abortion, IVF, cloning, or stem cell research—as requiring a mental component of planning, a verbal component of requesting or directing, and a physical component of doing or causing another to provide relevant procedures, thus magnifying the karmic repercussions. The valuation of the destruction of a nascent human life as representing a high-level karmic violation is based not on modern bioethical markers of life's beginning, personhood, or stage of pregnancy, but on the belief that an individual *jīva*'s karmic path is significantly advanced to warrant rebirth as a five-sensed human being.

Third, in light of these consequences, the primary vow of nonviolence is a guiding principle in Jain reproductive ethics. However, nonviolence does not function as a flat prohibition of all violence. In the case of abortion, for instance, Jain medical professionals measure the violence of abortion alongside related harms, such as death of the mother or future suffering of a child. To a lesser extent, some lay Jains also consider the relational context of a mother's emotional or financial well-being as a possible justification for abortion. In the case of stem cells, cloning, and gene editing, lay Jains seem to accept the destruction, manipulation, or duplication of cells if that harm can benefit five-sensed humans and animals, though destruction of fully developed living beings for the same purpose is less tenable.

Fourth, collateral costs are factored into the violence of an action. The Jain views cited above frequently identify unintended costs within reproductive issues. For instance, abortion may involve the direct and indirect approval or participation of medical professionals, family, or community members. Procreating exacts a cost upon other planetary lives in society and the environment, and these costs should be considered prior to reproduction. IVF raises concerns of justice for low-income egg/sperm donors and gender equality, creates excess embryos, and can lead to pregnancy complications such as multi-fetal implantation and selective reduction.

Some lay Jains, commenting on stem cell research, cloning, or gene editing, suggest limiting research to essential therapeutic benefits only and also limiting the numbers of beings involved in such research (e.g., utilizing only one stem cell line rather than many). The proactive pursuit of self-administered preventative care, as well as the high value placed on enduring afflictions, may also restrain the need for one to utilize treatments derived from stem cell research or gene editing technologies.

Fifth, women are largely considered valuable and educated members of society, though their treatment differs across texts, time, geography, and role in either a mendicant or lay community. Traditional mendicant manuals present women as sources of attachment to avoid, even as they are the vital progenitors of Jinas and other illumined Jain figures. In the modern period, Jain women have the highest degrees of literacy in India, regularly pursue education through the lay or mendicant path, and have low reproductive rates. Although women exist within wider social-cultural expectations, there are efforts with the Jain community as a whole to challenge certain contemporary aspects of gender inequity.

In considering these multifaceted Jain views, mendicant perspectives often emphasize a paramount ideal of restraint, even if it cannot be practiced fully, while other Jains—including intermediate mendicants, medical professionals, and lay Jains living outside of India—strive to interpret Jain principles in new contexts for which there is often neither textual guidance nor historical precedent, requiring flexible practice. The lack of a unified outlook or prescriptive paradigm, however, does not mean that the Jain tradition has no contributions to make toward these issues. On the contrary, the preliminary Jain principles of application outlined here offer a productive starting point for engaging the complex issues of reproductive ethics through the values of an equally complex tradition.

# 6

# Wages of Life

Medical care is a part of lived experience addressed by Jains throughout antiquity up to the present. In chapter 4, we detailed evolving textual views of medicine, highlighting an early duty to care that became increasingly regulated and manifested in the changing attitudes toward medical treatment, growing medical knowledge among mendicants, and emerging guidelines for seeking medical care from laypeople. By the medieval period, Jain mendicants had created their own formal medical manuals that contributed to the wider literary traditions of Indian medicine.

How might the perspectives of modern Jains resonate with or diverge from these evolving textual accounts? And what, if any, Jain insights might inform an engagement with modern bioethical issues that emerge during the course of life? In this chapter, we examine key bioethical concepts in the physician-patient relationship, including nonmaleficence, beneficence, autonomy, and truth. We also explore contemporary Jain views on the causes of illness, and ethical attitudes toward vaccinations and antibiotic use, surgery and human dissection, and research trials and access to care.

Concurrent with these issues, we investigate how contemporary Jain medical professionals maintain their Jain identity alongside competing values of medicine, science, and society, and we pay special attention to Jain views on animals used for food and biomedical studies. We conclude with a list of seven provisional principles of application for considering ethical issues in standard medical care during one's lifetime.

## THE PHYSICIAN-PATIENT RELATIONSHIP

As noted in chapter 3, Śvetāmbara texts on lay conduct from the sixteenth century onward generally refer to medicine (*vidyā*) as one of seven acceptable occupations (*upāya*) that can be practiced with lesser or greater degrees of purity (Williams

1963, 121–22).[1] But how do lay Jain medical professionals understand the vocation of medicine today? To start, we will examine Jain approaches to key bioethical terms that guide physician-patient relationships, such as *nonmaleficence, beneficence, autonomy*, and *truth*.

### *Considering Nonviolence and Compassion alongside Nonmaleficence and Beneficence*

Survey respondents understood medicine to be a less violent career according to their tradition, but also a way to offer positive care. When asked to choose the influences on their decision to pursue a medical career, the strongest responses included "My personal desire to help people" (42%, $n = 36$), "The tradition of Jains taking careers that are not overtly violent" (36%), "My personal desire to help people, informed by Jain values" (36%), and "My Jain parents, grandparents, or elders because of their commitments to Jain values" (17%).

The tension between avoiding violence and positive acts of care is reflected in the contemporary bioethical terms *nonmaleficence* and *beneficence. Nonmaleficence* refers to not harming others, or inflicting the least harm possible. This principle acknowledges that we can make the lives of other beings worse, and so we should, as stated in later versions of the Hippocratic Oath, "first, do no harm (*primum non nocere*)." Beneficence is a positive action to promote the welfare of other beings, based on the recognition that we can sometimes make the lives of other beings better.

Although Jain texts do not use these same terms, in chapter 3 we examined the role of nonviolence in Jainism in relation to both restraining action and positive acts of compassion. The relation between these two approaches is complex. For instance, if "compassion" signifies passion-filled attachment to social relationships, its exercise could be at odds with the ultimate aims of mendicant life to restrain such bonds. If "compassion" describes a critical insight that each embodied being is vulnerable to pain, violence, and destruction, its exercise may be a positive sign of attaining the right worldview.

The fact that survey respondents identified helping others as a primary motivation for their occupational path, even above medicine's designation as a less violent occupation, suggests that Jain medical professionals understand compassion to be a positive virtue for laypeople. Likewise, when asked, "As a patient, which do you value more?," a slight majority of respondents chose "A doctor who emphasizes compassionate communication over medical expertise" (36%, $n = 36$) than chose the reverse answer, "A doctor who emphasizes medical expertise over compassionate communication" (31%). A small group were unsure (14%), and another portion chose "Other" (19%), all of whom described a desire for both qualities equally. The positive assessment of compassion in these responses may signify a modern medical disposition among Jains that privileges beneficence over nonmaleficence.

*Entangled Autonomy*

The term *autonomy* was established as one of four principles of biomedical ethics by Tom Beauchamp and James Childress in their 1979 landmark text, *Principles of Biomedica*, along with nonmaleficence, beneficence, and justice. In bioethics, autonomy is often defined as self-governance, or the decision-making capacity to exercise one's values and path of life, especially pertaining to healthcare privacy and informed consent to accept or reject certain treatments or procedures. In practice, however, autonomy is more complex.

Some bioethicists interpret autonomy merely as freedom from external interference, which can overlook the need to respect mutual autonomy on both sides of the physician-patient relationship (Stirrat and Gill 2005). Others instrumentalize autonomy as the tool by which one ensures one's own well-being, an interpretation that can overlook how one might make an autonomous choice seemingly against one's own well-being, such as refusing life-sustaining treatment (Varelius 2006). Childress refined his own concept of autonomy to an act of ensuring the "conditions of autonomous choice" (1990, 12) by facilitating four criteria of decision-making capacity whereby an individual (1) *understands* information; (2) *appreciates* the relevance of information, including risks or benefits, to their own situation; (3) *reasons* in light of their own values, free of internal and external constraints; and (4) *communicates* a choice (Palmer and Harmell 2016).

Confronted with this snapshot of debates over the meaning and application of autonomy in bioethical contexts, what, if anything, might Jainism contribute to the concept of self-governance? As a tradition that emphasizes the karmic consequences of bodily, verbal, and mental conduct of self-governing *jīva*s, Jainism places a high value on individual freedom within a matrix of causal relations. Although the specific term *autonomy* does not appear in traditional Jain texts, some modern Jains have attempted to explain the concept through a Jain lens. In the well-known diaspora book *Jain Way of Life* (2007), Yogendra Jain—a US-based engineer specializing in telecom and medical devices, and former vice president of JAINA—links autonomy to three core Jain principles. First, he states that the vow of nonviolence (*ahiṃsā*) "promotes the autonomy of life of every living being. If you understand and believe that every [*jīva*] is autonomous, you will never trample on its right to live" (2007, 3). Jain's interpretation here demonstrates that *ahiṃsā* extends social consideration to every being possessing a *jīva*. Second, Jain asserts that the doctrine of non-one-sidedness (*anekānta-vāda*) "strengthens the autonomy of thought of every individual," explaining, "If you perceive every being as a thinking individual, you will not trample on his or her thoughts and emotions" (3).[2] In this case, Jain seems to suggest that employing *anekantā-vāda* reveals others' autonomy as deserving of respect. Third, Jain claims that the vow of nonattachment (*aparigraha*) "supports the autonomy of self-control, of striving to balance our personal consumption of things by rationalizing between our needs and desires. If you ultimately feel that you own nothing and no one, you will not trample the ecology on which our survival depends" (3). With this point, Jain equates *aparigraha* restraints toward goods and beings with a self-determining autonomy.

In another view, African-born Jain businessman Atul Shah, the CEO and founder of the British consulting firm Diverse Ethics, asserts that "over-valuing of independence and personal autonomy leads us to neglect interdependence—the essence of social cohesion" (Rankin and Shah 2008, 19). Rather than claim autonomy as compatible with Jainism, Shah rejects any isolated individualism implied in autonomy, opting for Jain ideals of "cooperation and common purpose" that place individuals in relations of responsiveness (35).

In the context of multireligious medicine, the Jain Society of Metropolitan Chicago, in conjunction with the Council for the World Parliament of Religions, identifies autonomy as a fundamental aspect of the Jain principle of nonviolence, even if the traditional language of Jainism does not explicitly articulate that term. Their jointly produced "Guidelines for Health Care Providers Interacting with Patients of the Jain Religion and Their Families" (2002) describes the principle of nonviolence as including the "preservation of life, sanctity of life, alleviation of suffering, which extends to respect of the patient's autonomy, while achieving best medical care without (harm) or with minimum harm; and always being honest and truthful in giving information" (3–4). In this view, autonomy becomes a mediating principle for non-Jain healthcare providers to understand nonviolence as both individual and relational.

These views present autonomy as a mode of self-governance possessed by all *jīvas* that is expressed, in part, by not harming other self-governing embodied beings. We might say that Jainism presents a form of "entangled autonomy" in which a *jīva*'s conduct toward self and others accrues numerous kinds of destructive and nondestructive karma that affect its own internal qualities and external circumstances (see chapter 2).

### *Truth as Subordinate to Nonviolence?*

In modern bioethics, truth is closely related to autonomy, since self-governing individuals cannot make choices aligned with their values without understanding relevant facts. There are many historical examples of forgoing truth to reap the benefits of deception within the modern medical context. Egregious instances of deceiving patients for the sake of producing knowledge—such as the deadly Nazi medical experiments on prisoners without their permission during World War II, or the infamous forty-year Tuskegee syphilis study that withheld available treatments from African American subjects—led to ethics reforms worldwide. The Nuremberg Code (1948) and the Declaration of Helsinki (1964) delineated requirements for voluntary "informed consent" in which patients must be aware of risks, benefits, and the ability to stop participation at any time. These reforms further clarified the priority of medical care for research participants *as patients* rather than merely as knowledge-producing subjects. After the violations of the Tuskegee study came to light in the United States, the 1974 National Research Act became law, creating a stricter standard for informed consent and requiring studies to be approved by institutional review boards to ensure that they meet ethical standards.

In ethics classes, a common thought experiment is often used to explore the morality of truth-telling between dominant accounts such as deontology and utilitarianism: If an individual with a lethal weapon comes to your house searching for a person whom you know to be inside, do you tell the visitor where to find them? Deontological advocates might stress that truth is a duty with no legitimate exception, while some utilitarian advocates might argue that lying in this case could preserve a life. Other theories, such as virtue ethics and feminist ethics of care, are often less suited to conceptual tests like this, since they explore moral decision making in alternative ways—for instance, imagining how a virtuous person might respond in this circumstance, or considering the relationship of the individuals involved, the social contexts of this threat, or if there were any third options. Most thought experiments, of course, do not invite this level of nuance, but merely illuminate a central question such as "Can deception ever be justified, and under what circumstances?"

As explained in chapter 3, truthfulness is one of the five vows in the Jain tradition, and as a vow it can be observed fully, as mendicants attempt to do, or partially, in the case of laity (TS 7.2). Truthfulness here refers to refraining from verbal activities that are informed by passions and therefore harm oneself, and from those that harm others. For laypeople, the vow of truthfulness is often described in relation to specific contexts in which they might be engaged, such as marriage and parental relations, business ownership, trade, and civic participation. Lay Jains are, thus, warned against providing wrong instruction, divulging secrets, forging documents, misusing entrusted funds, or sharing confidential thoughts of others ($TS^{Dig}$ 7.26[3]), as noted in chapter 3. Even verbally encouraging someone to cause harm, or insulting or embarrassing others, are seen as a violation of the vow (Williams 1963, 71–78).

Since the vow of truthfulness is subordinate to the primary vow of nonviolence, it does have flexibility in the textual tradition, as noted in chapter 3. If truth is bound to cause harm, it should not be revealed. While staying silent is preferable for mendicants, laity may even utter falsehoods in order to prevent violence. Certain texts also make concessions for violating the vow of truthfulness in order to secure the strength of the Jain mendicant community, as indicated in chapter 4.

As we will show below in relation to modern Jain attitudes toward clinical research trials, the Jain medical professionals in our survey seem to place a high value on truth-telling in medicine, advocating informed consent. However, some respondents were prepared to accept placebo deception within randomized clinical research trials for the sake of future benefits of research.

### *Competing Values among Jain Medical Professionals*

Do Jain medical professionals depend more on Jain values or on the professional requirements of their medical training for their ethical decision making? Although one can identify points of compatibility between Jain philosophical concepts and biomedical principles such as nonmaleficence, beneficence, autonomy, and truth, the Jain context rests on the acceptance of particular beliefs, guidelines, and goals, developed over the past twenty-five hundred years. Modern medicine, on the other hand, has its own systemic expectations, aims, laws, and recommendations. Additionally, authoritative bodies continually review and create regulations relating to medicine at the institutional, state, federal, and global levels, straining to articulate universal values that will extend across regional, economic, and cultural differences.

The Jain medical professionals in our survey seem to balance a commitment to Jain values with other sources of knowledge and value such as clinical experience, legal and medical standards, and cultural sources. We assessed respondents' exposure to Jain values through several different questions. When asked how they "primarily learned about the ethical principles of Jainism," respondents could choose all applicable answers from a provided list. The greatest sources included (1) guest lectures by visiting Jain scholars (50%, $n = 36$), (2) family (47%), (3) *pāṭhaśālā* classes (42%), (4) reading Jain scriptures or historical Jain texts in translation (English, German, French, etc.) on my own (39%), (5) guest lectures by monks and nuns (33%), and (6) guest lectures by visiting Jain laypeople (31%), among ten other possible sources. Importantly, no respondent selected the option "I have never really learned about Jain ethical principles" (0%, $n = 36$).

While all respondents were exposed to Jain ethical values in some way, they varied in their degree of dedication to Jain ethical practices, beliefs, and ritual practices. More professionals considered themselves very dedicated (v) or somewhat dedicated (sw) to Jain ethical practices (v 71%, sw 21%, $n = 42$) than to Jain beliefs (v 57%, sw 31%, $n = 42$) or ritual practices (v 14%, sw 33%, $n = 42$). These commitments are not relegated merely to the private sphere, as many respondents also affirmed that Jain principles had influenced their opinions toward work-related biomedical issues, especially regarding (1) honesty in business practices, (2) dietary choices at work, (3) animal research, (4) animal testing, and (5) conflict resolution practices (figure 11).

What is important to note at present is the way that survey respondents attempt to hold their identity as Jains and medical professionals together. Over half of respondents felt it was very important (vi) or moderately important (mi) for *colleagues* to know they were Jain (vi 33%, mi 24%; $n = 42$), while fewer thought it was very or moderately important for their *patients* or *students* to know (vi 17%, mi 21%; $n = 42$).

Like many medical and healthcare professionals, the majority of survey respondents had encountered an ethical dilemma in the course of their work (67%,

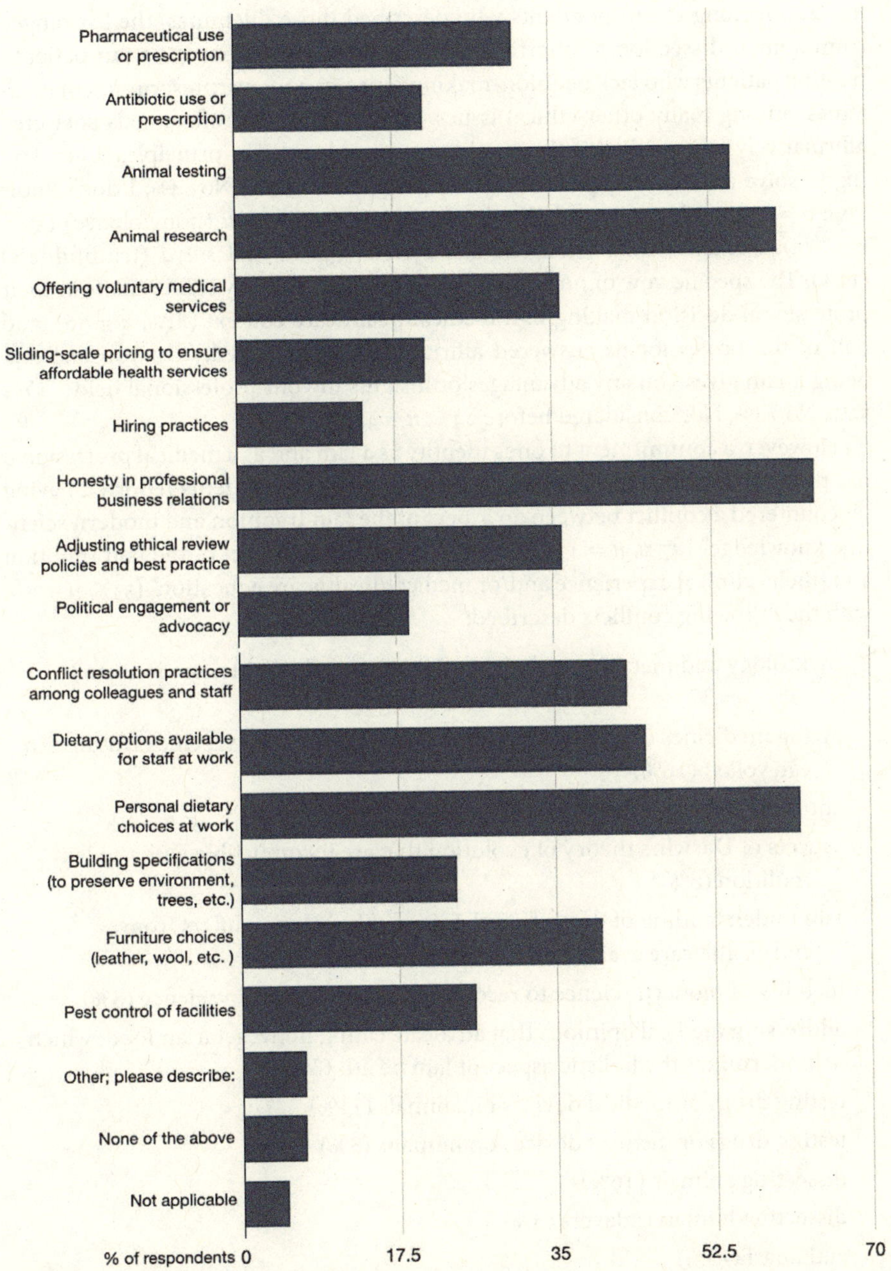


FIGURE 11. Responses of Jain medical professionals ($n = 42$) to the question "Has your commitment to Jain principles influenced your professional decision (in a work-related situation) regarding any of the following? Choose all that apply."

*n* = 42). Among the respondents who described those dilemmas, the list ranged from animal dissection to abortion services, counseling nonvegetarian patients, treating patients who lack decision-making capacity, and overprescription of medicines, among many other ethical issues. The majority of professionals answered affirmatively when asked if they had "ever considered Jain principles when trying to solve an ethical question in [their] work" (Yes 74%, No 14%, I don't know 12%; *n* = 42), with the most helpful principles being *ahiṃsā* (nonviolence) (33%, *n* = 42), *anekānta-vāda* (non-one-sided view) (31%), and *satya* (truthfulness) (19%). The specific vow of nonviolence also influenced many respondents in their professional decision making in a medical/healthcare context (81%, *n* = 36), and half of the professionals answered affirmatively when asked, "Do you feel that being a Jain gives you any advantages or insights in your professional field?" (Yes 52%, No 24%, Not considered before 24%; *n* = 42).

However, a commitment to one's identity as a Jain and as a medical professional did pose some conflicts. A significant percentage of respondents reported having "encountered a conflict between an aspect of the Jain tradition and modern scientific knowledge" (47%, *n* = 43), as well as "between an aspect of the Jain tradition and [their] clinical experience and/or medical/healthcare education" (53%, *n* = 39), with the following conflicts described:

mythology and metaphysics (such as Jain geography, reincarnation, etc.) (5%, *n* = 37)

giving medicines of animal origin (meat, fish, or gelatin; vaccines cultured in egg yolks) (16%)

abortion and contraception (8%)

aspects of Darwin's theory of evolution that are incompatible with the Jain tradition (8%)[4]

Jain understanding of death (*saṃthāra/sallekhanā*) as it differs from end-of-life care available in modern medicine (11%)[5]

inability of modern science to recognize the depths of Jain science (8%)

addressing medical opinions that advocate eating nonvegetarian food, which undermines the holistic aspect of Jain health (3%)

testing drugs or medical devices on animals (11%)

testing drugs or medical devices on humans (3%)

dissecting animals (16%)

dissecting human cadavers (3%)

euthanasia (3%)

how to advise patients on whether to kill mosquitoes or not (3%)

Jains are not well informed about being organ donors (3%)

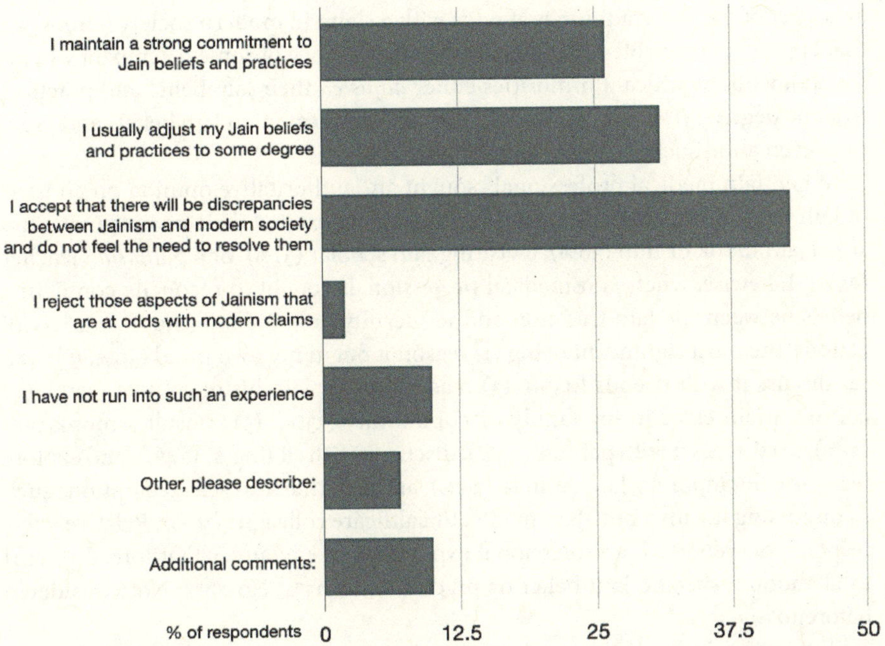


FIGURE 12. Responses of Jain medical professionals ($n = 42$) to the survey item "When an aspect of the Jain tradition is at odds with a claim in modern society . . . (Choose all that apply)."

While only one-tenth of respondents affirmed that "my commitment to Jain principles has put my professional career at risk at least one time" (10%, $n = 42$), a significant minority of Jain medical professionals had been chastised for their Jain beliefs or practices in a professional setting. These experiences ranged from rarely being teased or made fun of (29%, $n = 42$) to frequently being teased or made fun of (10%), and from rarely being assertively bullied (2%, $n = 42$) to frequently being assertively bullied (17%). Among those who described the incidents, they involved "having compassion for animals; viewing them as conscious entities," "vegetarian diet and avoiding alcohol," "being told I was short [in stature] because I did not eat meat," and failing "an Advanced Trauma Life Support class [offered by the American College of Surgeons] when I refused to use animals." Four additional responses referred to Jain diet or vegetarianism.

Additionally, a small percentage of professionals answered positively the question "When someone asks you about your religious tradition, have you ever told them you were a more prominent Indian tradition (Hindu or Buddhist, for example), for the sake of ease?" (14%, $n = 42$), suggesting some lack of familiarity with Jainism among non-Jain peers.[6]

Jain medical professionals appear to have developed several strategies to navigate between Jain beliefs and medical knowledge. Presented the statement "When an aspect of the Jain tradition is at odds with a claim in modern society (choose all that apply)," many professionals accepted the presence of some discrepancy (43%, $n = 42$), while significant minorities either *adjusted* their Jain belief and practices to some degree (31%) or *maintained* a strong commitment to Jain beliefs and practices even amid such tensions (26%) (figure 12).

When Jain medical professionals sought an "authoritative opinion on an issue of Jain belief or practice," they most commonly consulted their parents (42%, $n = 36$), a Jain monk or nun (36%), a visiting Jain scholar (31%), or a *pāṭhaśālā* teacher (25%). Likewise, when Jain medical professionals sought to reconcile conflicting beliefs between the Jain tradition and modernity, respondents chose a variety of actions, the most significant being (1) reason it out in my own mind (50%, $n = 42$), (2) discuss it with friends (43%), (3) read a specific Jain historical text (33%), (4) consult a Jain elder in my family or community (33%), (5) consult a monk/nun (31%), (6) discuss it with parents (24%), discuss it with sibling(s) (24%), and explore texts by contemporary Jain authors (24%), among other, less selected options such as discussing it with a non-Jain medical/healthcare colleague (19%). Relatively few respondents reported "a professional experience or encounter that forced [them] to abandon a specific Jain belief or practice" (Yes 13%, No 78%, Not considered before 10%; $n = 40$).

The use of individual reason in negotiating conflicting systems of meaning is highly valued by Jain medical professionals. Respondents believed it is "very important to use independent reasoning and critical thought to evaluate" both the claims of modern science (93%, $n = 42$) and the claims of Jainism (81%, $n = 42$). Many respondents claimed to be considerably more informed by clinical experience than by Jain sources, and to be equally or more informed by non-Jain legal and cultural sources than by Jain sources (figure 13).

Additionally, when asked to describe their current ethical framework or the principles they use when evaluating dilemmas in their professional life, participants who responded (47%, $n = 36$) described diverse concepts. Many principles stemmed from within the Jain tradition, such as nonviolence, non-one-sidedness, pursuing positive karma, truthfulness, non-stealing, and right thought, speech, and bodily conduct (60%, $n = 20$), but several participants referenced clinical sources such as medical training on ethics, responsibility, and autonomy (25%), or one's own individual reasoning (15%). A strong majority of respondents agreed that "medical/healthcare students and clinicians need more training in practical ethics to anticipate situations that arise in a clinical context" (78%, $n = 36$).

In summary, while the Jain medical professionals in our survey were very committed to Jain beliefs and practices, they were also adept at balancing clinical, medical, legal, and cultural sources of input into their reasoning. Jain principles provide guidance in ethical dilemmas, even as they also contribute to ethical dilemmas, which are then adjudicated by adjusting, maintaining, or (rarely) rejecting Jain

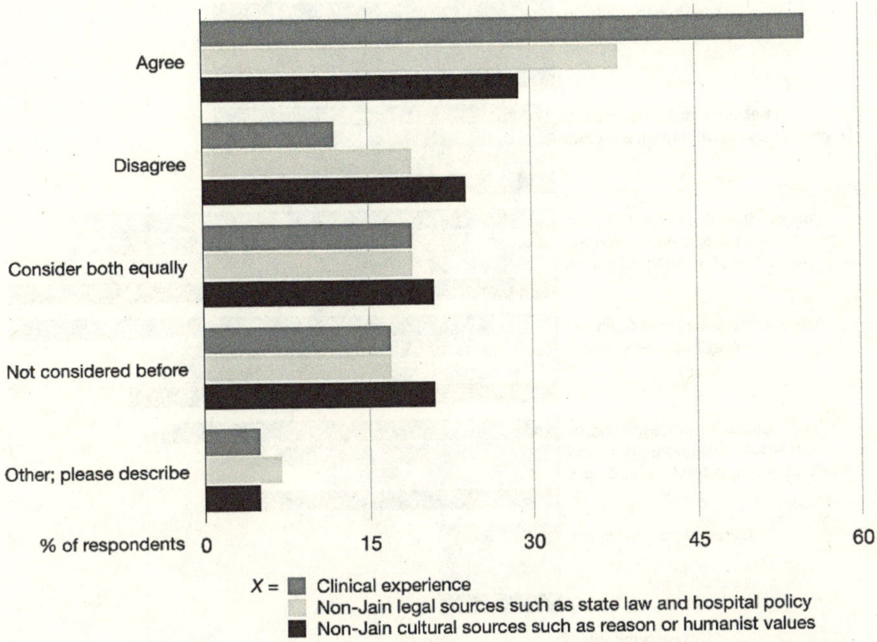


FIGURE 13. Responses of Jain medical professionals ($n = 42$) to "*X* informs my understanding of medicine/healthcare more than Jain sources." This graph is a composite of responses to three statements: (1) "Clinical experience informs my understanding of medicine/healthcare more than Jain sources"; (2) "Non-Jain legal sources such as state law and hospital policy inform my understanding of medicine/healthcare more than Jain sources"; and (3) "Non-Jain cultural sources such as reason or humanist values inform my understanding of medicine/healthcare more than Jain sources."

values, or by tolerating dissonance. Many respondents turned to their own reason, personal relationships, or specific texts for insight when such conflicts arose.

## CLINICAL CONSIDERATIONS AMONG JAIN MEDICAL PROFESSIONALS

The earliest portions of the Śvetāmbara canon had strong prohibitions against mendicants using medicines and various treatments that would either (1) harm other beings or (2) generate damaging attachments to one's body or comfort (see chapter 4). However, a duty to care for ill fellow mendicants soon emerged, gradually becoming a regulated expectation that resulted in the eventual acceptance of medical care from lay Jains if needed. In this section, we look at contemporary Jain views on the causes of illness and consider Jain views on vaccinations and antibiotics, surgery and human dissection, clinical research trials, and treating mendicants.

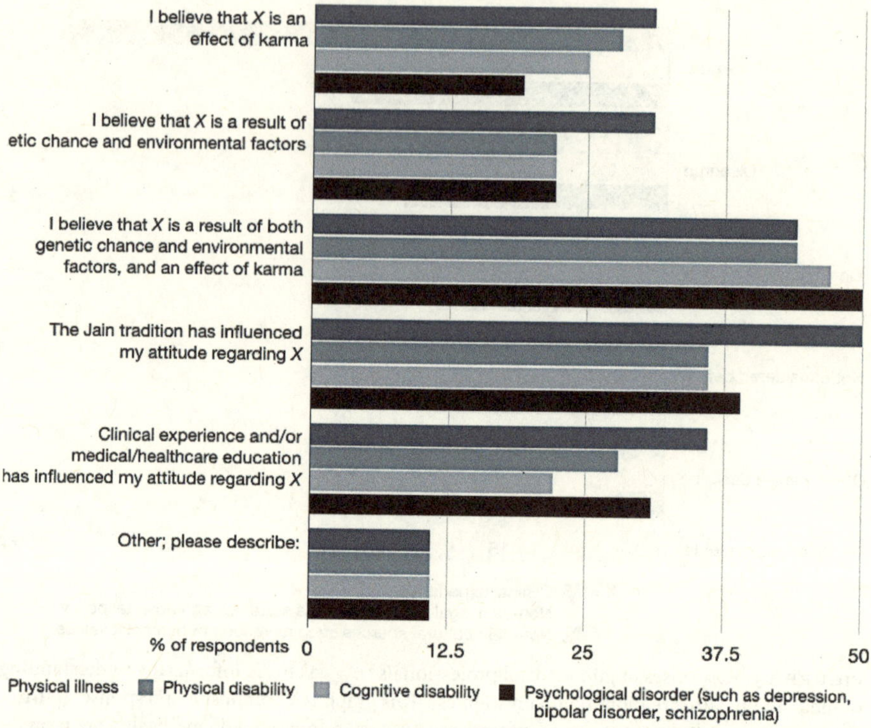


FIGURE 14. Responses of Jain medical professionals ($n = 36$) to four questions: (1) "When you encounter someone with a physical illness, how do you understand that? Choose all that apply"; (2) "When you encounter someone with a physical disability, how do you understand that? Choose all that apply"; (3) "When you encounter someone with a mental/cognitive disability, how do you understand that? Choose all that apply"; and (4) "When you encounter someone with a psychological disorder (such as depression, bipolar disorder, schizophrenia, etc.), how do you understand that? Choose all that apply."

### *Causes of Illness*

As stated in chapter 4, Jain texts attribute physical illnesses to several causes, including various kinds of nondestructive karma, bodily disturbances related to the three humors, lifestyle and behavioral choices, external factors like malevolent powers and curses, and the decline in physical vitality associated with old age. Mental illnesses are related to lifestyle and behavioral choices, imbalances in the three humors, possession by a *yakṣa*, and deluding karma.

The Jain medical professionals in our survey also attribute illness, disability, and psychological disorders to diverse causes. For instance, a greater number of respondents attributed physical illness to *joint causation* between genetic variation, environmental factors, and karma (50%, $n = 36$) than to either environmental factors alone (44%) or karma alone (31%) (figure 14). At the same time, a greater number attributed physical disability (pd) and cognitive disability (cd) to environmental factors alone (pd 44%; cd 47%) than to karma alone (pd 22%; cd 22%) or to a mix of genes, environment, and karma (pd 36%; cd 36%).

While our survey did not delineate cognitive disability from mental illness, this would be a rich area of future research as there seems to be variation as to how contemporary Jains approach mental illness. Some attribute mental illnesses, such as depression, to careless action, evil thoughts, or wrong worldview (Baya 2006, 124; Jain 2003, 66). Ācārya Tulsī, in his analysis of Jain Prekṣā meditation for health, offers the general claim that "the chief cause of bodily and mental illness is the wrong working of the parts of the physical organism," which can be rebalanced through Jain meditative postures (*āsana*) of standing, sitting, and lying motionless, along with Prekṣā breathing (1994, 128). "It is said that a healthy mind can live only in a healthy body," Tulsī writes. "Even if this be a partial truth, it is an established fact that, with the regular practice of [Jain meditative postures], changes occur both in the body and the mind" (130).

Several Jains writing in the Young Jains of America (YJA) publication *Young Minds* reject or bypass these causal explanations, seeing them as a barrier for South Asian youths that prevents individuals from seeking help. Amit Shah writes: "Many of our elders and their generation believe in the idea that, 'Therapy is meant for those who are crazy, and you are not crazy' and, 'What happens in life, will make you stronger'. In other situations, the unspoken belief is, 'Don't ask, Don't tell, and Don't Share' because this brings shame on us" (2017). In an article pointedly titled "What to Do When Your Parents Don't Understand Your Mental Health," Sachin Doshi—a YJA member and Mental Health America staffer—provides numerous mental health resources, noting that "unfortunately, seeking professional help—while never a sign of weakness—isn't always an option when you grow up in a South Asian household" (2018). Dhvani Mehta, writing for both YJA and Mann Mukti—a nonprofit organization fostering stigma-free conversations on mental health for South Asian youth—explains that Jainism provides her tools of "serenity, discipline, and knowledge" that help her live with depression and encourage her to "let other young Jains know that they are not alone in their battle against mental illness" (2018).

In our survey, a considerable number of respondents felt that clinical experience and medical education had influenced their attitude toward the causes of illness and disability, but a significantly greater number claimed that the Jain tradition had influenced their view (figure 14).

Modern Jain medical professionals retain a belief that karma plays a role in illness, not on its own, but in combination with genetic inheritance and environmental factors. Physical and cognitive disabilities, however, are attributed more to environmental factors than to either karmic or genetic influences.

*Vaccinations and Antibiotics*

Vaccines and antibiotics seem to present two unique challenges for Jains. The first is a conflict of interest between different kinds of living beings. The second is an evolving philosophical tension as to whether karma is accrued by any physical action at all or only by those acts motivated by a mental intent to harm. We will attend to both of these challenges as they apply to each of the forthcoming clinical concerns.

Vaccines contain a weakened or partial strain of the virus they aim to treat. When injected into the body, a vaccine produces antibodies that build immunity. Modern vaccine production includes the growth and harvesting of the virus, or a portion thereof, in cell cultures from bacteria, yeast, or animal-based cell lines. Additional animal-derived ingredients can be used in growth mediums or as vaccine preservatives (e.g., gelatin, enzymes, muscle tissue, blood), and vaccines are typically tested on animals prior to approval ("How Vaccines Work").

The term *antibiotic* was coined in 1941 by the microbiologist Selman Waksman to describe any molecule that destroys bacteria or inhibits their growth (Clardy et al. 2009). Early antibiotic discoveries, such as penicillin and streptomycin, were produced naturally by fungi and soil bacteria, respectively, which are today produced en masse as a growth medium. Antibiotics are also tested on animals. Accordingly, using a Jain account of one- through five-sensed living beings, both vaccines and antibiotics (1) utilize living beings in the substance itself; (2) require testing on living beings; and (3) when effective, destroy minute living beings deemed harmful to a patient's well-being.

The consideration of even minute life-forms was a unique and central aspect of early Jain manuals of mendicant conduct and remains a significant consideration for modern Jain mendicants and laity. The canonical *Daśavaikālika-sūtra* uniquely describes eight subtle (*sūkṣma*)[7] living entities that mendicants should be aware of, including moisture (*sneha*), subtle blossoms (*puṣpa-sūkṣma*), (subtle) life-forms (*prāṇa*),[8] insects (*uttiṅga*),[9] mould (*panaka*),[10] seeds (*bīja*), (minute) plants (*harita*),[11] and subtle eggs (*aṇḍa-sūkṣma*), to all of which mendicants should extend compassion (*dayā*) (DVS 8.13–15). Mendicant texts also recognized that certain medical treatments and settings could inflict less harm upon minute kinds of beings than others. Granoff examines a case in the *Bṛhatkalpa-bhāṣya* in which monks consider whether to take an ill fellow mendicant to see a doctor (2014, 240). One factor in their decision making is that if the patient dies at the doctor's home, innumerable living beings will be killed when the physician's space is cleaned, a karmic harm that would be caused or approved of by the mendicants; the mendicants' lodging, on the other hand, could at least be washed with water filtered of living beings (*prāsuka*), demonstrating an attempt to act with the lowest overall loss of life.

Modern Jains also attempt to account for minute forms of life. We will here focus on the modern interpretations of viruses and bacteria, since these are the minute beings harmed by vaccinations and antibiotics. Drawing upon Jain canonical and postcanonical accounts of living beings, J.C. Sikdar classifies both viruses and bacteria as *nigoda*s (1964, 354–55; 1974, 39, 88–89, 94–95, 98, 263; 1975, 12, 14; see chapter 2). Bacteria, along with some fungi, according to Sikdar, are like other plants and animals in that they are made of cells (*arbuda*)[12] and function through metabolic processes; they are distinguished from other living beings by their heterotrophic quality, meaning their inability to produce food through carbon fixation, and derive nutrition instead from the "sap" or "humours" of other beings, or from decaying matter (1975, 13–14). Surendra Bothra, in his manual for modern Jains titled *Ahimsa: The Science of Peace*, locates bacteria and viruses in the category of immobile beings (*sthāvara*), claiming that "in modern terminology the [*sthāvara*] category of life-forms would probably be termed as mono-cellular organisms . . . [such as] bacteria and virus[es]" (2004, 17). He assigns Jain terms to bacteria based on the stage of evolution in which they developed, where they live, and what they feed on. For example, bacteria nourished by carbon compounds formed from condensed vapors might be considered air-bodied beings, photosynthesizing bacteria that rely on the sun may be fire-bodied beings, and bacteria that grow in colonies are like plant beings (19–21). He further notes that viruses "share plant characteristics" (21).

As explored in chapter 3, mendicants and lay Jains have different levels of responsibilities toward different life-forms, with mendicants avoiding *sūkṣma-hiṃsā*, or "subtle violence," even toward one-sensed beings that may be difficult to perceive, and laypeople avoiding *sthūla-hiṃsā*, or "gross violence," toward mobile beings with two or more senses that are easier to detect (Williams 1963, 65–66).

The respondents in our survey consisted of lay Jains rather than mendicants. The majority of Jain medical professionals seemed to have little discomfort when considering vaccination. Most felt that mandatory vaccination presented little or no violation of Jain principles (73%, $n$ = 37), though some did not know (16%). Those who selected "Other" (8%) raised concerns about vaccines being tested on animals and containing animal ingredients, or affirmed their value as "a preventative measure necessary for well-being," akin to beneficence-based obligations. In sum, the primary concern of Jain medical professionals regarding vaccinations was their possible negative effect on animals who would be used for research or harmed to procure ingredients for the vaccine.

Respondents' views on antibiotics were more mixed and frequently centered on the tension between physical harm and mental intent. When presented the statement "I consider antibiotics that may kill one-sensed organisms a form of violence," one-third of respondents agreed (30%, $n$ = 36), though a larger portion disagreed (42%). A small contingent did not know (6%), had not considered the question before (11%), or selected "Other" (8%), with comments including (1) that the sacrifice of one-sensed beings is done to benefit five-sensed beings, (2) that the goal of healing neutralizes violation, and (3) that there is debate as to

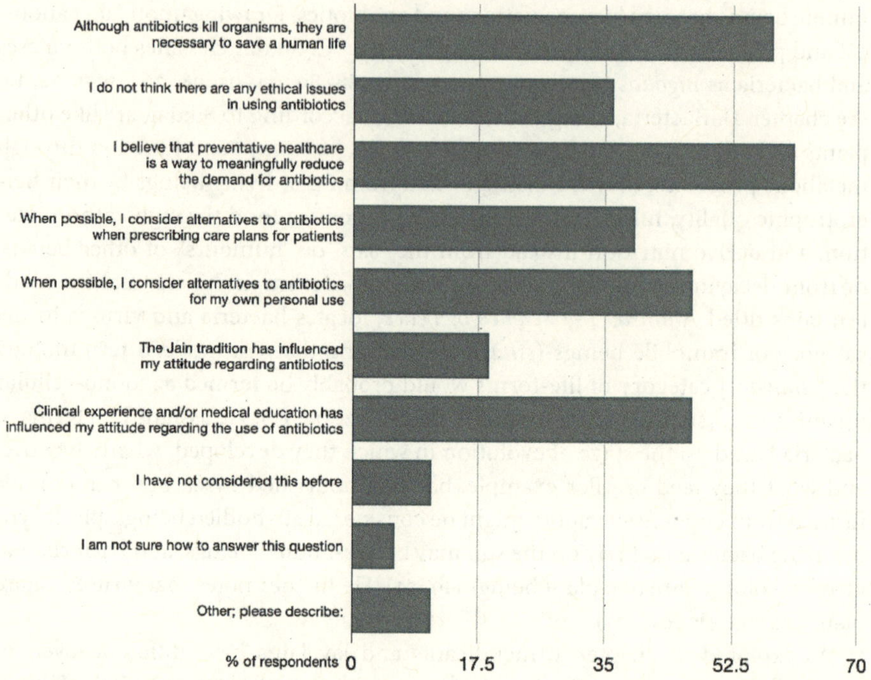


FIGURE 15. Responses of Jain medical professionals ($n = 36$) to the question "Which of the following statements [regarding antibiotics] is/are most true for you? Choose all that apply."

what constitutes a one-sensed being. When asked to elaborate upon their position regarding antibiotics, respondents emphasized preventative care to reduce the demand for antibiotics (61%, $n = 36$) and acknowledged that antibiotics—while killing one-sensed beings—were sometimes necessary to save human life (58%) (figure 15).

Considering the intended benefit of an act reflects a key development in Jain attitudes toward harm generally and medical harm specifically (see chapters 3 and 4, respectively). The above answers suggest that a majority of respondents are aware that antibiotic use can be detrimental to other living beings. However, desires such as healing or preserving human life may justify their use.

At the same time, many respondents saw personal and professional value in preventative care to avoid antibiotics altogether, or to consider alternative treatments when possible. For instance, while a sizable minority did not see any ethical issues in using antibiotics (36%, $n = 36$), a greater number of participants considered alternatives to antibiotics when prescribing patient care (39%), as well as in their personal healthcare (47%) (figure 15). As we will address in the next chapter's examination of death and dying, the Jain medical professionals we surveyed stated that they would accept antibiotics (36%, $n = 36$) as a form of life-sustaining treatment above all other listed interventions, such as blood transfusion (31%), dialysis (28%), and CPR (25%), although these data suggest that more than 60 percent of respondents may not accept antibiotics.

The issue of antibiotics is also debated among Jains themselves in various social forums. One Jain blogger creatively described antibiotics as a form of v iolence done in self-defense (*virodhī-hiṃsā*), but stated that the best defense is keeping oneself as healthy as possible (Sanglikar 2016).[13] In an online discussion thread titled "Does Jainism Allow the Usage of Antibiotics?," Jains were in disagreement. One respondent commented that Jainism neither allows nor disallows their use, but left it to individuals to discern the best way to reduce harm in their daily life: "Though [harm] of one-sense living-beings . . . is permissible for household[er]s," the blogger writes, "they are supposed to exercise due caution to minimize their *hiṃsā*" (Jain 2016). Another blog response claimed that antibiotic use by mendicants differs by sect (Dhanki 2017), while others asserted that monks can never take such medications (Jain 2017). Jain physician Manibhai Mehta, in an interview with the *Los Angeles Times*, describes the "fine line" of antibiotic use between "whether you want to save the patient . . . or the small creatures. You have to choose between the two" (Loar 1996), suggesting that there is a choice to consider between two harms. Monks, however, face no such dilemma, he asserts: "Monks won't take antibiotics. They will let the sickness go away by itself . . . [or] [t]hey just let their lives go by, because they would not want to harm those bacteria" (Loar 1996). In spite of this stated ideal, the textual tradition mapped in chapter 4 shows that mendicants have varied historically in their approach to medicine, and as we will demonstrate shortly, many contemporary mendicants do seek medical care.

When a Jain physician decides to use antibiotics, according to Mehta, "then you [the physician] should repent for it" (Loar 1996). Likewise, in a document titled "Caring for the Jain Patient," utilized by the UK-based Ashford and St. Peter's healthcare system, Jain attitudes toward medicine were noted, including views on antibiotics. "Some [Jains] may prefer not to take antibiotics because of the prohibition against harming any form of life," the document advises, but "if antibiotics are essential they would probably be accepted, but with regret" ("Caring" n.d.). Among contemporary practitioners, a significant minority of survey respondents affirmed that they had "practiced *pratikramaṇa* (the ritual of repentance or seeking forgiveness) after [they had] engaged in a medical procedure or practice for which [they] had ethical uncertainty" (22%, $n = 36$).[14]

On one hand, accepting harm "with regret," or conducting a ritual of repentance, may seem like a token gesture for humans who are ultimately going to use whatever resources they deem essential. On the other hand, regret signifies the Jain tradition's unique acknowledgment of living beings, including minute one-sensed beings, whose destruction constitutes a karmic harm, and whose pain and demise can often be prevented.

The various contemporary responses detailed above—both from medical professionals and within the broader lay Jain community—emerge from a view that the universe is permeated with numerous life-forms whom one must acknowledge if there is any chance of dialing back the use and injury of those beings. Utilizing antibiotics is not forbidden, but the practice is viewed through calculations of karmic cost, medical benefit, and preventative healthcare. How mendicants and lay Jains view their responsibility toward one-sensed beings often differs, and one's context and stage of life might also factor into decision making.

### *Human Surgery and Dissection*

In Jain texts on lay conduct, vocations that rely on mutilation (*nirlañchana*)—such as gelding of bulls and other animals, branding, tail docking, cutting off of ears and dewlaps, and nose piercing of livestock—are discouraged (Williams 1963, 120; YŚ 3.111). Apart from harming the living beings, whose skin is pierced, cutting into their flesh can also harm groups of *nigoda*s that inhabit the flesh of animals and humans in particularly high concentrations, as noted in chapter 2. On the other hand, medicine (*vidyā*), which includes surgery, is classified as an acceptable occupation for laity (see chapters 3 and 4). Texts for laity attempt to articulate and justify these accommodations—for example, that one can slice into skin if this is done with due care (*sāpekṣa*)—that is, without the mental intention to harm, and/or with the positive mental intention to heal. Williams discusses various attitudes toward cutting of flesh (*chavi-ccheda*) in Jain texts,[15] for example that lancing a boil or a swelling for the purpose of relieving suffering is acceptable, though cutting for the purpose of mutilating prisoners, enemies, animals, trees, or other one-sensed beings is still a violation (1963, 68). Padmanabh Jaini notes that occupational violence, such as that done by surgery, falls under the category of the so-called *ārambhajā-hiṃsā*, since it occurs as a result of practicing an occupation that is considered acceptable by the tradition (2001/1979, 170–71).

The overwhelming majority of Jain professionals in our survey did not consider "cutting into the human body for minor or major surgery a violation of Jain principles" (83%, $n = 35$). Additional comments describe a notable distinction, asserting that (group *a*) surgical harm is regrettable, but it results in a meaningful benefit for a five-sensed being (40%, $n = 5$); or (group *b*) surgical harm is no harm at all because the intention is to heal (and, according to one comment, heal with the least damage to other beings as possible) (60%, $n = 5$). Put another way, group *a* still factors the *physical* harms to other beings into their calculation, whereas group *b* seems to give precedence to the *mental* state. These distinctions certainly require more research, but they reflect persistent tensions over the violence of physical harm and mental intention that continually inform Jain ethical attitudes among mendicants and laity.

Only a small portion of respondents felt that *human* dissection—meaning cutting into skin posthumously for educational and/or research purposes—violates

Jain principles (11%, $n = 35$). The majority felt that postmortem human dissection poses no violation (71%).[16] Likewise, Jain respondents do not appear to share a view articulated by certain interpretations of Islam, Christianity, and Judaism that dissection violates a divinely gifted body (Aramesh 2009; Notzer et al. 2006). It is unclear precisely why Jain medical professionals accept human dissection, as we did not ask them that question specifically. Yet one could infer that, like surgery, cutting into flesh for the purposes of human dissection is acceptable with regret, or merely accepted, if the mental intent is to benefit five-sensed beings.

### *Clinical Research Trials and Access to Care*

Jain attitudes toward human research—namely studies with higher risk such as clinical trials or experimental treatments—offer insight into the challenges of entangled autonomy and competing values of truthfulness alongside the value of nonviolence. When presented the statement "I consider randomized controlled clinical trials (RCTs; where certain vulnerable/terminal patients receive placebos, standard medication, or no intervention) a violation of Jain principles," respondents diverged in their opinions. Nearly half of respondents disagreed that RCTs violate Jain principles (47%, $n = 36$), while a small minority agreed that RCTs constitute a violation (14%). A significant percentage either did not know (22%) or had not considered the issue before (11%). Additional comments included "Patients have a right to know," "You cannot torment somebody to save someone else in the future," and "If the patient is fully aware of the principles of the trial and agrees, I think it is okay to take part in RCT; there is no one 'playing god' in this situation."

One of the ongoing ethical challenges in clinical trials is determining the priority between *therapeutic* and *nontherapeutic* research. Therapeutic research aims to produce generalizable medical knowledge with an expectation that the subject-patient will also medically benefit from the drugs or procedures being investigated, contrasted with nontherapeutic research aimed to produce generalizable knowledge alone.

Ethical guidelines and medical codes weigh the production of new knowledge against an absolute requirement that research subjects benefit from their participation (Glantz et al. 2010). Some research, for instance, may only have the *possibility* of benefit but take too long to aid a patient with a terminal illness; likewise, some research subjects—especially in remote, underserved, or poor communities nationally or abroad—may not be able to access or afford treatment when a trial is complete, raising questions as to what constitutes a fair benefit. Is access to a drug the only value gained by clinical trials, or might communities benefit from infrastructure, training, or being paid for research ("Fair Benefits" 2002)? Must an individual receive a benefit in the present moment, or could future generations of a specific community—as in disease research among indigenous tribes—count as community benefit (Fitzpatrick et al. 2016)? Justice-related concerns of coercion quickly emerge when vulnerable individuals are offered a nonmedical benefit—

such as a payment, a future benefit, or a communal benefit—for participation that carries risk of any kind (Brody 2010). Even the common procedure of paying donors for blood plasma donation in the United States generates ongoing debates alongside evidence that paid donations exploit poor communities where individuals need quick cash (Farrugia et al. 2015; Shaefer and Ochoa 2018).

Jain medical professionals were not necessarily averse to research risk in general, as the majority disagreed (56%, $n$ = 36) that "the high risk of experimental treatments in general is a violation of Jain principles," though a minority agreed (11%), did not know (22%), or had not considered the issue before (8%). Interestingly, two additional comments note that a patient's longevity-determining karma (*āyu-karman*) plays a role in illness outcome (see chapters 2 and 7); another states that karma, combined with informed consent, removes any ethical question.

Regarding the ethics of clinical human research trials, most respondents placed a relatively high value on medical benefit for participants. When asked to identify their positions on RCTs (when subjects may receive placebos, standard medication, or no intervention), survey respondents could choose multiple positions from a provided list. One-third of participants believed that RCTs can be justified only "if all vulnerable/terminal patients are eventually given free access and transit to any treatment deemed successful" (33%, $n$ = 36). At the same time, a quarter of respondents felt that trials can be justified "because of future patients who will hopefully benefit from the sacrifice of these vulnerable/terminal research subjects" (22%), and a significant minority felt that RCTs cannot be justified "because it involves a form of deception to vulnerable/terminal patients" (19%).

Respondents reported that their attitudes on RCTs were more highly influenced by clinical experience and medical education (33%, $n$ = 36) than by the Jain tradition (14%). These various attitudes suggest that a minority of Jain medical professionals place their ethical obligation of truth above possible benefit in human research; but a larger portion of respondents feel that medical benefit to the individual, or even to future generations, may justify deception (such as placebo) so long as participants are aware of and consent to the study design.

Jain medical professionals also valued universal access to healthcare. When asked to elaborate their view on the topic, a majority affirmed that "all people should have equal access to all of their healthcare needs" (57%, $n$ = 37). Among competing economic models regarding access (Sreenivasan 2007), the Jains in our survey favored a "basic decent minimum" of care provided to all people, with individual patients given the option to pay for specialty services above that threshold (35%, $n$ = 37), considerably more than they endorsed the "libertarian" model in which patients receive only those services they can pay for (5%). More respondents felt that it is the government's responsibility to provide healthcare for the most vulnerable members of society by utilizing taxes (43%, $n$ = 37) than considered this the responsibility of private organizations (11%).

These views on healthcare access were only slightly more informed by the Jain tradition (24%, $n = 37$) than by clinical experience or medical education (22%). The vast majority of healthcare professionals we surveyed (75%, $n = 36$) had offered free medical services as a nurse, doctor, administrator, or assistant either for people (63%, $n = 27$), for animals (4%), or for both people and animals (30%). Several respondents reported that their commitment to Jain principles had influenced their professional decision to offer free medical services (36%, $n = 42$) or sliding-scale pricing (21%) to ensure affordable health services.

*Treating Medicants*

Jainism has rarely been dramatized in film. However, the critically acclaimed movie *Ship of Theseus* (2012) depicts a fictionalized Jain monk who, after spending years fighting against animal testing, is confronted with accepting medications tested on animals in order to receive a liver transplant. The film invites viewers into the monk's decision making in a personal way. Should he accept the medication?

Even as mendicant attitudes in textual sources gradually reflect a more favorable view of medicine as necessary to maintain the community and one's body for austerities (see chapter 4), an indifference to bodily care and pain, and the refusal of treatment, is still seen as having merit among contemporary Jain mendicants. In N. Shāntā's study of female mendicants (*sādhvī*) in India, one nun suggested that a more experienced mendicant may offer guidance on whether to seek or eschew medical care:

> [O]n the one hand, one must avoid for oneself and for others anything that is violent or causes suffering, and neglect[ing] an illness or a wound may be a form of *hiṃsā*; on the other hand, is it not necessary [for a mendicant] to proceed to *kāyotsarga* [and] the abandonment of the body? At this point the wisdom and spirit of discernment and long experience of the *ācārya* or *guruṇi* or the senior *sādhvī*s have a decisive importance . . . [regarding] the advisability or not of following some treatment or consulting a doctor. (1997, 562)

Shāntā notes that nuns in India at the beginning of the twentieth century were "inclined to put up with suffering and illness without paying much heed to it and to walk in a heroic manner to the end, without complaint . . . [as] part of the process of purification"; yet contemporary nuns "are not only cared for and visit the doctor, but they may also enter hospital, follow a course of treatment there and even undergo an operation" (1997, 563).[17] If a nun falls ill, this may affect group wandering. According to Shāntā, if illness is short lived, the whole group may pause their wandering to stay with the sick nun; otherwise, only a few other nuns might stay with her. It may also be possible for a nun to stay with a layperson during her illness. A nun who cannot lead a wandering lifestyle because of an illness may further transgress this obligation, and "if she is unable to walk, then, when the time comes to move on, she is transported in a sedan-chair or palanquin" (564). Still, Shāntā makes it clear that accepting any of these treatments, as well as accepting special care from fellow nuns or transgressing obligations—such as being carried or waited upon—requires the sick nun to perform atonements (*prāyaścitta*) for all the violations of *ahiṃsā* that have occurred (563–64).[18]

The case of mendicant demon (*bhūta*) possession, and associated mental disturbances, provides another example of mendicants seeking treatment. As described in chapter 4, mental illness, including possession, is not always seen as a failing of the mendicant, but rather can be attributed to outside forces affecting that individual to which the wider mendicant community may need to respond. Vallely asserts that "when [mendicants] fall sick, they usually do take medicine. . . . And when *bhūta*s strike [in possession], they seek the help of ritual exorcists," alongside other modes of healing (2011, 71). In Vallely's research with Terāpanthī nuns, possession treatments included examining the afflicted woman's past lives, engaging in acts of austerity such as fasting and prayer, and, in the case of one nun-in-training, fasting to death by *sallekhanā* (2002a, 72–74; see chapter 7).[19] Vallely describes another nun suffering from possession who was not spared responsibility for her affliction; after being sent back to her family, she was instructed that she could return to the order only if she undertook the vow of fasting unto death to demonstrate a maturing spirituality—which she was not prepared to do (130).

In a tangible example of medicant attitudes to dental care, a 2007 study of the oral hygiene of 180 Śvetāmbara Terāpanthī Jain monks in India revealed signs of periodontal disease in nearly every mendicant, due to malnourishment as well as to the fact that most did not brush their teeth in keeping with mendicant rules, nor visit a dentist for checkups or treatment (Jain et al. 2009).

Prevention remains a key medical model for mendicants, as we saw above in lay attitudes toward antibiotics. In his book *Lord Mahavira's Scripture of Health* (2001), Ācārya Mahāprajña rarely acknowledges medicine at all, but instead mines Jain texts that address activities supporting well-being, such as diet, breath exercises, adequate sleep, fasting, and yogic exercises, along with textual references to psychological dispositions, emotions, and the restraint of passions that shape one's lifestyle. The specific details of medication are sidestepped in favor of prevention.

The majority of Jain medical professionals in our survey reported serving relatively few lay Jain patients in their practice overall. Most claimed that only 0–5% of their patients were Jain (60%, $n = 42$), though a few served larger populations of 5–20% (14%) or 40–60% (2%). Some were not aware of how many patients were Jain (10%) or chose Not applicable (12%) or Other (2%).[20]

However, a portion of respondents treated Jain mendicants—including fully ordained mendicants (in India) or intermediate mendicants (*samaṇs*/*samaṇīs*)—by offering medical treatment (17%, $n = 42$) or prescribing medication (14%). These physicians were also asked if there were "any special considerations or changes to your care that you had to implement to treat or prescribe medication for a Jain mendicant." A third of respondents reported no change in care (36%, $n = 14$), while the rest (64%) noted various changes, such as checking labels for animal-derived ingredients in medicines, avoiding over-the-counter medicines known to contain animal products, offering natural remedies, or prescribing once-daily medication that is not taken at night (since mendicants take no food or water after sunset).

One respondent noted that Digambara monks in India will not take medicine, while another said that some, but not all, mendicants will accept medicinal treatment. One physician described chronic health issues among mendicants related to poor diet for which more education was needed among monks and nuns, and another described their experience treating Jain mendicants for acute conditions such as coma, surgery after traumatic brain injury, and coronary angioplasty, which suggests that certain mendicants will accept intensive and emergency care when needed.

As we will explore in the next chapter, the ideal way for a mendicant to die in the Jain tradition is to forgo medical care, as well as food and fluids, when the body is no longer able to maintain the vows appropriately. The act of fasting unto death, though practiced by relatively few mendicants and even fewer lay Jains, is highly valorized as a preeminent expression of nonviolence; this ultimate disregard for medicine and the body when it can no longer serve the goals of one's *jīva* is an act of great karmic merit. Nevertheless, many Jains—both lay and mendicant—accept the benefits provided by clinical medicine during the regular course of life, while navigating unique Jain concerns such as conflicts of interest between living beings, and the karmic impact of medicine based on physical consequences and mental intentions.

## THE ETHICS OF ANIMAL USE

Jainism is distinctive among world philosophical and religious traditions for its sustained ethical commitment toward animals. This commitment is doubly intriguing because it exists alongside the unapologetic Jain affirmation that being human is a privileged birth-form separate from animals and plants (Vallely 2014, 29). At the same time, Anne Vallely explains, "the animal in Jainism, though ontologically distinct, is on the same existential trajectory as the human, and its claims to life are no less valid than those of any other sentient being" (39). Although, in the Jain worldview, only humans can attain liberation, this transcendent capacity is dependent on one's right worldview, knowledge, and conduct toward other living beings. As Vallely puts it, "human exceptionalism *resides singularly in its demonstration*, through ethical behavior and practices of bodily detachment" that take other beings into account (2020, 563; emphasis added; see also chapter 3).

Consequently, "the exceptionalism [that Jainism] claims for humans is weak and conditional, and its ethic of reverence for life is strong and absolute" (564).

This complex ethical sensibility between humans and animals is found within the Jain texts since the earliest canonical sources, in part as a response to dominant practices of the time, including Vedic rituals of animal sacrifice (Doniger 2009, 192; Kapadia 2010/1933; Williams 1963, 54). While the early Jain mendicant texts declare all violations of living beings, including nonhuman kinds, to result in karma, the degree of karmic burden is eventually established in the tradition as being based on two primary calculations: first, that the greater the degree of passions motivating an activity, the more karma is acquired; and second, as indicated above, that the higher the number of senses a violated being possesses—from one to five—the greater the karma that accrues to the one causing injury (see chapters 2 and 3).

### *The Special Significance of Five-Sensed Animals*

Although all one- through five-sensed beings are, as Naomi Appleton describes, "fellow travelers in the cycle of rebirth and redeath" (2014, 24), injuring five-sensed beings incurs the greatest karmic burden. Humans and some five-sensed animals born in a womb are endowed with mind (*manas*), enabling them to actively reflect on merits and demerits of their actions. As Dundas states, animals can practice austerities, develop compassion, observe the principle of nonviolence, and progress on the spiritual path (2002a, 106–7). While Jain narratives often depict humans being reborn in animal form as a consequence of violent or foolish actions, animals are also moral exemplars. A popular tale found in the *Jñātṛdharma-kathā* (Pkt. *Nāyādhamma-kahāo*)[21] describes a lay Jain disciple of Mahāvīra who becomes so fixated on building a pool outside his home that when he dies he becomes a frog within it. Yet, as a frog, he recalls his past material obsessions, and takes up his lay vows again. When he is later crushed by a horse while attempting to hear a sermon by Mahāvīra, the frog attains rebirth as a heavenly being and, eventually, liberation (JK 1.13; Appleton 2014, 26).

Moreover, remembering one's past embodiments as various animals is described as a powerful deterrent to violence and an encouragement to enter the path of renunciation. In the *Uttarādhyayana-sūtra*, Prince Mṛgāputra provides a dramatic account of the violence he experienced in his previous lives in animal forms: he was bound and killed as an antelope, caught by hooks and nets, scraped, and killed as a fish, and trapped and killed as a bird (US 19.63–65).

Beyond such cautionary tales, Mahāvīra's own virtues are likened to the qualities of animals (KS 5.118), and the great assembly (*samavasaraṇa*) said to occur when a Jina achieves perfect knowledge (*kevala-jñāna*) includes five-sensed animals with a mind who can also understand the teachings of the Jina (Wiley 2006b, 250; see also Balbir 1994a; Caillat and Kumar 1981, 44–47; Deshpande 2011, 186; Dundas 1996, 141).

### *Euthanasia and Five-Sensed Animals*

Jains have historically avoided keeping pets, seeing it as an endorsement of animal use that also restricts the freedom of a living being. This uneasiness with pet culture is just one of many ways, according to Christopher Chapple, that Jainism "avoids sentimentalizing animals" (2006, 248). Though some diaspora Jains do live with companion animals today, it remains a point of creative debate among Jains as to how to reduce the violence inherent in domestication—by reflecting on one's motivation for living with an animal, adopting rather than supporting breeders, feeding plant-based diets, and increasing a pet's freedom whenever possible ("Jainism View" 2019).

In the Jain view, every living being is entitled to work through its karmic burden in its own way, and to receive the fruits of dying well. In Jain-run animal shelters, or *pañjrapol*s, Jains are not to euthanize animals, since doing so injures both the person who commits or approves of the act and the animal itself. In his *Puruṣārtha-siddhyupaya*, Amṛtacandrasūri clearly states that killing, even out of compassion (*anukampā*), is an error. In this context, Amṛtacandrasūri is arguing against a rival view that one could kill living beings who naturally kill many others (*bahu-sattva-ghātin*) in order to save the lives of those preyed upon; likewise one cannot kill an animal to prevent its own great suffering (*bahu-duḥkha*) (PSU 83–85; Granoff 1992a, 29; Williams 1963, 65). Amṛtacandrasūri specifically rejects the claim that killing a living being will relieve that being from suffering (*duḥkha-vicchitti*) (PSU 85). In his commentary on this passage, Ajit Prasada explains: "The pain and suffering which a living being has to endure and go through is inevitable. . . . It must be undergone now, or hereafter, in this life or the next" (1933a, 42).[22] But that does not mean that one does nothing. Prasada writes:

> One may help the distressed by nursing or helping otherwise. Veterinary hospitals should take as much care of [animals] as other hospitals do for humanity. . . . There should be no fee charged for medicine, attendance, or surgical operation. This is the primary duty of individual citizens, municipal corporations, and of the State. (42)

At Jain-run hospitals, animals who can be treated and released are; those who cannot be released will stay in the hospital, receiving treatment or palliative care, in order to work through their karmic burden. It is not uncommon to see an animal with a custom-made prosthesis or bird-size cast in these hospitals, nor is it unusual to see an animal disfigured or enduring terminal injury near the end of life.

Jainism presents a cosmos "where all creaturely life has agency [and] Jains do not claim an unequivocal right to decide on another body's behalf, especially regarding death" (Donaldson 2015, 56). Although there are valuable criticisms of *pañjrapol* institutions that are overcrowded and in need of greater oversight (Evans 2013), Jains do have a long tradition of medical treatment and comfort care for animals, charitable giving to animal causes (*jīva-dāya*), and compulsory vegetarianism.[23]

### *Contemporary Animal Use and Welfare*

In 2018, approximately 335 million tons of animal meat were produced worldwide—from an estimated seventy-four billion cows, pigs, chickens, goats, and sheep ("Livestock Slaughter" 2018). In the United States, food animals make up the overwhelming majority of the ten billion animals slaughtered each year, a figure that does not include the estimated fifty billion fish and shellfish killed each year for consumption; nor does it count horses, rabbits, or the 150 million industry-documented animals who die each year before making it to slaughter ("Farm Animal"). The estimated one million animals used for research each year constitutes 0.0001 percent of that ten billion total, though mice—who make up the majority of vivisection subjects—are not counted in these totals ("USDA" n.d.).

Very few governmental protections exist for animals worldwide. These legal precedents provide an important starting point for considering the ethics of animal use, since these laws determine what actions are legally permissible. The United States has some of the weakest protection laws for animals among high-income nations. The 1966 Animal Welfare Act (AWA), amended most recently in 2013, excludes all farmed animals as well as mice, who make up the majority of animal research subjects. The AWA offers no regulations on how research animals can be used but only industry-established standards for basic housing, care, and transport (Cardon et al. 2012). The Humane Methods of Livestock Slaughter Act, originally passed in 1958, states that animals be rendered unconscious before slaughter, but excludes birds, rabbits, and fish, who represent the majority of animals consumed in the United States. The Twenty-Eight Hour Law, enacted in 1873 and revised in 1994, requires only that animals transported for slaughter be let out for food, water, and exercise every twenty-eight hours. The law does not address overcrowding or transport in extreme temperatures, and it does not apply to birds. In early 2017, the US Department of Agriculture further obscured animal deaths by removing public access to tens of thousands of reports that document the numbers of animals kept by nearly eight thousand research labs, companies, zoos, circuses, and animal transporters—and whether those animals are being treated humanely under existing laws.

A few select countries have significantly increased their animal welfare standards since 2000. According to World Animal Protection's current index, Austria, Switzerland, the United Kingdom, Germany, Sweden, and the Netherlands rate highest for improved animal welfare ("Animal Protection Index" n.d.). Austria, for instance, banned wild animals in circuses, primates in research, and fur farming. The United Kingdom has introduced harsher fines and penalties for violations of animal welfare, and the Netherlands has prohibited all great ape testing and extended "duty of care" provisions to farmed animals. The European Union has prohibited some of the worst practices of industrial farming, such as veal crates, battery cages for hens, and gestation crates for sows after the first four weeks, though it is important to note that none of these countries has seriously questioned the use of animals for mass food production.

### *Jainism, Animals, and Food*

Jain texts are particularly attuned to the reality of using animals for food, medicine, and labor, and we primarily address the first two categories in this and the next section.

The Jain attitude toward animals-as-meat must be understood in relation to the more general assertion that food requires violence, and that craving for it leads to the three other instincts of fear, reproduction, and accumulation of goods for future use, all of which constitute the roots of violence (*hiṃsā*) (GJK 134–38; Jaini 2010e, 284; see chapter 3). As Paul Dundas puts it, eating is "a dangerous activity which can determine the sort of person an individual is and becomes" (2000, 112).

Mendicant prohibitions against eating garlic, onions, carrots, potatoes, honey, butter, and even high-seed vegetables such as eggplants are due to the great number of *nigoda*s related to those foods (BhS 7.3§299b–300a; YŚ 3.34–46; Williams 1963, 52–55; see chapters 2 and 3). Likewise, eating meat not only destroys a two- to five-sensed being, but also kills innumerable one-sensed beings that live in flesh through cutting, cooking, and consumption, described by Hemacandra "like provisions on the road leading to hell" (YŚ 3.33, trans. Qvarnström).

Scholars identify rare examples of Jains consuming meat in unique circumstances, such as when it was provided as alms to a mendicant (and the animal had not been killed specifically for that purpose), or when a layperson was sick, or during famine (Dundas 2000, 101; 2002a, 177; Ohira 1994, 18–19). In these cases, meat eating may have been accepted but not permitted per se, since its consumption would still equate to great karmic cost, though Jains have refuted these historical examples (Kapadia 2010/1933).

The first rigid prohibition of mendicants eating meat in all circumstances may have originated with Pūjyapāda (Ohira 1994, 18–19), and the first systematic defense of Jain vegetarianism was likely made by Haribhadra in the *Aṣṭaka-prakaraṇa* (eighth century CE), to be developed in greater detail about a thousand years later in the *Dvātriṃśad-dvātriṃśikā* by Yaśovijaya (seventeenth century CE) (Dundas 2000, 102). Hemacandra expresses particular disdain for meat eating and animal sacrifice justified in the Hindu law book *Manu-smṛti*,[24] which he renames the *"hiṃsā-śāstra"* for its perceived erosion of compassion (Williams 1963, 70; YŚ 2.33–49, 3.20–31).

Today Jainism is frequently considered an ancient vegetarian tradition. Chapple describes vegetarianism as the "Ethical Non-Negotiable" for Jains (2013, 83), while Laidlaw asserts, "As it is presented for external consumption, Jainism is more or less a campaign for vegetarianism" (1995, 99). Still, it is not sufficient to equate early Jain food ethics with modern vegetarianism, since Jain ethics emphasizes the karmic burden of ingesting *any* living being, not just animals, with some *nigoda*-laden root vegetables exacting a higher karmic cost than other plants. Food cravings are terminated only in the twelfth *guṇa-sthāna* when all deluding (*mohanīya*) karmas are destroyed, attesting to the ingrained quality of this instinct and its persistent role in activity (Jaini 2010e, 292; see chapter 3). When lay Jains practice voluntary forms of fasting (Jaini 2001/1979, 217–21), they acknowledge the self-control of Mahāvīra, whose mendicant diet consisted only of rice, pounded jujube, and legumes, and those eaten only rarely (ĀS 1.8.4.4–7). Food, it is emphasized, should be eaten to sustain life rather than for its pleasant taste (US 35.17).[25]

In light of this food philosophy, mendicants are limited in their regular food intake; Digambaras typically take one meal per day, while Śvetāmbaras may collect food two or three times daily (Jaini 2001/1979, 40–41). The food is meant to come from lay Jains who, at least according to mendicant texts, had merely been preparing a meal for themselves when mendicants came in search of their daily sustenance. The provided food should not contain any of the prohibited foods listed above (Jaini 2010e, 284–85).

Modern lay Jains also avoid meat, though their diet is not as restrictive as mendicants'. In India, where there is greater familiarity with and access to "Jain food," many will avoid roots, eggs, and honey as well; in diaspora countries, many Jains abstain from these additional items at home or during holidays.

Today, a growing segment of modern Jains—primarily in diaspora countries—advocate a vegan diet—avoiding use and consumption of dairy, as well as meat, eggs, leather, or fur—as a contemporary expression of nonviolence. Groups such as US-based Vegan Jains and UK-based Jain Vegans host events to educate Jains about the cruelty of modern dairy in terms of forced impregnation, removal of female calves, and killing of male calves, as well as the effects on workers and the environment. As of 2018, Young Jains of America serve only vegan meals at their biennial conference and the large Jain Center of Southern California also announced that it would serve only vegan meals in its temple kitchen. The 2019 "Jain Declaration on the Climate Crisis," issued by JAINA, acknowledges that care of animals is closely tied to climate issues, calling for an end to government subsidies of industrial agriculture, protection of species from deforestation and exploitation, and requesting that Jain communities take specific actions that jointly impact climate and animals in their personal and temple practices ("Jain Declaration"). These efforts reflect the unique Jain view that food has impacts beyond nutrition. Ācārya Mahāprajña describes food as one of the six vitalities, or *paryāptis*,[26] on which well-being depends, a "basic foundation of life" that, if maintained properly, will enable one to "overcome the obstructions in the way of our health" (2001, 44–45), both personally and socially.

All the Jain medical professionals in our survey practiced a Jain diet of some kind, the majority being lacto vegetarian (eating dairy products but no meat or eggs) (61%, $n = 36$) and smaller percentages being ovo-lacto vegetarian (eating eggs and dairy products) (19%), vegan (abstaining from meat, dairy products, eggs, leather, and fur) (17%), or Jain vegetarian (no meat, eggs, garlic, onion, or root vegetables) (6%). No respondents selected pescatarian (eats fish) or omnivore (eats meat, dairy, and vegetables). When asked, "Does the Jain tradition influence the kind of diet or dietary needs you prescribe to your patients (in light of medical trends that suggest meat, milk for vitamin D, eggs for protein, certain vegetables or supplements)?," participants answered Yes (59%, $n = 37$), No (32%), I have not considered this before (8%), Not applicable (8%), or Other (16%). Some gave specific examples of their dietary prescriptions:

"I will not prescribe meat, eggs, etc. [but will prescribe] vegetables, fruits."

"I advocate a plant-based diet and let [patients] make their own decision."

"I do not prescribe meat or eggs for protein, and I encourage eating less [food overall] based on Jain methods of partial fasting."

"[I] emphasize vegetables, fruits and lentils as sources of protein."

"I would not advise intake of meat, eggs, fish, etc.; for cancer patients I strongly recommend they discontinue meat."

"I usually highlight vegetarian options."

"I will rarely mention meat but always suggest vegetarian choices to increase food intake."

"[S]ubstitute red meat with vegetarian source of protein."

"I am more aware of nutritional deficiencies in vegetarian and vegan diets and try to address those."

"[The Jain tradition] was an influence for my study of the medical science of a vegan diet."

"I never recommend anything as a diet that I don't practice; I explain the reason that it is something I do not believe in. I have had [occasions] where my patients are surprised and intrigued and admire it."

Recall that most survey respondents claimed that only 0–5 percent of their patients were Jain (60%, $n = 42$). Presented the question "Are there any special considerations or changes to your care that you had to implement to treat or prescribe medication to a lay Jain patient?," those who described the changes (62%, $n = 42$) emphasized diet-related issues (38%)—such as offering specific Jain-friendly foods to deal with a vitamin deficiency, or adjusting prescription timing for periods of fasting or pre-sunset—while the remainder (62%) described attempts to seek Jain-friendly medication that involves less harm to living beings, such as natural remedies, treatments that avoid animal-tested pharmaceuticals, tablets rather than capsules made from gelatin or shellfish, and alternatives to fish oil supplements. Relatedly, a significant minority of survey respondents reported that they presently incorporated alternative, āyurvedic medicine into their healthcare practice (28%, $n = 36$) or would like to do so in the future (14%).

### *Jainism, Animals, and Medicine*

Animal research is a contested issue in contemporary biomedical ethics, often framed as either pro-animal or pro-science, with little space between. Ethicist

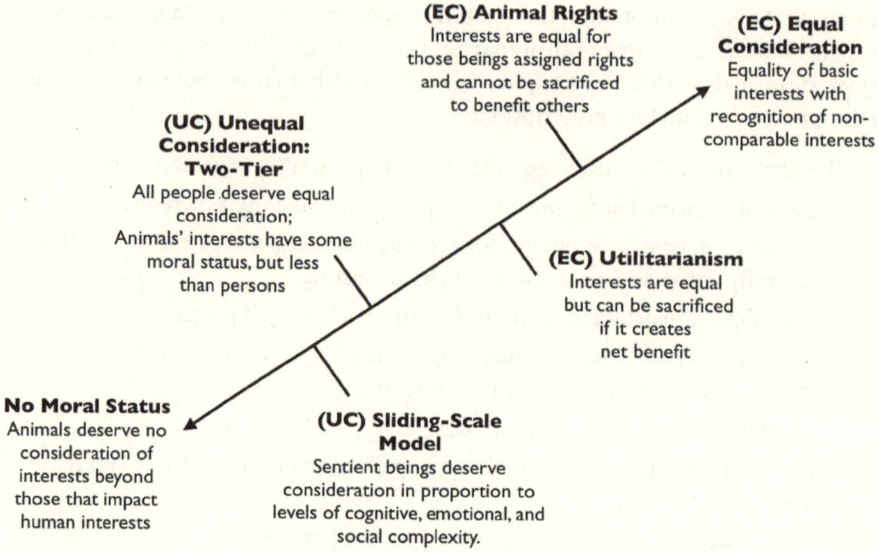
(EC) Animal Rights
Interests are equal for those beings assigned rights and cannot be sacrificed to benefit others
(EC) Equal Consideration
Equality of basic interests with recognition of non-comparable interests
(UC) Unequal Consideration: Two-Tier
All people deserve equal consideration; Animals' interests have some moral status, but less than persons
(EC) Utilitarianism
Interests are equal but can be sacrificed if it creates net benefit
No Moral Status
Animals deserve no consideration of interests beyond those that impact human interests
(UC) Sliding-Scale Model
Sentient beings deserve consideration in proportion to levels of cognitive, emotional, and social complexity.

FIGURE 16. A diagram of selected bioethical positions regarding moral consideration due to animals. Credit: B. Donaldson (adapted from DeGrazia et al. 2010).

David DeGrazia offers a continuum of views (figure 16)—applicable for vertebrate mammals—that exceeds this binary snapshot (2011, 305–13). On one end of the contemporary spectrum is the "no-status" view, meaning that animals' interests have no moral significance unless their injury affects human interests. On the other end of the spectrum is "equal consideration," meaning that all "sentient beings have equal moral status at the level of basic consideration" regardless of species, though individual groups may also have "noncomparable interests" (DeGrazia 2010, 308). An example of this in a biomedical context is that one may extend equal consideration to a mouse for basic interests of pain, fear, suffering, kinship, and autonomy, but also accept that death, when it comes to a mouse, is less traumatic, and hence noncomparable to that of a human (Yeates 2010; Carbone 2004).

Degrazia describes two different standards of equal consideration. (1) Utilitarian views consider the interests of sentient beings equally, but may sacrifice the pleasure/pain interests of some of these beings when doing so benefits the pleasure/pain interests of the majority. For example, capturing and killing ten primates for Ebola research might be justified if it will save a certain number of other animals and people; likewise, a utilitarian view might justify removing a community of people inhabiting a vulnerable ecosystem if doing so would preserve numerous plants, animals, and microorganisms. (2) Animal rights positions strive to assign and protect specific rights to certain living beings, usually those who are most like humans or most entangled in human life. Recent efforts to assign legal rights to nonhuman primates are an example of these efforts. Ideally, these legal rights could not be sacrificed even when it might benefit the majority.

Another point on the continuum is "unequal consideration," in which animals' interests have some moral status, but less than those of persons; this may be a "two-tier theory," in which persons deserve full and equal consideration while other sentient beings require meaningful, but less-than-equal, consideration, or a "sliding-scale model" in which sentient beings deserve consideration in relation to their cognitive, emotional, and social sensitivities (DeGrazia 2011, 308).

DeGrazia asserts that any serious engagement with bioethics must reject the "no status" view, arguing that no real ethical judgments can be made if a target population has already been deemed fundamentally usable and killable without relevant justification. However, the "equal consideration" and "unequal consideration" views offer valid ethical options, according to DeGrazia, that can clarify what is ethically at stake. For instance, those who endorse an animal rights approach of equal consideration might accept observation-based forms of animal research such as Jane Goodall's work with the primates of Tanzania, or might accept medical research that had *direct benefit* to the animal subjects themselves, such as in a veterinary hospital. Conversely, those who advocate unequal consideration may support varying levels of restrictions on animal use. For example, testing on animals for cosmetics and personal products may be deemed unacceptable, as is now the case in the European Union, Norway, Israel, and India, while medical testing is still accepted. Additionally, people who land on different spots of this continuum may find overlapping consensus on increased regulatory and financial support for complete or partial replacement models, such as computer-based models; organs on chips; synthetic skin; or use of animals "down the phylogenetic scale," as in replacing a chimpanzee with a guinea pig or fish (Marks 2012). As DeGrazia cautions, "we must remember that particular benefits from animal studies are only *possible and hoped for*; whereas the harms to animals are typically immediate and certain," and multiple studies have produced no benefit while exacting great harm (2011, 309; original emphasis).

Jain medical professionals in our survey had considerable agreement on their discomfort with animals used in medicine. The majority of respondents agreed that *animal testing* is a form of violence (81%, $n$ = 36), while small minorities disagreed (8%), did not know (3%), had not considered it before (3%), or selected "Other" (6%). Likewise, a majority considered *animal dissection* for educational and/or research purposes a form of violence (61%)—versus only 11% who felt that human dissection constitutes a form of harm—while a slightly more significant minority disagreed (17%), did not know (11%), had not considered it before (6%), or chose "Other" (6%).

Although only one-quarter of respondents had participated in animal testing as part of their medical/healthcare training (25%, $n$ = 36), a larger percentage had either "declined to test on animals, advocated against testing on animals, or suggested alternatives to animal testing in [their] medical/healthcare training or work" (39%, $n$ = 36). In spite of opposition to dissection, nearly three-quarters of respondents had dissected an animal as part their medical training (72%, $n$ = 36).

Jain views will not map easily onto DeGrazia's continuum, especially considering the differences between mendicant and lay perspectives. However, it can still be fruitful to consider resonances, differences, or gaps between these bioethical positions and Jain perspectives. When it comes to animals as *food*, Jains seem to inhabit an equal consideration view more akin to an animal rights position, insofar as they reject the sacrifice of animals even when their flesh might satisfy a human need or desire. Jain lay philosophy actually extends moral consideration further than most "rights" frameworks to include all two- through five-sensed beings regardless of their similarity or difference to humans. As discussed above, Jains diverge in their views on using animals for dairy production, and in practice many lay Jains living in diaspora make some exceptions for honey and eggs.

What about animals in research? Respondents to our survey might land between equal and unequal consideration on DeGrazia's continuum. When asked to elaborate their views on animal testing, introduced above, the greatest number of participants affirmed that animal testing can never be justified (39%, $n = 36$). But many also felt that it may be justified when the results benefit animals themselves (31%) or when the results contribute to the medical advancement of humans (31%). Few felt that animals can ethically be used for safety tests on household products or cosmetics (6%). A greater number of respondents claimed that their view on animal research was more influenced by the Jain tradition (36%) than by their clinical experience or medical education (25%). A minority affirmed that though they personally disagreed with animal testing, it was a necessary part of their occupational training or responsibilities (22%) (figure 17).

Some might argue that the Jain understanding of living beings is so unique that it cannot be translated into bioethical discourse with others who do not share the same worldview. One could also reason that the Jain history of renunciation may justify a retreat from these ethical dilemmas rather than an active exploration of them. However, the medical professionals in our survey already bring their values into ethical dilemmas encountered in their personal and professional lives. When presented the statement "I feel that the Jain framework of one- to five-sensed beings is a meaningful framework to make practical ethical decisions in my *personal* (as opposed to my professional) day-to-day life," the vast majority agreed (83% [strongly agree 36%/agree 47%], $n = 36$) and no participants disagreed. A slightly lower percentage, but still a majority, agreed when asked if the framework of one- to five-sensed living beings "is a meaningful framework to make practical ethical decisions in my *professional* (as opposed to my personal) day-to-day life" (61% [strongly agree 21%/agree 40%], $n = 35$), with others selecting I don't know (6%), I somewhat disagree (11%), I have not considered before (16%), or Other (6%). Likewise, the majority of respondents affirmed that "the Jain vow of nonviolence has influenced my professional decision making in a medical/healthcare context" (80% [strongly agree 36%/agree 44%], $n = 35$).

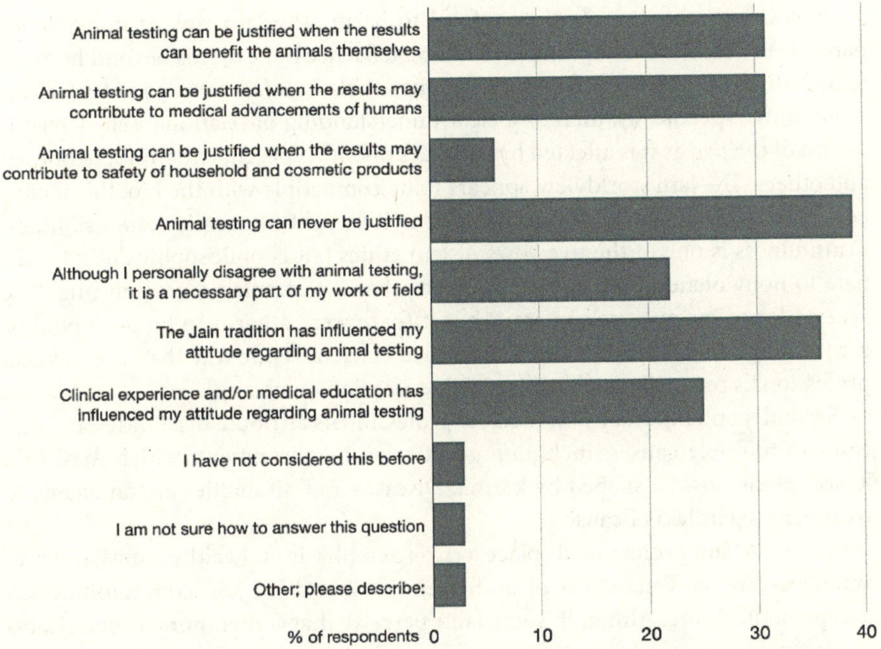


FIGURE 17. Responses of Jain medical professionals ($n = 36$) to the question "Which of the following statements [regarding animal testing] is/are most true for you? Choose all that apply."

We return to Vallely's description at the start of this section of human privilege as characterized by right conduct and restraint toward other living beings. The Jain view of animals in research seems to sit between a pro-animal view that takes the suffering of other beings very seriously and a pro-science view that privileges human endeavors and well-being based on the large number of healthcare professionals within the global Jain community. With a foot in both of these worlds, Jains may be able to uniquely contribute to ethical conversations regarding animal use in medicine, science, and society.[27]

## JAIN PRINCIPLES OF APPLICATION FOR STANDARD MEDICAL CARE

What provisional Jain principles of application can we deduce from this chapter's analysis of Jain philosophy, medical history, and contemporary attitudes in relation to vaccinations and antibiotics, surgery and human dissection, clinical research trials, and animal ethics?

First, the physician-patient relationship in Jainism places a strong emphasis on beneficence-based obligations, entangled autonomy, and contextual truthfulness. Jain medical professionals in our survey privileged the duty to improve the welfare of others more than an absolute refusal to harm. The Jain vow of nonviolence parallels the bioethical imperative of nonmaleficence but extends beyond humans to include all one- through five-sensed beings. Although Jain texts do not reference "autonomy" specifically, there is a clear understanding of relational self-determination of the *jīva* as it is affected by activities of body, speech, and mind, of oneself and others. The Jain worldview appears to be compatible with the bioethical concept of autonomy, but Jains typically define it in light of karmic responsibilities. Truthfulness is one of the five vows of Jain ethics but is philosophically subordinate to nonviolence. In theory, this means that a particular deception might be accepted, not for one's self interest, but if there were a harm to be prevented or great enough benefit to be gained. Informed consent is one way that Jain medical professionals reconcile truth-telling with deceptions such as placebo.

Second, contemporary Jain medical professionals attribute disabilities and diseases to multiple causes, including genetics and environment, which may, to a lesser extent, also be shaped by karma. Diseases and disabilities are amenable to treatment regardless of cause.

Third, lay Jain professionals place a strong emphasis on healthy habits and preventative care, and members of both mendicant and lay Jain communities will accept medical care. Although some Jains perceive that contemporary mendicants eschew medicine in all forms, there are several contemporary examples of at least some mendicants receiving treatment for acute, chronic, or emergency healthcare needs. When lay Jain medical professionals treat mendicants, some describe special considerations such as prescribing nonanimal medications, or medications that do not interfere with periods of fasting.

Fourth, when there is a conflict of interest between one- through five-sensed beings—such as in vaccinations, antibiotics, or surgery—Jain medical professionals will typically privilege the being with the higher number of senses. However, this may not be the case in every situation—such as the end of life—or with every Jain—such as the distinction between mendicants and lay Jains. Regardless, personally forgoing medical care that injures other beings is a meaningful karmic virtue. When the interests of five-sensed beings collide, Jains are more resistant to accepting that harm. The majority of respondents were aware of the background violence endured by one- through five-sensed beings in pharmaceutical ingredients, animal testing, and research trials, and a portion identified opportunities to decrease that harm on other one- through five-sensed beings in medicine.

Fifth, lay Jain medical professionals do consider mental intent in their calculations of harm, reflecting the textual developments whereby mental intent (and/or degree of motivating passion) impacts the karma accrued in a given action. For some, the cost is counted, accepted with regret, and repented for. For others, there may be no perceived harm at all if the intent was to heal.

Sixth, when viewed through a modern bioethical framework, Jain principles for animal ethics seem to parallel an equal consideration approach within the mendicant ideal, including the rejection of sacrifice and the widespread practice of vegetarianism; Jain principles also overlap an unequal consideration approach in other ethical areas based on a sliding scale of one- through five-sensed beings. Although many Jain professionals accept some harms to five-sensed animals in medicine, refusing to harm animals personally, recommending a meat-reduced diet to patients, and prescribing animal-free or non-animal-tested medications are ways to lessen harm.

Finally, Jain medical professionals in our survey frequently consider Jain values alongside clinical, legal, and medical standards, with the majority accepting that tensions may persist between these sources that must be navigated through independent reasoning. Although not all Jains are equally dedicated to Jain ethical practices, beliefs, and ritual activities, the majority of medical professionals in our survey wanted their colleagues to know they were Jain. The Jain values that provided the most guidance for these professionals in clinical settings included nonviolence, non-one-sidedness, and truthfulness, respectively. Jain healthcare providers privileged clinical experience and non-Jain sources in their occupational knowledge, but sought guidance from Jains or Jain sources considerably more than from non-Jain colleagues during ethical dilemmas.

Overall, Jain medical professionals present a positive view of preserving the health and well-being of the body. Our survey reveals that Jain medical professionals retain a sense of Jain identity and ethical orientation in their work, opening the door for possible multicultural discourse and debates in bioethics among Jain studies scholars, practitioners, and clinicians.

# 7

# Calculations of Death

Hundreds of memorials (*niṣidhi*) in the form of carved stones, pillars, images, and temples are found at the Jain pilgrimage site of Śravaṇa Beḷgoḷa in the southern Indian state of Karnataka, commemorating Jains—both mendicant and lay—who pursued a unique form of voluntary religious death through fasting, called *sallekhanā* (also *saṃstāra, samādhi-maraṇa*), considered a wise way of dying in the Jain tradition (Wiley 2009, 201).[1] According to some Digambara sources, at a time of great famine, Candragupta Maurya (320–293 BCE), who founded the Mauryan empire of ancient India, accompanied his Jain preceptor Bhadrabāhu, along with members of the northern Jain mendicant community, from Pāṭaliputra to Śravaṇa Beḷgoḷa after renouncing his kingdom and wealth. In Śravaṇa Beḷgoḷa, Bhadrabāhu performed the ritual of *sallekhanā*, and a pair of rock-cut footprints mark the place where he is thought to have died. After living for another twelve years, Candragupta Maurya is also believed to have died there by fasting unto death (Caillat 1977, 64; Lalwani 1997, 88; Singh 1975, 64–65).

Jain texts deal at great length with the physical certainty of death and its spiritual significance. Like rebirth, death is a critical transition in a much longer journey within the Jain account of life, and maintaining equanimity as death approaches is considered to carry great significance, playing a determinative role in one's future existence.[2] The inevitability of old age and death motivates both mendicants and lay Jains to strive for right worldview and shed their karmic attachments in order to ensure a better rebirth—and perhaps, one day, liberation from the relentless cycles of repeated embodied existence and suffering (ĀS 1.3.1.3).

In this chapter, we explore the Jain understanding of death alongside modern bioethical definitions and legal precedents—primarily in the United States but also globally—that illuminate current tensions and debates in end-of-life issues. We explore the wise and voluntary death of *sallekhanā* in Jainism, and various Jain attitudes toward organ donation, life-sustaining treatment, advance directives, euthanasia, physician aid-in-dying, and refusal of food and fluids. We conclude with five provisional principles of application through which Jain thought and practice might contribute to bioethical discourses and clinical practices related to death and dying well.

## DEFINING DEATH IN THE JAIN TRADITION

The Jain medical treatise *Kalyāṇa-kāraka* describes the current life span—during the present epoch of time (*kali-yuga*)—to be one hundred years, divided into four stages of childhood (*śiśu*), adolescence (*yuvan*), adulthood (*madhyama*), and old age (*vṛddha*) (KK 2.8). Walther Schubring describes the second half of the ten-times-ten years of a normal human life as "a decline of the senses, loquacity, bending of the body, expectation of death, and the last bed" (2000/1962, 150; see also chapter 2). As many as forty-eight kinds of death are described in Jain texts (Settar 2016/1986, xv, 9). We will examine several of these varieties later in the chapter. At present, we will briefly identify key elements for understanding death in the Jain tradition, namely the decisive role of longevity-determining karma, death as a motivation for religious practice, and Jain funeral practices.

### *The Role of the Longevity-Determining Karma*

Death itself is defined in the Jain tradition as the destruction of longevity-determining karma (*āyu-karman*) (Settar 2017/1990, 8). The nondestructive (*aghātiyā*) karma that governs the kind of embodiment a *jīva* will experience is of four types: longevity-determining karma decides life span, while name-, status-, and feeling-determining karmas govern birth form, status, and feelings, respectively (see chapter 2). As indicated in chapter 2, longevity-determining karma is unique in two ways: (1) by determining the life span, it sets the framework for the operation of all the other nondestructive karmas; and (2) unlike the other three nondestructive karmas, which bind to the *jīva* continuously, longevity-determining karma is said to be fixed *only one time* in a given life span, and to come to fruition in the life that immediately follows. The binding of the karma is understood to occur sometime during the last third of life,[3] and without any knowledge on the part of the individual (BhS 7.6§304a–b; Jaini 2001/1979, 126). This doctrine has implications for how an individual Jain may view the later years of their life. As Jaini explains, "by earnestly adhering to the path of proper conduct, a Jaina can hope, during the latter portion of his [*sic*] life, to greatly influence the determination of his āyu-karma and thus the character of his entire next existence" (2001/1979, 126).

The rise of longevity-determining karma energizes the body throughout the duration assigned in the previous life. Death occurs when some event interrupts the ten vitalities (*prāṇa*) responsible for strength, respiration, and the senses (see chapter 2). However, as Wiley emphasizes, the ultimate cause of death is the destruction of longevity-determining karma, which severs the *jīva*'s vitality of life span, allowing another longevity-determining karma to rise in its place (2000a, 307; see chapter 2).

### *Death as Motivation for Religious Practice*

Religious practice is considered the best way to influence one's longevity-determining karma, and Jainism understands death as a motivating factor in strengthening one's dedication to it as well as in initially propelling one onto the spiritual path. A ubiquitous theme in Jain narratives is that of the layperson who realizes the inevitability of decay and death and turns from the obsessive attachments of daily life toward right worldview, knowledge, and conduct. The realization of death can apply to one's present impending demise or to past experiences of death in earlier rebirths. As we described in chapter 6, the *Uttarādhyayana-sūtra* recounts the story of Prince Mṛgāputra, who remembers his gruesome earlier deaths. Having realized that life is full of suffering, including birth, old age, illness, and death, he petitions his parents for permission to leave the royal court and pursue the *śramaṇa* path (US 19.14–15).

Since developing a clear awareness of death and the transitoriness of life is such an important motivation for spiritual efforts, mendicants and laity are urged to see the body as perpetually in decline. To cultivate the proper attitude toward life and death, the Jain practitioners are to meditate regularly on the twelve mental reflections (*anuprekṣā*) of humanity's existence in the universe, including the realizations that we are helpless against death, that everything is transitory, that the cycle of rebirths is full of sorrow, that the body is afflicted, and that ultimately each individual must struggle alone (TS 9.7; Jaini 2001/1979, 248; see chapter 3). These meditative practices (*dhyāna*) are designed to reveal the unsatisfactoriness of embodied life and thereby prompt one to develop a sense of disillusionment with the world and an aspiration to seek a way beyond it (*saṃvega*).[4] Emphasizing that the experience of mortality is faced by each living being alone, with no familial or social relations being able to prevent death and suffering, is aimed at reminding individuals to seize the lifetime at hand, renounce their attachments, and strive to transcend the cycle of rebirths (US 13.22–23). Stated succinctly in the *Ācārāṅga-sūtra*, "Knowing birth and death (*jāti-maraṇa*), one should firmly walk on the path (*saṃkramaṇa*) [to liberation]" (ĀS 1.2.3.4).

### *Jain Funeral Rituals*

Anne Vallely states that funerary rituals were not part of traditional Jainism, possibly because of the belief that rebirth of the deceased in a new life-form happens almost immediately (see chapters 2 and 5; see Jaini 1991b, 189), but that many lay Jains now nevertheless practice them (Vallely 2011, 70–71; see also Sangave 1959, 360–61). Robert Williams asserts that textual sources do not reference Jain funerary rites before the fifteenth century (1963, xxiv; see also Flügel 2010, 46–49). Phyllis Granoff, however, argues that "medieval Jain religious practices at least in so far as they concern the dead and the dying did not deviate as sharply as has been thought from Hindu practices of the same period: Jains and Hindus alike prepared people for dying, ensured them the best possible rebirth through rituals conducted on their behalf and honored them by building them memorial monuments" (1994, 183; see also Dundas 2011; Flügel 2010, 46–47, and Flügel 2018, 123–25). Schubring writes that ordinarily the dead bodies were cremated (2000/1962, 290).[5]

Peter Flügel points out that apart from examples in narrative literature, comprehensive prescriptions for conducting funerary rituals and related ceremonies for deceased Jain mendicants do not exist in any text. He lists seven different rituals and ceremonies that are included in the mortuary practices for mendicants: (1) voluntary death (*sallekhanā*), (2) removal of the dead body (*nirharaṇa*),[6] (3) funeral ceremonies in relation to cremation (*dāha-saṃskāra*), (4) collection of the bone relics (*asthi-saṃcayana*), (5) disposal of the bone relics (*asthi-visarjana*) or construction of a funerary monument (*stupa/samādhi*),[7] (6) commemoration (*smṛti*), and (7) veneration (*vandanā*) and/or worship (*pūjā*) (2018, 120–22). In contrast to the funerary rituals for laity, funerals for mendicants have a celebratory character, since it is believed that the deceased has moved on to a good rebirth in the heavenly realm (125–26).

Contemporary Jain laity, Flügel notes, observe a broad variety of funerary rites "that represent variations of Brāhmaṇical custom" (2010, 60; see also Sangave 1959, 361). In his extensive sociological account of Jains in India in the mid-twentieth century, Vilas Sangave describes the diversity of regional funerary practices wherein some Jain communities may go immediately to the temple while others wait for various durations; some families may observe an "unclean" period of ten to thirteen days after the death of a relative before having a social gathering to commemorate the dead; and some may practice monthly or annual memorials while others do not (1959, 360–62). Flügel writes that the dead body of a common Jain layperson is "carried in a lying posture, covered from head to toe by a shroud, by male family members to the funeral pyre, on a simple bier (*siḍī* or *sīḍī*) constructed out of bamboo sticks that are laid out in the form of a ladder, as its name indicates (*siḍī* = *sīṛhī*), and is cremated with slight variations in a standard modern Hindu fashion" (2018, 125).[8] According to the "Guidelines for Healthcare Providers Interacting with Patients of the Jain Religion and Their Families," prepared by the Metropolitan Chicago Healthcare Council, Jain postmortem practices (perhaps in this case particularly as observed by the US Jain communities) involve washing and dressing the body after death, accompanied by prayers and possibly a lit lamp in the room with the body of the deceased. The process of cremation may be open to the community (2002).[9]

Christopher Chapple explains that these various social rites "are not performed for the benefit of the dead but to encourage devotion to Jaina ritual and ethical observances" among the surviving community (2010, 205). As indicated above, counterexamples exist, however, and Granoff writes that "both texts and inscriptions indicate that Jains in fact both prayed for the dead and to the dead" (Granoff 1992b; see also Flügel 2018, 129). Maintaining various forms of relationships with the dead certainly seems to have a place in Jain communities, and is considered potentially beneficial for the parties involved. For example, even approving (*anumodana*) of the spiritual path of the deceased mendicant can, according to Flügel, accrue karmic merit. "Like the obligatory *kāyostarga* meditation, performed by mendicants after abandonment of the corpse of a deceased monk or nun, cremation rites performed by the laity are believed to offer opportunities for self-transformation, if they indeed result in an intensification of the personal realization of the Jaina perspective on the transience of worldly existence in contrast to the immortality of the soul" (2018, 128, see also 122). This shows that just as the Jain path invites discipline and restraint in preparing for one's own death, how one responds to the death of others is part of religious practice and may therefore be a valuable opportunity for spiritual advancement.

## DEFINING DEATH IN MODERN MEDICINE

The definition of death remains an enduring dilemma in biomedical ethics. Prior to the advent of mechanical ventilation in the 1950s, death was determined by the cessation of respiration and heartbeat. This heart-lung definition could be detected by checking the pulse and observing the breath; if these ceased, the brain and other organs stopped functioning in quick succession.

### *Determining Death and the Dead Donor Rule*

The development of the positive-pressure mechanical ventilator allowed physicians to maintain respiration and thus circulation, supporting patients as they recuperated from disease or injury. This technology also preserved vital signs in patients unlikely to recover, as in the case of traumatic brain injury, creating new dilemmas. If a patient is alive due to circulatory support—even if their brain has suffered irreversible injury—are they dead or alive? This question is critical, since removing organs for transplant or withdrawing life-sustaining treatments from a living patient would constitute killing, a grave breach of a physician's oath to "do no harm" (Bendorf et al. 2013). If those patients are dead, procuring organs and removing support pose no moral hurdle.

Consequently, ventilation technology necessitated a revised definition of death within the global medical community. In 1968, an ad hoc committee of the Harvard Medical School issued a report that introduced the criterion for "brain death." The report detailed a series of tests to identify the permanent cessation of functioning throughout the *whole brain*, what they called "irreversible coma." According to the committee, if a patient receives this diagnosis, "death is to be declared and then the respirator turned off" ("A Definition of Irreversible Coma" 1968, 338). "Brain death" was to be considered "death," even if heart and lung function was maintained mechanically.

These guidelines were formalized in the United States through the Uniform Determination of Death Act (1980), drafted by the National Conference of Commissioners on Uniform State Laws, and that model legislation was soon after published in a report developed by the President's Commission for the Study of Ethical Problems in Medicine and Biomedical and Behavioral Research ("Defining Death" 1981). In addition to retaining the heart-lung criteria, the Uniform Determination of Death Act stated that death could also be determined by "irreversible cessation of all functions of the entire brain, *including the brain stem*" (1980, 5; emphasis added). To clarify clinical diagnostics, the American Academy of Neurology (AAN) released a checklist for physicians in 1995—reaffirmed in 2010, 2014, and 2017—to standardize the determination of death by cessation of the whole-brain and brainstem criteria (Wijdicks et al. 2010).

The Uniform Determination of Death, along with the AAN criteria to assess cessation of the whole brain plus the brainstem, remains the standard in the United States and most European countries. The United Kingdom developed its own formulation in 1976, designating death of the *brainstem* alone as sufficient to terminate breathing and consciousness (Oram and Murphy 2011). India and Canada similarly use brainstem criteria; physicians in these countries can declare death without "whole-brain" confirmation (Dhanwate 2014; Gardiner et al. 2012; Smith 2012).

Although these two different criteria seem relatively straightforward, the category of "brain death" continues to generate controversy. At the bedside, many families are unclear on the meaning of brain death as it relates to death, especially when a patient's body appears to breathe, feels warm to the touch, and may display physical movements or vocalizations ("Controversies" 2009). Some clinicians and critics have persistently disputed whether brain death, in fact, constitutes the death of a human person (Verheijde and Rady 2014). Additionally, organ transplantation protocol requires that a patient be pronounced dead—known as "the Dead Donor Rule"—before organs are procured, though some physicians believe that this diagnosis can be made prior to whole-brain death, thereby increasing transplant success (Sade 2011). Perhaps most importantly, rare cases of patients recovering after being misdiagnosed with brain death, or being diagnosed too quickly after injury, invite a reconsideration of the consensus (Greenberg 2014). In an attempt to standardize the guidelines for determining brain death, the World Health Organization held several forums and published "International Guidelines for the Determination of Death" (2012), which establish minimum clinical standards, as well as additional test protocols, for assessing brain function.

An important lingering debate centers on the "higher-brain death" criteria (Smith 2012). Distinct from whole-brain or brainstem criteria, which identify death as the loss of an organism's integrated bodily function, some advocates claim that loss of the "higher" cerebral cortex—the part of the brain that enables our sense of *personhood*—should be sufficient to determine death. In cases of traumatic brain injury, the portion of one's brain that corresponds to waking awareness, speech, vision, and motor function has been seriously damaged, but the parts of the hypothalamus and brainstem that maintain regulative functions—such as sleeping and waking cycles, body temperature, breathing, digestion, blood pressure, and heart rate—remain intact. In this "vegetative state" (increasingly called "unresponsive wakefulness syndrome") the markers of personhood are difficult, or impossible, to discern, leading some to equate such a state with death. The state can be temporary or persistent. In a "persistent vegetative state," the body is technically alive but one's personality and ability to engage in the world are nonfunctional, creating a situation in which, as described by philosopher Jeff McMahan, "you could be survived by your organism" (2006, 48).

In spite of arguments to include higher-brain death in the medical definition of death, the neurological criteria of whole-brain death remain standard in most countries, and brainstem death in a select few. Yet the definition of death is not only a medical decision, but an interdisciplinary question (Bagheri 2007; Lewis et al. 2018). As bioethicists Charles Culver and Bernard Gert have argued, "defining death is primarily a philosophical task" (2006, 313), for which medicine requires cultural and religious insights to more adequately engage our collective understanding of what constitutes a meaningful life of the body and mind—and, subsequently, what constitutes its death.

### *Contemporary Jain Views on the Biomedical Definitions of Death*

In our survey of Jain medical professionals, when asked, "Which do you feel is the most adequate definition of death? Choose those that apply," the greatest number of participants chose heart and lung criteria (44%, $n = 36$), followed by whole-brain death, including integrated function of the cortex and brainstem (33%); and higher-brain death, including loss of cognitive function in the cortex (19%). Still, there was also considerable ambiguity, with a significant minority of participants selecting "I need more information to adequately understand these definitions of death" (25%), "I have not considered this before" (25%), or "Other; please describe" (11%). Explanatory comments included the following:

> "[W]e don't know for sure."
> "Depends on the decision for which you need the definition."
> "Death of the body or death of the soul?"

Moreover, when asked if they believed that "someone diagnosed to be in a vegetative state (or unresponsive wakefulness syndrome) should be considered dead," the majority of Jain medical professionals felt that such patients should not be presumed dead (42%, $n = 36$), while smaller minorities felt they should be considered dead (25%), had not considered it before (25%), or did not know (8%). Their view of the vegetative state/unresponsive wakefulness syndrome was more informed by respondents' medical/healthcare education (33%, $n$ = 36) than by clinical experience (19%) or the Jain tradition (14%). A significant minority felt that clinical experience, medical education, and the Jain tradition influenced them equally in their view of a persistent vegetative state (17%).

Relatedly, when asked, "Do you feel that cognitive abilities are synonymous with consciousness, that is, if one loses cognitive abilities, they have lost consciousness?," the majority disagreed (56%, $n$ = 36), while fewer respondents agreed (14%) or had not considered it before (25%). When asked if the Jain tradition influenced their view on the relationship between cognitive abilities and consciousness, respondents selected Yes (42%, $n$ = 36), No (44%), or Not applicable (11%).

Although longevity-determining karma was not an option on the survey, none of the participants referred to the exhaustion of karma within their comments, which could suggest that this technical aspect of death in the Jain tradition may not be widely discussed, or may not be perceived as in conflict with medical definitions. At the same time, not all respondents were satisfied with the provided survey options to capture their understanding of death.

### *Contemporary Jain Views on Organ Donation*

While Jain professionals varied in their definitions of death, the majority of participants viewed organ donation from dead donors favorably. Nearly 64 percent of participants ($n$ = 35) were registered donors, and over 90 percent of those donors lived in opt-in countries; 11% had elected not to opt in, while a small minority either did not know if they were donors (6%) or had not considered the issue before (9%). When asked, "Does the Jain tradition influence your view on whether or not to donate your organs?," participants responded Yes (44%, $n$ = 36), No (47%), or Not applicable (8%). Asked to describe their "prime reason either for being an organ donor or for not being a donor," pro-donation respondents' answers ($n$ = 24) fell along three primary lines: (1) helping another individual (with no mention of family ties); (2) a lesser desire to serve medical students and the advancement of medicine; and (3) a desire for one's material body to be of use after death (figure 18). One answer equated the decision of organ donation with "being Jain," while another considered it a karmically beneficial act of compassion. Anti-donation responses ($n$ = 3) included going against one's conscience, violating a dead body, and uncertainty of the karmic ramifications (figure 18).

The positive orientation to organ donation among Jain medical professionals is significant, given that massive organ donation shortages persist worldwide (Beard and Osterkamp 2013) and organ donations from ethnic minorities are especially needed (Sharif 2013). Because of shortages in the United States, for example, from 2003 to 2013 the number of patients on a waiting list for kidney transplantation doubled to approximately one hundred thousand patients, with wait times extended to

## Pro-donation Reasoning

- "to help someone"
- "to help someone in need; charity of life"
- "to help [a] needy person"
- "it will help another human being—will save or improve his/her life"
- "I [would] like to help living [people] as well as the dying and dead"
- "something I can give to someone in need"
- "helping someone in need"
- "my organs will be of use to another"
- "help someone even after I die"
- "I would like to help others if I can"
- "help other fellow beings"
- "giving somebody a better life after Soul has left it"
- "potential to save other lives"
- "it benefits the recipient"
- "[offering] the use of my organ for someone else"
- "helps the medical community advance"
- "help medical students"
- "to be of use"
- "my body is useless to me after death; it should serve a purpose to others"
- "life serving life; if my organs can sustain other life, why not?"
- "my organs are only useful to the slow decay ... of the environment if I do not donate [them]"
- "the body will be cremated and if the organs can improve someone's quality of life it should be donated; consider it a *karuna daan* [*karuṇā-dāna* = gift of compassion]"
- "being Jain"
- "a dead person has no soul, so the organ donated is not any violence"

## Anti-donation Reasoning

- "I don't want to be an organ donor; my conscious[ness] won't permit [it]"
- "it could be source of violation to the dead body"
- "I don't know that life that will survive due to my organ donation will lead to a life [that] increases more karmas or brings peace to other souls and lessens karma"

FIGURE 18. Responses of Jain medical professionals ($n = 27$) to the question "What is your prime reason either for being an organ donor or for not being an organ donor?"

4.5 years; consequently, nearly five thousand patients die while awaiting a kidney transplant from a dead donor every year (Wu et al. 2017, 1287). Certain studies also show that religious concerns can negatively impact decisions to donate. In their research on organ donation and religion, Michael Oliver and colleagues describe various conflicting religious commitments: the importance of altruism in Islam and Judaism competing with requirements for burying a complete body within twenty-four hours after death, the value of compassion in Buddhism competing with the possibility of disrupting lingering consciousness that may persist for days after death, and the requirement for an intact body within Hindu funerary rites competing with a strong emphasis on selfless giving, among others (2011). While the reasoning for organ donation among Jain survey respondents is not uniform, the overwhelmingly positive orientation to the practice suggests that Jain medical professionals have fewer competing values at play.

Whether other lay Jains also view organ donation positively requires further investigation. A 2013 report from Mumbai shows that 85 percent of corneas donated for transplant and 95 percent of skin donations came from the state of Gujarat, namely from a community of Gujaratis from Kutch, and from the Jain community (Debroy 2013). The local liaison for soliciting donations, Kusum Vira, credited the communities for their positive perspective on donation, describing their "religion-backed ideology that perceived donation as an ultimate form of charity" (Debroy 2013). One possible factor for the positive view of donation may be the fact that rebirth happens almost instantaneously in Jainism, so as soon as the *jīva* leaves the body, only the nonliving body remains (see chapters 2 and 5). Investigating other reasons for this communal support may provide insights for efforts to increase donations among religious communities in India and abroad.

## VARIETIES OF DEATH IN THE JAIN TRADITION

As noted above, Jains have detailed at least forty-eight different kinds of death,[10] several of which we will consider here according to (1) timeliness and (2) manner of death.

### *Timely or Premature Death*

Jain texts state that deaths can be timely or untimely. A timely death (*kāla-mṛtyu*) refers to a fully experienced life span that is exhausted at an appropriate time, while an untimely death (*akāla-mṛtyu*) depicts a premature end (Settar 2017/1990, 9). Wiley explains that in the case of human beings in our part of the cosmos, longevity-determining karma can be bound tightly or loosely depending on whether an individual has strong or weak mental effort/resolve (*adhyavasāya/adhyavasāna*) at the time of death. A strong mental effort/resolve causes this specific kind of karma to bind tightly so that the determined amount (rather than length; see chapter 2) of life (*sthiti*) is *not subject to reduction* in any circumstances (*anapavartanīya-āyu*), and, thus, life cannot end prematurely. A weak mental effort/determination results in loosely bound longevity-determining karma, the duration of which *may be subject to reduction* in certain cases (*apavartanīya-āyu*) (2021). Wiley notes that most mendicant authorities assert that all beings born in the present epoch in this part of the cosmos bind longevity-determining karma that is subject to reduction, meaning that it is always possible for death to be untimely (2000a, 49–52, 310–11).[11]

### *Manner of Death*

There are several ways to classify the different manners of death listed in Jain texts (Settar 2017/1990, 15). For our purposes, we will examine forms of death shared by all beings, as well as deaths considered wise or unwise and involuntary or voluntary.

The moment of death that each of us will experience when our body ceases to function is called *tadbhava-maraṇa*, representing that which we ordinarily refer to as "death" (Wiley 2000a, 312). In the Jain tradition, this event is followed by rebirth into another body. Each of the forty-eight kinds of death is considered *tadbhava-maraṇa* (Settar 2017/1990, 9, 11). The moment of death can occur due to the presence (*upakrama*) of efficient external causes (*nimitta*) or without them (*nirupakrama*) (Wiley 2000a, 49–52; see chapter 2).[12] For example, an efficient external cause might be disease, being killed with a weapon, or falling victim to a natural disaster. This kind of death could be considered timely or untimely. As discussed above, tightly bound longevity-determining karma ensures that life can never end prematurely, and that holds even in the presence of external efficient causes (Wiley 2000a, 49–50).

Every being will also undergo death as a slow loss of vitality that does not reach the level of awareness. This continuous process of perpetual death is called *nitya-maraṇa*, also known as *āvīci-maraṇa*, meaning death like the disappearance of a wave. The Digambara text *Bhagavatī-ārādhanā* (Pkt. *Bhagavaī-ārāhaṇa*; first to second centuries CE) written by Śivārya (also called Śivakoṭi)—one of the primary Jain treatises devoted to the subject of death—describes this gradual form of dying with a story: The Cakravartin emperor Sanatkumāra is visited by heavenly beings who inform him of his approaching death. When he asks how they could perceive his loss of *āyu*, the guests fill a bowl with water and dip in a fly whisk to sprinkle water on the crowd gathered there. With each dip of the whisk the water level lowers, though so gradually that none can detect the decrease during the process. "Just as the loss of water cannot be assessed by observing the movement of the whisk," they explain, "the loss of lifespan cannot be realized from the tick of every second of time" (Settar 2017/1990, 9; Wiley 2000a, 312–13).

As indicated above, the manner of death is also classified as unwise or wise, as well as voluntary (*sakāma-maraṇa*) or involuntary (*akāma-maraṇa*). We will discuss these kinds of death in the next three sections.

*Unwise Voluntary and Involuntary Death.* S. Settar states that unwise deaths (*bāla-maraṇa*) can be voluntary or involuntary (2017/1990, 10–11). An unwise *voluntary* death is described as death conditioned by a desire to die (*icchā-pravṛtta*). These deaths are usually violent in nature. They result in the accumulation of inauspicious kinds of karma, and may lead to a low type of rebirth (Wiley 2000a, 329; Jaini 2001/1979, 228). The *Bhagavatī-sūtra* describes twelve forms of unwise death, including jumping from a mountain or tree, drowning oneself, self-immolation,[13] ingesting poison, killing oneself by using a weapon, hanging oneself, and allowing oneself to be eaten by vultures (BhS 2.1§118a; Wiley 2000a, 329; see also ĀS 2.10.13; cf. ĀS 1.7.4.2). The *Sthānāṅga-sūtra* describes a similar list of deaths condemned by Mahāvīra (SthS 2.4.411). All of these deaths are considered untimely not only because they prematurely exhaust longevity-determining karma, but also because the body is terminated while it is not yet a hindrance to spiritual progress (Wiley 2000a, 329).

According to Settar, an unwise *involuntary* death (*anicchā-pravṛtta*) involves the desire to prolong life or active resistance to death when it comes (2017/1990, 10). Wiley notes that this kind of death might be unavoidable in the case of deaths of very young persons (2002a, 330). We have not been able to determine whether dying in an unwise and involuntary manner primarily concerns mental dispositions at the time of death or whether it is also associated with self-directed physical violence. Wiley notes that this type of death is not accompanied by violent acts (2002a, 330). She classifies the first four kinds of unwise death that are listed in the *Bhagavatī-sūtra* before the types mentioned above (BhS 2.1§118a) as involuntary and interprets them as reflecting mental states at the time of dying. These are (1) "weariness" (*valan-maraṇa*) (Deleu 1996/1970, 89), which is variously explained as "death while straying from restraint, of one whose mind is attached because it is afflicted by the condition of being desirous of enjoyment or pleasure" (Wiley 2002a, 330–31, explaining Abhayadevasūri's commentary), "to die after abandoning ascetic-discipline in a disturbed state of mind due to pain caused by afflictions" (Bothra 2004, 160; see also Deo 1954–1955, 202), and death "in consequence of moral weakness" (Caillat 1977, 49); (2) "incapacity" (*vaśārta-maraṇa*) (Deleu 1996/1970, 89), which is described as being "afflicted by the power of the senses" (Wiley 2002a, 331), "to die after succumbing to indulgence in mundane sensual pleasures" (Bothra 2004, 160; see also Deo 1954–1955, 202), and "physical weakness" (Caillat 1977, 49); (3) "an interior dart" (*antaḥśalya-maraṇa*) (Deleu 1996/1970, 89), which is explained as "death of one . . . who is subject to transgressions" (Wiley 2002a, 331), and as dying "without confession" (Caillat 1977, 49; see also Deo 1954–1955, 203); and finally, (4) "the desire for a certain rebirth" (*tadbhava-maraṇa*) (Deleu 1996/1970, 89), which according to Wiley may include a wish to be reborn either as a human or a heavenly being (2002a, 331). S.B. Deo, on the other hand, explains it as the death that occurs "at the time of which the person does a karman [i.e., action] due to which he [*sic*] gets the same rebirth" (1954–1955, 202; cf. Bothra 2004, 160). In contrast to Wiley's interpretation, Colette Caillat, describes all these as conditions in consequence of which individuals kill themselves and so highlights them as causes rather than only mental states at the time of death (49; see also Settar 2017/1990, 10, cf. 11). Jozef Deleu similarly designates the first three kinds of death on the list as "suicide"; however, it must be noted that he also defines them as voluntary rather than involuntary (1996/1970, 89–90). In any case, death in these "unwise" circumstances can also result in an undesirable rebirth, since they do not attract the auspicious kinds of longevity-determining karma (Wiley 2000a, 330).

*Wise Voluntary Death:* Sallekhanā. Wise voluntary death (*paṇḍita-maraṇa*) within Jainism is achieved through fasting (*anaśana*) and is today often referred to as *saṃthāra* (Skt. *saṃstāra*, lit. "deathbed") or *samādhi-maraṇa* (lit. "meditative death") by Śvetāmbaras, and as *sallekhanā* (also *saṃlekhanā*, Pkt. *saṃlehaṇā*) by

Digambaras. The term *sallekhanā* derives from the Sanskrit verbal root *likh-*, with the prefix *sam-*, meaning "to scratch out or scrape." The "scratching out" refers to the thinning of the physical body through the restriction of nourishment, as well as of the karmic body through the restriction of the passions (Wiley 2000a, 316; Williams, 1963, 166). Chapple describes his experience observing this fast in 1989 while visiting a Jain university in Ladnun, Rajasthan. During his stay, an eighty-year-old nun of the Terāpanthī Śvetāmbara sect by the name of Kesharji had taken the vow of fasting unto death twenty-eight days prior, after being unsuccessfully treated for advanced kidney disease. The community of nuns—as well as the Terāpanthī leader Ācārya Tulsī—had gathered to encourage Kesharji on her fast in a calm but joyful gathering that venerated the nun's life and efforts toward a peaceful death, which took place twelve days after Chapple's visit (1993, 104–6). Other scholars have also witnessed or recounted various aspects of this kind of ritual death within the Jain community (Braun 2008; Deo 1954–1955, 420, fn. 217, 562, fn. 433; Jaini 2001/1979, 1; Renou and Renou 1951; Vallely 2002a, 132–36).

Three kinds of wise voluntary deaths are listed in Śvetāmbara and Digambara texts: (1) fasting to death with the care and companionship of others (*bhakta-pratyākhyāna-maraṇa*), during which mendicants support the practitioner's resolve to forgo nourishment (*bhakta*) by telling religious stories of other exemplars, reciting prayers, and uplifting the vows; (2) fasting to death by aiding oneself but without others (*iṅgiṇī-maraṇa* or *itvara-maraṇa*) with limited movement allowed; and (3) fasting to death without any movement or self-aid (*prāyopagamana-maraṇa*) (Settar 2017/1990, 12–13; Soni 2014, 6–8; Wiley 2000a, 314). The *Ācārāṅga-sūtra* and the *Bhagavatī-ārādhanā* describe all three of these deaths; the *Bhagavatī-sūtra* mentions the first and third (ĀS 1.7.5.1–1.7.8.25;[14] BhĀ 28; BhS 2.1§118a; see also US 5.32).[15]

In the early texts, these deaths are prescribed only for mendicants who have had years of experience practicing vows and austerities and, thus, possess right knowledge of the relationship between the *jīva* and transient body, and control over the passions (Caillat 1977, 53–54, 57–60).[16] However, later texts tend to be more flexible with regard to the requirement of lengthy prior ascetic training (62–64). For example, while still demanding "preparatory purification," Caillat observes that "preparation for death is milder" and "considerably shortened" in the Śvetāmbara *Prakīrṇaka-sūtra*s (Pkt. *Paiṇṇa-sutta*) (1977, 63).[17] "They do not insist on the necessity of a hard, lifelong training; this, apparently, could be replaced by the ceremonial which they teach" (62). The *Prakīrṇaka-sūtra*s include several texts explaining preparations for death, including how to renounce food, maintain consciousness, and assume the vows (Kamptz 1929; Wiley 2009, xxiv). The *Bhagavatī-ārādhanā* acknowledges a possibility of attaining a "perfect death," even without prior spiritual preparation; however, it emphasizes that such occasions are not standard and sometimes even interprets them as a result of previously accumulated auspicious karma (Soni 2014, 3–4)

Later texts, further, open the practice to laypeople. Already in the early Śvetāmbara canon some laypeople are seen as surpassing mendicants in control as death approaches (US 5.19–32), and narratives of laity fasting unto death are found in the canonical *Upāsaka-daśāḥ* (Caillat 1977, 56–57; Jaini 2001/1979, 233–40; Wiley 2000a, 318). Caillat writes that with regard to fasting unto death, *Prakīrṇaka-sūtras* "apparently make no basic difference between the lay-follower and the monk, whose case they examine jointly" (1977, 62). In line with this, Umāsvāti states in the *Śrāvaka-prajñapti* that the practice of fasting unto death is not restricted to mendicants (Williams 1963, 166), and in his *Tattvārtha-sūtra*, authoritative for all Jains, he asserts that at the end of life the householder undergoes *saṃlekhanā* ($TS^{Dig}$ 7.22[18]). In the Digambara tradition, the *Bhagavatī-ārādhanā*, cited above, explains various attainments (*ārādhanā*) that are available at the end of life for both mendicants and laity (BhĀ 2; Soni 2014, 2). Williams notes that texts on lay conduct (*śrāvaka-ācāra*) describe the fast unto death as a supplement to the twelve lay vows, with some Digambaras incorporating it into the twelfth vow (1963, 166).[19] Among the Śvetāmbara texts on lay conduct, Williams points out Devagupta's *Navapada-prakaraṇa* (eleventh century CE) as the only one that treats *sallekhanā* in detail, describing the three forms of voluntary death permissible for a Jain (1963, 166).[20]

Additionally, later Jain texts introduce the importance of a teacher overseeing the process of fasting unto death (Caillat 1977, 115; Dundas 2002a, 180). Jaini points out that today, only mendicants are usually allowed to undertake the fast unto death on their own accord, whereas mendicants administer the vow to laity, except in cases of emergency (Jaini 2001/1979, 231; Wiley 2000a, 319, fn. 45). "Jainas are quick to point out," Jaini says, "the difference between such a practice and that of common suicide, wherein a person tells no one of his [*sic*] deed and commits it in secret" (2001/1979, 231). The role of the mendicant who administers the vow is to assess whether the lay aspirant possesses sufficient control and spiritual level to undertake the fast (232; Wiley 2000a, 324, 326–28).

Fasting unto death is believed to bring positive spiritual results. While the earliest canonical sources indicate that "there might be no future rebirth" for mendicants who pursue such a mode of dying (Wiley 2000a, 316), the *Bhagavatī-sūtra* states that ending one's life with a wise kind of death reduces the length of wandering in *saṃsāra* (BhS 2.1§118a; see also Caillat 1977, 63). In one specific story, Mahāvīra suggests that the person who had fasted unto death would be first reborn as a heavenly being and then attain liberation as a human being in a part of the cosmos where liberation is always possible (BhS 2.1§120a; see also Jaini 2001/1979, 240). The author of the *Bhagavatī-ārādhanā*, Śivāraya, promises liberation in seven or eight births for those who, even once, die in a state of equanimity (*samādhi*) (Jain 2015, 21).

*Sallekhanā* can be undertaken by Jain mendicants and laity only in certain circumstances, and the process requires several specific steps. In the early canonical sources, mendicants are advised to pursue fasting unto death when they can no longer maintain their vows or austerities, being too weak due to factors such as disease (Wiley 2000a, 314). The *Ratnakaraṇḍa-śrāvakācāra*, a text on lay conduct, authored by Samantabhadra, describes the valid circumstances as calamity (*upasarga*), severe famine (*durbhikṣā*), old age (*jarā*), or terminal illness (*niḥpratīkāra-rujā*) (RŚ 5.1). With old age are associated physical weakness, blindness, the inability to walk, senility, and so on (Wiley 2000a, 322). Samantabhadra details the unfolding process of *sallekhanā* by, first, giving up all attachments and possessiveness as well as desire and enmity. The aspirant then confesses all transgressions (*ālocanā*), and forgives friends and family for any wrongdoings while also seeking forgiveness from them (*kṣāmaṇā*) (RŚ 5.3–5). At that point the individual begins a ritual fast in three stages that involve the gradual reduction, first of solid food, then of fatty liquids (*snigdha-pāna*) such as milk or yogurt, then of acidic liquids (*khara-pāna*) such as juice, until finally even water is abandoned (RŚ 5.6–7; see also Jaini 2001/1979, 230–31 and Wiley 2000a, 320–21). It was typically at the water-only stage, when death seems imminent, that a lay aspirant would take the great vows, including the vow of unlimited fasting, since traditionally these vows could not be rescinded once taken (RŚ 5.4; Jaini 2001/1979, 231; Wiley 2000a, 321). The aspirant should then keep the mind focused on the *pañca-namaskāra-mantra* and the five supreme beings (*pañca-parameṣṭhin*) until the arrival of death (see chapter 3).[21]

Texts of both traditions list five violations (*aticāra*) of the vow of *sallekhanā*. These are (1) desire for rebirth as a human being (*iha-loka-āśaṃsā*); (2) desire for rebirth as a heavenly being (*para-loka-āśaṃsā*); (3) desire to continue living (*jivita-āśaṃsā*); (4) desire to die (*maraṇa-āśaṃsā*); and (5) desire for sensual pleasures (*kāma-bhoga-āśaṃsā*; Dig. *nidāna*) (Jaini 2001/1979, 230–31; Williams 1963, 170; see also TS$^{Dig}$ 9.33[22]). Samantabhadra lists the first one as fear (*bhaya*) (RŚ 5.8). Franklin Edgerton locates these Jain restrictions in opposition to the spiritual value of dying wishes in certain Hindu and Buddhist practices (1927, 226–32). In the Jain tradition, Edgerton asserts, "you can wish for anything to which your ascetic practice entitles you, nothing more," without paying a high karmic price (229).

Giving in to desires is considered a waste of previous religious practice. According to the *Bhagavatī-ārādhanā*, maintaining the mastery of worldview, knowledge, conduct, and asceticism (*ārādhanā*) has tremendous power at life's end; a lifelong path of austere conduct will be in vain if one fails, while a lifelong path of mistakes will be transformed into perfection for one who succeeds (BhĀ 15, 17; see also Jaini 2001/1979, 232–33; Wiley 2000a, 325; Williams 1963, 172). Hemacandra's *Triṣaṣṭiśalākāpuruṣa-caritra* give several examples of people falling to the temptation of desires, frequently made as wishes to vanquish one's enemy.[23] For example, King Parvata, after a great loss on the battlefield to his rival King Vindhyaśakti, becomes a mendicant under a Jain teacher. Although he performs extremely difficult austerities, Parvata secretly wishes to kill Vindhyaśakti in a future rebirth, undermining the benefits of his restraints. After fasting unto death, Parvata is reborn as a heavenly being; however, the text describes his dying desire as bartering "his great penance . . . like bartering a jewel for chaff" (TC 4.2.185–88, trans. Johnson). Although these wishes can be made or resisted at any time during life, psychological longing during the approach of death is considered particularly detrimental to the equanimity required for a wise death, as indicated above, and both mendicants and laity are instructed to avoid such violations.

Jain texts establish that animals are also able to undergo a wise death. A well-known story among Jains is that of Mahāvīra's encounter with the angry snake Caṇḍakauśika, born a serpent because of his persistent rage in previous lives. After unsuccessfully trying to strike and kill Mahāvīra, the Jina helps the snake remember his past existences. Upon recollecting these past lives of anger, the story concludes, the snake's "heart changed and the seeds of equanimity for all beings began to sprout in him. He sat motionless and performed *santhara* [i.e., *sallekhanā*]" (Vallely 2002a, 35–37).[24] Another prominent tale describes one of Mahāvīra's previous lives as a lion, a karmic consequence of an earlier life in which he viciously killed a lion. One day, while hunting, the lion (future Mahāvīra) was eating prey he had just killed when two Jain monks came upon the scene and, sensing that the lion was amenable to their teaching, conveyed to him the truth of nonviolence and karma, reminding him of his previous lives. The lion recollected his past existences and, moved by the Jain teaching, assumed the minor vows. He then undertook the voluntary fast unto death, and was later reborn as the twenty-fourth Jina, Mahāvīra (Jaini 2010d, 262–63; De Clercq 2013, 148–49).[25]

Death through fasting is the most well-documented end-of-life practice within the Jain tradition, though it is not undertaken with great frequency (Dundas 2002a, 180–81; Jaini 2001/1979, 227–33; Settar 1989, 2017; Tukol 1976; Wiley 2000a, 326–28). It is estimated that approximately two hundred lay Jains and mendicants undertake the death fast each year in India (McCarthy 2015). The *Times of India* has reported on one unique community of Jains living outside Mumbai that has recorded four hundred acts of voluntary death over a seven-year period, although this is a notable exception (Chhapia 2015). In spite of its relative rarity, the practice looms undeniably large in the textual imagination of the tradition and community.

Because of its perceived similarity to suicide, the practice of *sallekhanā* has drawn criticism historically and in the present, such that Jains have felt the need to defend the practice. Pūjyapāda, for example, claimed that *sallekhanā* was distinct from suicide because it lacks the passions present in those who violently end their life (SSi 7.22§705; Bhargava 1968, 139–41; Williams 1963, 171). Among modern commentators, T.K. Tukol offered a detailed response to critics in his 1976 book *Sallekhanā Is Not Suicide*. In 2006, a case was brought before the Rajasthan High Court in which petitioner Nikhil Soni argued that the Jain fast unto death should be viewed as suicide according to Indian law—specifically Article 21, which safeguards the right to life but not the right to die. Soni alleged instances of abuse in which individuals may have been pressured into completing the fast (Braun 2008, 922; Sharma 2015). In 2015, the court banned the practice, making *sallekhanā* or its abetment punishable according to the Indian penal code. However, the court suspended this judgment in August of the same year after nationwide protests by Jains, and the case is currently under review (Mahapatra 2015; Sethi 2019).

*Wise Involuntary Death.* There is one last manner of death that is wise, but not voluntary, called *paṇḍita-paṇḍita-maraṇa*. This death is attained in the fourteenth *guṇa-sthāna* by *kevalins*, those who have reached omniscience and exhausted all destructive karmas in the twelfth *guṇa-sthāna*. The Śvetāmbara and Digambara sources disagree about whether *kevalins* consume any food upon reaching this advanced stage. According to Digambaras, *kevalins* no longer need food in order to sustain their bodies and therefore also do not perform any fasts. Śvetāmbaras, on the other hand, who maintain that *kevalins* continue to eat, describe them as sometimes undertaking different kinds of fasts, including the fast unto death. These fasts are, however, not prompted by the same reasons that motivate laity, such as reducing the amount of destructive types of karma or keeping in a state of equanimity as death approaches, since they have already eliminated all passions and destructive karmas. "Since *kevalins* are omniscient," Wiley explains, "they know in advance when they will die and they stop eating food by mouth (*kavalāhāra*) when it is no longer needed to sustain the body." This occurs along with the cessastion of all gross and subtle activities that occurs in the last two *guṇasthānas* (Wiley 2000a, 331–33; see chapter 3).

## DYING WELL IN MODERN MEDICINE

While the orthodox Jain tradition places central emphasis on dying in a state of calm awareness for the sake of an auspicious rebirth and eventual liberation, modern medicine is also grappling with what it means to die well. What, if anything, might the Jain community offer contemporary debates about end-of-life decision making? Similarly, how do contemporary Jains within and beyond the medical community reflect on end-of-life dilemmas that may not be addressed by the historical practice of a voluntary fast unto death?

The litigation surrounding *sallekhanā* in the Rajasthan High Court brought a rare practice of the minority Jain community into the public spotlight. On one hand, the case raises the question of whether an individual has the right to bring about their own death. On the other hand, the case invites needed conversation about the diverse and personal values of dying well that cannot be answered by medicine or law alone.

### *Refusing Life-Sustaining Treatment, and Advance Directives*

In her analysis of the Indian court case, bioethicist Whitny Braun argues that *sallekhanā* should be legally protected on the grounds of religious freedom and autonomy (2008, 913). The choice to fast unto death involves two decisions: the first to forgo additional treatment, the second to forgo nutrition and water. Indeed, at least according to US law, the right to refuse life-sustaining treatment rests on firm precedent, notably the landmark cases of Karen Quinlan and Nancy Cruzan.

In 1975, twenty-one-year-old Karen Quinlan lost consciousness and stopped breathing at a party after consuming alcohol and Quaaludes. She lapsed into a coma followed by a persistent vegetative/unresponsive wakefulness state, caused by irreversible brain damage due to respiratory failure. Quinlan's parents felt that the mechanical ventilator constituted an extraordinary means of prolonging her life and requested its removal. When doctors refused, under threat from prosecutors that the act would constitute homicide and a breach of the Hippocratic Oath, the Quinlans filed for a court order to remove the ventilator in the New Jersey Supreme Court. Ultimately, the court held that the right to privacy—in this case, the right of a patient to make a private decision regarding the future of her life—was broad enough to include the Quinlans' refusal (on their daughter's behalf) of life-sustaining treatment, and ordered that the ventilator be removed. To everyone's surprise, Quinlan continued to breathe after the vent was removed and her parents never attempted to withdraw her feeding tube. She survived for nine more years in a nursing facility until her death from respiratory failure in 1985.

Another key legal decision related to the refusal of medical treatment was in the later case of Nancy Cruzan. In 1983, at the age of twenty-five, Cruzan lost control of her car while driving at night near Carthage, Missouri. Paramedics found her thrown from the vehicle, face-down in a water-filled ditch and without vital signs, but managed to resuscitate her. After three weeks in a coma, Cruzan was diagnosed as being in a persistent vegetative/unresponsive wakefulness state and placed on a surgical feeding tube.

In 1988, Cruzan's parents requested that the feeding tube be removed. The physicians refused to do so without a court order, because the tube removal would cause Cruzan's death. The Missouri court granted the order to remove Cruzan's feeding tube on the basis that one could withdraw treatment that promises no chance of meaningful recovery, and that Nancy had effectively instructed such withdrawal when she told a friend, prior to the accident, that she would not want to continue living if she ever had severe impairments. The case was appealed, however, and the Missouri Supreme Court reversed the lower court's decision on the grounds that no third party could refuse treatment for another person without a living will or clear evidence of personal wishes. The Cruzans appealed to the US Supreme Court, which ruled 5–4 that competent individuals may refuse medical treatment under the Due Process Clause of the Fourteenth Amendment. However, in the case of *incompetent individuals* such as Nancy, their decision sided with the

Missouri court's requirement for a "higher standard" of evidence of a patient's previous wishes. The Cruzans gathered additional evidence of Nancy's preference not to live on life support and successfully won a court order to have their daughter's feeding tube removed in December 1990; she died two weeks later, almost eight years after her accident.

The Cruzan decision was instrumental in establishing what was required for a third party to refuse treatment for an incompetent patient. Without clear evidence of a patient's wishes, the state's interest to preserve life outweighed an individual's right to refuse treatment. In the United States, this decision generated increased interest in living wills and other advance directives and motivated support for the Patient Self-Determination Act (PSDA) passed by Congress in 1990, which requires many hospitals, hospices, and nursing facilities to provide information about advance directives upon admission.

In the United States today, advance directives for end-of-life care include naming a surrogate decision maker and opting for one or two important documents. The first is a do-not-resuscitate (DNR) order signed by a physician; this is a direct medical order for emergency personnel and healthcare providers not to perform cardiopulmonary resuscitation (CPR) if a patient is unconscious or if their heartbeat or breathing stops, but it does not include details about other end-of-life wishes. The second is a "POLST form," which addresses issues left out of the DNR (POLST stands for Physician Orders for Life-Sustaining Treatment; however, the "P" can refer to any medical professional or care provider and sometimes stands for Patient, Professional, Preferences, or Palliative). Often printed on bright pink paper and available in most but not all states, the POLST is signed by a physician after conversations with a patient who is elderly, seriously ill, frail, or near the end of life. The document is a formal medical order that offers greater detail on whether the patient desires CPR in the event they stop breathing or their heart stops; it also describes the conditions under which they want to be taken to the hospital or left where they are, the types of life-prolonging interventions they would want, their desires for pain management, and if they want a feeding tube and for how long.[26] Without a DNR or POLST, hospital staff and emergency technicians are required to resuscitate someone who is not breathing or lacks a heartbeat and transport them to a hospital. They cannot stop these efforts without a medical order.[27]

A related advance directive effort known as "Five Wishes" was begun in Florida in 1996, intended to make the legal, emotional, and spiritual wishes of a patient known in straightforward language. The first two wishes include legal documents and/or medical orders:

Wish 1: A designated decision maker if a patient becomes incapacitated

Wish 2: Treatment a patient wants or does not want (e.g., if a patient is found breathing/not breathing, if a patient wants to stay where they are or go to the hospital)

The remaining three wishes address additional personal desires at the end of life:

Wish 3: Desired comfort level through pain management, bathing, grooming, hospice care options, etc.

Wish 4: Desires for how others should treat the patient (e.g., to be kept at home, to have someone pray or offer other actions at the patient's bedside)

Wish 5: Desires for what loved ones should know regarding the patient's feelings, forgiveness, arrangements for funerals, memorial services, burial, cremation, etc.

*Contemporary Jain Views on Life-Sustaining Treatment.* The majority of Jain medical professionals in our survey wanted the ability to refuse life-sustaining treatment. When asked, "What is most true for your own personal end-of-life care?," the majority stated that they would choose a DNR order if they went into cardiac or respiratory failure (69%, $n = 36$), while a small minority wanted "doctors to do all they can to keep me alive at the end of life" (3%). The remainder did not know (6%), had not considered it before (8%), or chose "Other" (14%). Among those who selected "Other," one participant stated they "prefer death with *samādhi* [the meditative state sought in *sallekhanā*]," and three stated that use of a DNR would depend on the specific situation.

About half of the Jain medical professionals felt that the Jain community as a whole was open to dialoguing about death, dying, and end-of-life care (47%, $n = 36$), though significant minorities disagreed (19%) or did not know (25%). Likewise, just over half of respondents in our survey had their own "living will or advance directive for end-of-life care" (56%, $n = 36$); 28 percent did not have a directive; 8 percent had not considered it; and two individuals included comments regarding their intention to pursue a directive in the future. When asked, "Do you encourage your patients, family, or friends to complete a living will or advance directive for end-of-life care? Choose all that apply," a significant percentage of participants had recommended advance directives for their patients (50%, $n = 36$), family (61%), or friends (47%).

These responses suggest that Jain medical professionals are acquainted with the ethical dilemmas that might arise when one's decision-making capacity is compromised. As with the previous question, many respondents desired the ability to forgo resuscitative treatments at the end of life. However, DNR is just one of many aspects of life-sustaining treatment, and living wills and other advance directives have frequently been criticized as being too vague, and for lacking specific guidance for third-party decision makers (Teno et al. 1997). When asked what specific life-sustaining treatments they would accept at the end of life, survey participants present a more complex picture (figure 19).

The largest percentage would accept antibiotics (36%, $n = 36$)[28] and blood transfusion (31%), while a significant minority would also accept CPR (25%), dialysis

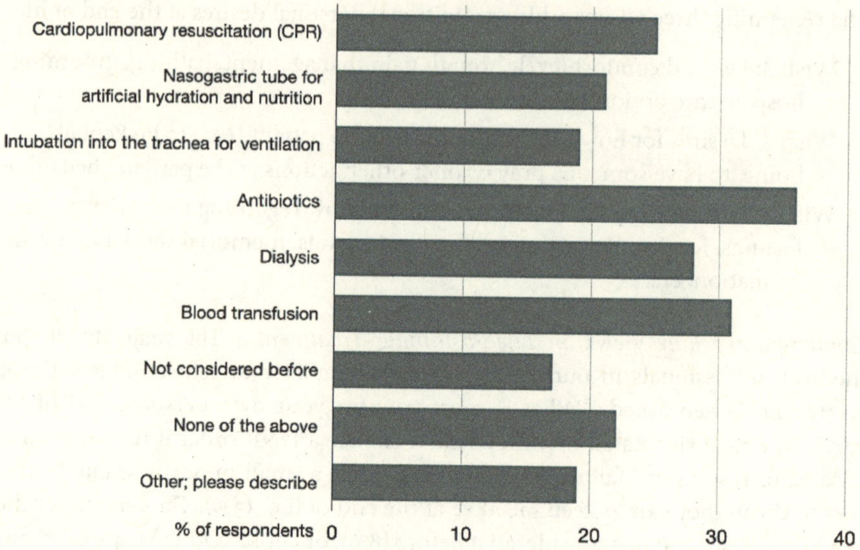


FIGURE 19. Responses of Jain medical professionals ($n = 36$) to the question "Which of the following life-sustaining treatments would you be willing to accept as part of your end-of-life care?"

(28%), feeding tube (19%), and intubation (19%). A similar minority would accept none of the available treatments (22%). Those who selected "Other" offered the following remarks:

"Depends on the situation; but in advanced age or poor baseline health I would choose DNR; prior to this such interventions may be acceptable."

"Depends on the situation."

"It will depend upon the circumstances as I may consider many options if I know it is for short term."

"If I know that I am dying, I do not want treatment of any kind."

"Die with dignity [through] *sallekhanā*."

"None of the above [treatments] contradict with Jain principles."

The Quinlan and Cruzan cases established that patients could forgo life-sustaining treatment and that third-party surrogates could also refuse this care so long as they could produce a living will, another advance directive, or convincing evidence of a patient's wishes before becoming incapacitated. In a clinical setting, the hierarchy of decision making revolves around a patient's autonomous choice, ideally expressed through informed consent or in a detailed advance directive for those who lack capacity. If no such document exists, the hierarchy of decision making falls to a surrogate decision maker who has some knowledge of the patient's wishes or values, as in the case of Nancy Cruzan's parents. Absent that knowledge, physicians and family members exercise substitutionary judgment using the "best interests" standard for the patient's well-being.

### *Euthanasia and Physician Aid-in-Dying*

The term *euthanasia* is derived from the Greek *eu-* and *thanatos*, meaning a good, happy, or easy death. Akin to the many types of death discussed in the Jain tradition, the good death of euthanasia can be active or passive, as well as voluntary or involuntary.

"Passive euthanasia" refers to an indirect action, typically a removal or withholding of care, rather than direct action. An example of *voluntary* passive euthanasia is when a competent patient exercises informed decision-making capacity to refuse life-sustaining treatment, which may include refusing food and fluids, as in the Quinlan and Cruzan cases above. What is morally and legally salient in voluntary passive euthanasia is that it constitutes a patient's *act of omission* in which an additional treatment is refused or removed, thereby "allowing" an underlying disease or condition to take its course, rather than a direct *act of commission* in which the act itself causes the death. *Involuntary* passive euthanasia, on the other hand, occurs when a physician withdraws a treatment without a patient's request or consent, such as unplugging a dialysis machine for a patient with kidney disease. Advance directives, including DNR and/or POLST forms, are intended to clarify a patient's wishes for precisely these times, so that surrogate decision makers and care staff can rely on those wishes to guide the maintaining, stoppage, or withdrawal of life-sustaining treatment.

"Active euthanasia" refers to a direct action that causes a patient's death. Sometimes referred to as a "gentle death" or "mercy killing," *voluntary* active euthanasia (VAE) requires a physician to act directly upon a patient who has requested that action—for instance, directly administering a lethal dose of medication to a patient who no longer wants to live. This form of euthanasia was brought into the public eye by Jack Kevorkian, a Michigan-based pathologist who claimed to have helped over a hundred patients end their lives in the 1990s. In the majority of these cases, Kevorkian utilized a machine he had built in which a patient would press a button to initiate the administration of a lethal drug, thereby "assisting" a patient in ending their own life. Because Michigan had no laws against assisted death on record, attempts to charge Kevorkian with illegal wrongdoing failed.

However, in 1998, Kevorkian released a video in which he removed the artifice of the machine and directly administered a lethal injection to Thomas Youk, a fifty-two-year-old man in the final stages of Lou Gehrig's disease. The video depicts Youk stating his informed consent, followed by Kevorkian giving a series of injections that swiftly stop Youk's heart. With this act, Kevorkian crossed an already murky legal line between aid-in-dying and the perceived killing of VAE. He was convicted of second degree murder in 1999, subsequently serving over eight years in prison. *Involuntary* active euthanasia takes place when a fatal action is intentionally initiated without a patient's request and consent. A common example of this kind of death is when a veterinarian euthanizes a companion pet without that animal's voluntary participation or consent in the decision.

Physician aid-in-dying (PAD), also sometimes called "physician-assisted suicide," does not fit neatly into the above euthanasia paradigm. It involves a physician making lethal means available that patients must administer to themselves at a time of their own choosing. Some have referred to it as "passive-assisted death," since the physician is not actively engaging in a direct fatal act. Kevorkian's machine—which required the patient to press a button—is an example of PAD.

*Dying Well as an Ongoing Moral and Legal Debate.* Every living being will undergo a death of some kind. The speculations of bioethicists and judges emerge from actual situations in which there is no clear guidance. In spite of considerable consensus on the value of autonomy in making individual end-of-life decisions, there is little agreement across or within cultures—legally or morally—about the accepted ways in which individuals can end their own life. At the same time, the ongoing advancement of life-sustaining technologies and treatments confronts us with longer lives characterized by ever-greater medical interventions that can obstruct our ability to die in accordance with our desires and values.

A select group of countries have laws that permit voluntary active euthanasia as a legally acceptable mode of dying for those experiencing unbearable pain or suffering. As of 2020, these countries include Belgium, Colombia, Japan, Luxembourg, and the Netherlands. The Netherlands, considered to have the most permissive laws regarding assisted death in the world, ruled in 1986 that "psychic suffering" be included in criteria for euthanasia, resulting in the sanctioned deaths of individuals with mental illness and depressive disorders. In 2014, Belgium expanded its euthanasia statute to include children undergoing unbearable suffering, and in 2016–17, three Belgian children were euthanized after a process involving their written request and psychological evaluation: a seventeen-year-old with muscular dystrophy, an eleven-year-old with cystic fibrosis, and a nine-year-old with a brain tumor (Embury-Dennis 2018). In all other countries, it is illegal for a physician to directly administer a lethal dose of medication to a competent patient who has requested and consented to the action. As in the Kevorkian case, such an act would be deemed murder, even though the same act, when it is done to companion animals, is frequently understood to provide a "merciful" death.

*Contemporary Jain Views on Euthanasia.* As we discussed in chapter 6, Jainism rejects the ultimate value of mercy killing for people and animals. The possible consequences of euthanasia within the orthodox Jain view are twofold: first, the one performing, causing another to perform, or approving of the performance of death would incur negative karma, inhibiting their own path toward liberation;

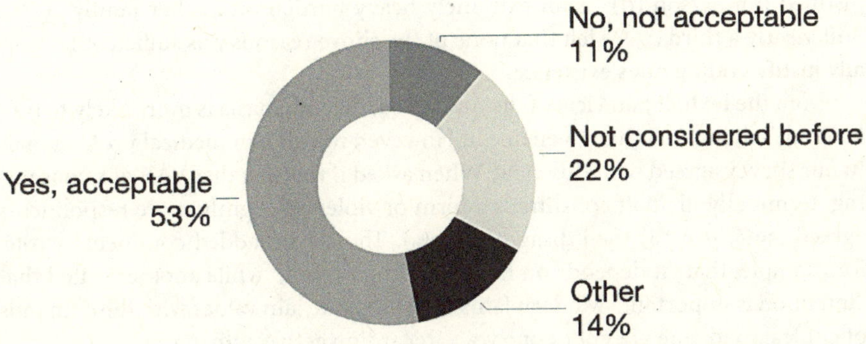


FIGURE 20. Responses of Jain medical professionals ($n$ = 36) to the question "Certain forms of palliative care (pain relief) can potentially shorten life by depressing respiration, among other side effects. Do you feel that such pain management techniques are acceptable if they may shorten life?"

and second, it would interfere in the path of another living being, who is considered to deserve the opportunity to work through their karmic burden in their own way and time. The consequences of this Jain perspective may strike some readers as callous or cruel, whereas many Jains see active euthanasia—whether voluntary or involuntary and whether of an animal or person—as a costly act of harm to another being's ongoing existence.

However, a majority (53%, $n$ = 36) of the Jain medical professionals we surveyed felt that palliative care, or aggressive pain medication to relieve suffering, is acceptable even if it might shorten a patient's life through depressed respiration or other side effects (figure 20). The other responses were divided among those who selected "No, it is not acceptable" (11%), those who had not considered it before (22%), and those who selected "Other" (11%). The latter included the following responses:

> "Only for terminal illness."
>
> "Acceptable if patient has consented."
>
> "Treatment depends on what the patient desires who is suffering."
>
> "If the intent of pain medication is patient comfort then I would discuss with the patient the possible consequences of shortening life and prescribe pain medication if the patient wishes."

Even more significant, a considerable number of respondents felt that a patient can make a morally correct decision to end their life in certain circumstances—for example, if that person (a) "is suffering a great deal with no hope of improvement" (47%, $n$ = 36) or (b) "has an incurable disease" (45%). A significant minority also felt that it is morally justified to end one's life if a person (c) "is ready to die (living has become a burden)" (25%). Relatively few felt that terminating one's life is justified if a person (d) "is an extremely heavy burden on his/her family" (6%). Still, nearly a third (27%) felt that none of the above reasons was sufficient to morally justify ending one's existence.

From the textual Jain view of the unwise death, euthanasia is more likely to prevent one's dying well than to enable it. However, not all Jain medical professionals in our survey agreed with this view. When asked if they felt that VAE of a consenting, terminally ill adult constitutes a form of violence, slightly more respondents agreed (39%, $n$ = 36) than disagreed (33%). Those who added comments wrote, for example, that "it depends on the will of the person," while another stated that "intention is important." Modern Jains who integrate Jain values with the demands of clinical medicine are not of one voice regarding active euthanasia.

*Contemporary Jain Views on Physician Aid-in-Dying.* A larger number of countries have legalized PAD than euthanasia. Worldwide, as of 2020, PAD is permitted under certain conditions in Belgium, Canada, Colombia, Germany, Japan, Luxembourg, the Netherlands, Switzerland, and certain states in Australia and the United States. As with VAE, advocates disagree on whom these laws should apply to. In Canada, for example, legislation is currently being debated that would open PAD to patients who have only mental illness and no underlying physical malady. In the United States, PAD is not legal at the federal level, though growing public support has enabled several states to successfully introduce so-called "death with dignity" laws permitting PAD under certain guidelines. As of 2020, California, Colorado, Hawaii, Maine, Montana, New Jersey, Oregon, Vermont, Washington, and the District of Columbia permit regulated forms of PAD, and advocates are committed to pursuing similar statutes in every state.

Opponents of PAD in the United States—including the Catholic Church and other religious organizations, some disability-rights groups, and certain medical ethicists, among others—raise legitimate concerns about assisted dying that state-based initiatives have tried to address. Chief among these issues is the contention that PAD is not a truly autonomous act because it requires the participation of a physician and pharmacy staff who must involve themselves in another's death, and thus contributes to a pervasive cheapening of human life at a social level, beyond mere personal decision making. Critics also see PAD as a "slippery slope" to sanctioning euthanasia for those who are depressed or lonely, for individuals with mental illness or physical disability, and for the elderly, the homeless, or anyone else society deems undesirable or useless. While advocates insist that only those who are truly suffering would pursue this avenue, it is worth considering whether a person who fails to have a "meaningful life" in the normative sense of regular happiness, family, friendships, meaningful work, being able-bodied, or being distress-free might be more inclined to explore assisted death if it were available, rather than the creative challenge and therapeutic interventions involved in coping and thriving with non-normative experiences that are not acknowledged or welcomed in media and society. Finally, critics argue that PAD contradicts the physician's oath to "do no harm" by enabling others to actively end life.

The 1994 Oregon Death with Dignity Act has served as a model for several states (and countries) attempting to address these concerns by permitting physicians or institutions to refuse participation, allowing only adults eighteen years and older with a terminal diagnosis of less than six months and demonstrated decision-making capacity to initiate PAD. The process also requires an oral and written letter of request from the patient, an evaluation by two physicians, referring the patient to counseling or psychiatric services if needed, and a mandatory waiting period between the request and the writing of a prescription.

Still, considerable controversy persists. Advocates note issues of access. Even if a state legalizes PAD, the ability of doctors, pharmacists, and institutions to opt out makes the "right" to PAD an empty one that many patients cannot actualize. In the Coachella Valley region of Southern California, for instance, three of the largest healthcare systems have opted out, making it difficult for patients to find a doctor who will write the prescription or a pharmacy to fill it (Aleccia 2017). Additionally, federal funds cannot be used for PAD, so patients on Medicare as well as patients of the Department of Veterans Affairs cannot have these costs covered. Opponents note examples of abuse. One 2008 study showed that one in six patients who sought and received prescriptions for lethal medication was clinically depressed (Ganzini et al. 2008).

Jain medical professionals in our survey had varied opinions on PAD. When asked if aid-in-dying is a form of violence, respondents diverged, with equal numbers of agreement and dispute (33% each). When asked, "Have you ever provided physician aid-in-dying (PAD) services or counseling at the end of someone's life in your medical/healthcare career?," a small minority answered affirmatively (11%, $n = 36$). The majority had not (64%), while the remainder chose "Not applicable" (25%).

### Sallekhanā *and US Policy: PAD versus VRFF and Terminal Sedation*

The Jain practice of *sallekhanā* does not fit into the category of aid-in-dying, though it rests on a similar commitment to autonomy and has a detailed set of regulations to ensure its responsible practice. Because it involves the gradual refusal of treatment, as well as solid food and liquid nourishment, *sallekhanā* could be described as a form of voluntary passive euthanasia in which a person is "allowed to die." Dilip Bobra, in his brief analysis of Jain bioethics, writes that "Jainism tries to answer the questions of physician-assisted suicide and 'death with dignity' by voluntarily making the decision to plan *sallekhanā*." He continues: "This is very similar to a non-written directive, after the opinion of [a] physician that there are no possible options of treatment" (2008).

This comparison opens an especially rich arena for Jains to engage with end-of-life practices and policy in India, the United States, and other diaspora countries that limit legal options for voluntary euthanasia. If we look to the United States as a case study, only two modes of voluntary euthanasia are legal at the federal level. The first form is the voluntary refusal of food and fluids (VRFF), also called voluntary stopping of eating and drinking (VSED). The second is terminal sedation.

The US Supreme Court has been unwilling to make PAD the law of the land, in part, because VRFF already exists as an alternative (Bernat et al. 1993; Quill and Byock 2000). According to the Court, VRFF is a preferable legal alternative to PAD because it is already enshrined in law under the right of competent patients to refuse or withdraw treatment. In one influential study of Oregon hospice nurses who cared for a patient who undertook VRFF, the majority of nurses rated their patient as having a "good death" using a provided scale, while only a small minority described the patient's experience as a "bad death" (Ganzini et al. 2003). Such studies suggest that patients can exercise their principled self-determination while medical staff can focus on providing palliative care rather than a lethal dose of medication. Per the court, VRFF is potentially less likely to be abused and is also seen to be reversible, in that patients can resume food and fluids at any time (Quill et al. 1997).

Terminal sedation is closely related to VRFF. When patients experience extreme pain that cannot be relieved by high doses of common pain medications, it is legal for a medical professional to continuously sedate the patient into an unconscious state; this is typically followed by the withdrawal of artificial nutrition and hydration, until the patient dies. From a legal perspective, terminal sedation acknowledges that the cause of death is the underlying disease rather than an active intervention of the doctor.

Some critics, however, claim that VRFF and terminal sedation are actually more problematic than either PAD or active euthanasia. VRFF opponents assert that physicians must still collaborate with patients in an act that is not altogether different from suicide (Jansen 2015; Jansen and Sulmasy 2002). Although many "death with dignity" advocates acknowledge that VRFF can be an effective and meaningful end-of-life choice for some patients, many emphasize the challenges and ambivalence of dying through dehydration for patients and families. In an influential public opinion piece, California physician Christopher Stookey described his own father's death by VRFF after seven days, documenting arm movements and accelerated breathing that seemed to indicate prolonged distress until his father lost consciousness on the sixth day. Stookey reasons, "The moment we'd decided to withhold fluids, my father was on a sure path to death. . . . Why did we have to wait 6 days to reach this point?" (2015).

Critics of terminal sedation claim that there are insufficient data on the suffering that patients undergo in an unconscious state (Rady and Verheijde 2012). Others also assert that terminal sedation poses greater risks of abuse than either PAD or active euthanasia, since it does not have the extensive consent process, and also results in a patient who will likely be incapacitated for several days prior to death (Orentlicher 2010). According to physician and attorney David Orentlicher, the approval of terminal sedation reflects the "Court's deference to symbolic considerations" that privilege the appearance of "allowing to die" over a treatment that is essentially active euthanasia (2010, 417). The informed consent process of PAD, Orentlicher argues, better exemplifies a physician's duty to relieve pain, in that it is preferable for patients for whom death is imminent and who do not wish to linger in an unconscious state in which pain and suffering may be undetectable to outside observers.

How might the Jain community weigh in on these end-of-life debates? The practice of *sallekhanā* is, at the surface, most similar to VRFF, which is legal in many countries under the right to refuse treatment. Indeed, the Supreme Court of India passed such a law in March 2018, permitting patients to refuse life-sustaining treatment through advance directives. Upon the announcement, a well-known Digambara monk, Taruṇ Sāgar, publicly praised the Court's decision, even as the nation's Catholic bishop denounced it. Taruṇ Sāgar, whose response was reported across national media outlets, stated: "Today, the Supreme Court has given a historical ruling, which has been a law in Jainism for ages. I thank the Supreme Court [for the verdict]" ("Passive Euthanasia Legalised" 2018).

Jain medical professionals, however, had diverse opinions on the modes of dying that should be available to patients at the end of life. Among respondents, 28 percent ($n = 36$) affirmed that "PAD should be available to any consenting, competent adult when terminal illness has been clinically diagnosed." A significant minority felt that PAD is never justified because of the karmic burden it places upon the physician (22%) or upon the patient (19%). Only 11 percent of participants believed that "PAD is completely different than *sallekhanā*," which suggests that most respondents see some overlap between the two processes (figure 21).

Interestingly, over half of respondents (53%, $n = 36$) agreed that *sallekhanā* "is a better alternative to PAD for Jains," while 36 percent felt that it is also a better alternative to PAD for *non-Jains*. The fact that Jains see *sallekhanā* as having value outside the Jain community suggests that voluntary fasting unto death can be appreciated by those who do not share the overall Jain worldview. US bioethicist Dena Davis asserted this very point over twenty-five years ago, stating that *sallekhanā* could help Western medical practitioners and patients "break our automatic association of starvation with moral evil" and offer "an image of food refusal that is associated with voluntariness, with the fulfillment of a life span, with the last chapter of a completed narrative" (1990). Likewise, Chapple asserts that the paradigm of legal "rights" related to death might be enriched by encountering Jain "rites" that reflect a unique understanding of the self in relation to the body, to other beings, and to an existence that extends beyond one lifetime (2016a). In the final section of this chapter, we reflect on five principles of application for dying and death. Some are unique to the Jain worldview, and others—primarily derived from the insights of *sallekhanā*—may offer common ground to support a Jain engagement with contemporary bioethical debates related to the end of life.

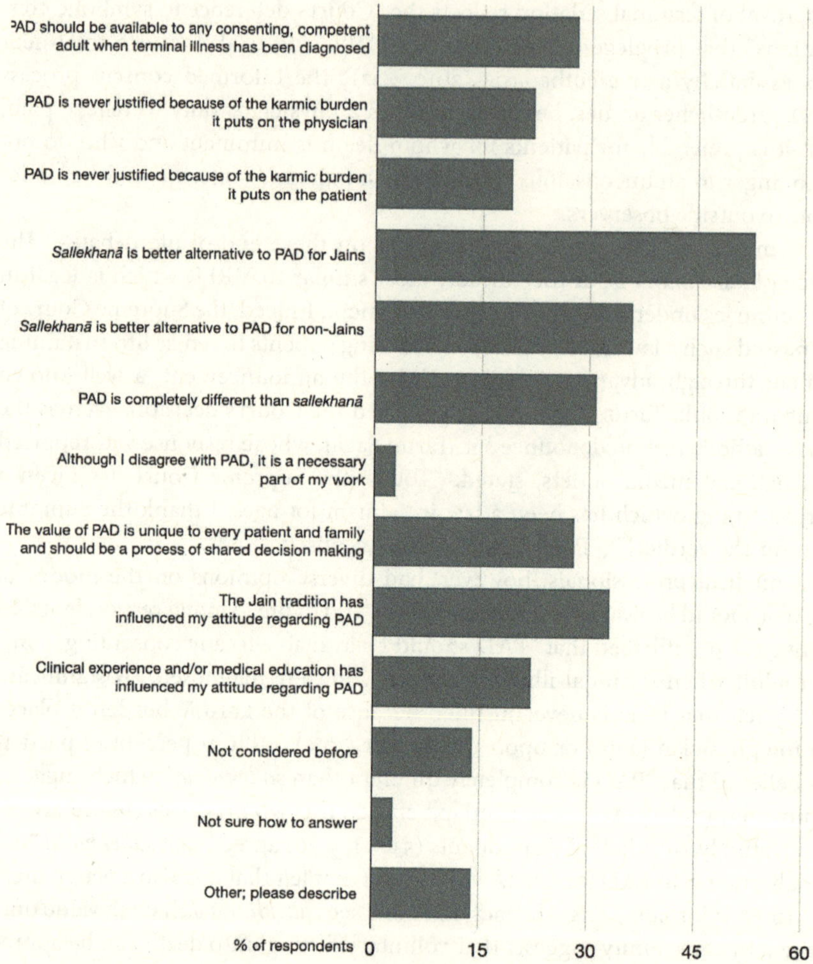


FIGURE 21. Responses of Jain medical professionals ($n = 36$) to the question "Which of the following statements [regarding physician aid-in-dying (PAD)] is/are most true for you? Choose all that apply."

## JAIN PRINCIPLES OF APPLICATION FOR DYING AND DEATH

Jains understand death, like rebirth, as a transition point within one's overall karmic journey, which may span innumerable lifetimes. The inevitability of old age and death provides motivation to strive for right worldview, knowledge, and conduct in order to shed karmic attachments and advance oneself toward a better rebirth, a possibility open to mendicants, laypeople, and even animals. While most of the Jain medical professionals in our survey identified with the currently prevailing medical definitions of death—namely heart-lung criteria, whole-brain death, or brainstem death—their overall support for organ donation as a Jain-inspired act of merit, their support of advance directives (for themselves and others) that enable them to forgo medical care, and their ambivalence with accepting certain life-sustaining treatments are suggestive of a keen awareness about dying wisely.

The wise and voluntary death of *sallekhanā* is widely seen as the ideal means by which a Jain can die well. The practice of *sallekhanā* looms large in the Jain imagination, defended in both historical and modern times as a value-laden mode of dying that is counter to the violent impulses of suicide. At the same time, while "mercy killing" is not accepted in the textual tradition, about one-third of Jain medical professionals in our survey viewed active euthanasia as well as physician aid-in-dying as morally and medically acceptable, demonstrating a departure from orthodox belief. Drawing upon the insights of *sallekhanā*, we identify five additional Jain principles of death and dying.

First, autonomy is a critical, but insufficient, criterion for end-of-life decisions. The act of *sallekhanā* always takes place within the bodily, environmental, and cognitive constraints of a given life. It requires a process of preparation and ideally takes place in a community that understands the person's wishes and supports their values. The practice of fasting is a way to expand autonomy by enlarging one's experience and understanding of the self through one's relationship to others.

Second, life-sustaining treatments are a meaningful aspect of end-of-life care. Dying is not an all-or-nothing process; the vow of *sallekhanā* contains many steps, prior to the final vow of unlimited fasting, in which one can weigh the costs and benefits of a specific treatment.

Third, maintaining awareness and agency is a valuable part of the dying process. The vow of fasting is an attempt to consciously approach death with awareness and determination, applying the values of one's life to the experience of dying. Efforts to enshrine POLST forms, as well as the "Five Wishes," resonate with this aspect of *sallekhanā* by creating a framework that requires discussion between patient, loved ones, and caregivers and involves a more holistic framework to think through the medical, emotional, and spiritual significance of death, especially as one advances in age or illness. The significant support of PAD by Jain medical professionals in our survey suggests that the required steps of informed decision making may be compatible with certain aspects of *sallekhanā*, insofar as they allow a patient to maintain awareness up to the moment of death. It is not clear whether terminal sedation would be theoretically welcomed by Jains, since it forces one into an unconscious state.

Fourth, limiting one's use of material resources at the end of life has personal and social benefits beyond "allocation" debates. The practice of *sallekhanā* reflects the real costs of living in a dynamic universe where life requires life. Forgoing food and water is an act of compassion for other life-forms that benefits oneself during life and at its end. Healthcare debates regarding the "allocation of resources" between those at the end of life and those who have a longer life ahead of them give way to a relational understanding of responsibility and care for self and others.

Fifth, and finally, it is a meaningful goal to approach death without fear. Meeting death with a calm state of mind is paramount in *sallekhanā*. Cultivating this state requires practice and community dialogue about our common experiences of aversions and attachments, which shape our attitudes toward identity, body, daily life, and death, and which perpetuate anxiety rather than equanimity.

Articulating these and other possible principles may be just as important within the Jain community as outside it. While Braun claims that "*sallekhanā* is being practiced in the United States," only a very few cases have been documented (2008, 923). In 1997, Vijay Bhade, a forty-three-year-old Jain mother and wife from West Virginia, undertook a final fast after six months of unsuccessful treatment for sarcoma (Chapple 2010, 206). Bhagwati Gada, a retired physician in Texas, undertook a short-term fast in 2013, after her colon cancer progressed to stage 4 and she declined further treatment (Eplett 2015). The "Guidelines for Healthcare Providers Interacting with Patients of the Jain Religion and Their Families" (2002), created by the Jain Society of Metropolitan Chicago in conjunction with the Council for the World Parliament of Religions, mention the practice of *sallekhanā* (called *santharo* in the guide), stating that it is a "personal choice done with the advice of a spiritual leader . . . generally done away from the hospital" ("Guidelines" 2002, 6). This view suggests that *sallekhanā* is a private practice that has little bearing on the clinical context.

Yet, with the recent litigation in Rajasthan regarding *sallekhanā*, the global Jain community may be poised to deepen their engagement with modern medicine regarding end-of-life care. Jains mobilized around the world to protest and overturn the High Court's 2015 ban and continue to lobby to safeguard the practice ("JAINA President's Message" 2017, 8). Videos and articles by Jain laypeople and mendicants have proliferated on the internet, offering detailed support for the end-of-life fast, which has also been featured in documentaries and a *National Geographic* special on unique death rituals.[29] It remains to be seen whether Jains will bring the traditional insights of a wise voluntary death into modern biomedical debates or maintain it as a religious ritual that takes place in the private sphere.

Among legal options for death in the United States, *sallekhanā* is most parallel to the voluntary refusal of food and fluids. Given that a significant number of respondents felt that *sallekhanā* could offer a meaningful alternative to physician aid-in-dying for Jains as well as non-Jains, Jains might have unique contributions to public discourses on end-of-life care. There is similar overlap with initiatives such as POLST or Five Wishes, which articulate and support holistic dying initiatives that understand medical decisions in light of one's physical, emotional, and spiritual fears, hopes, and aspirations. Uniquely, Jains also extend these conversations into wider consideration of the many one- through five-sensed beings in existence who are affirmed when use of medicines, food, fluids, and water is dialed back.

# Epilogue

## *Multiple Voices and Future Directions in Jain Bioethics*

In this book we have explored the "cumulative tradition" of Jainism by mapping multiple Jain principles for, and perspectives about, contemporary bioethics. Our aim was to pay close attention to the diversity of Jain voices as an essential task in avoiding the perception that Jainism is a homogeneous tradition that speaks with a single voice. To this end, we outlined the development of the doctrines in textual sources over time, and highlighted the distinction between mendicants and laity, sectarian perspectives, and Jains living in India and in the diaspora.

In part 1 we strove to identify textually supported principles that would represent the complexity of Jainism as a self-contained, alternative philosophical worldview, with its own internal logic. We focused primarily on its evolving metaphysical, ethical, and soteriological frameworks as well as its rich history of encounters with medicine, which are conceptual areas that we found to be most relevant for bioethical discussions.

In part 2 we drew from traditional textual sources and contemporary Jain voices to explore various approaches to specific bioethical issues. While there is no direct line between Jain philosophy as expounded in the traditional texts and modern practice for many of the bioethical issues that we examined in the book, contemporary Jains have thought about most of the issues either personally, professionally, or academically. The survey that we conducted with medical professionals was particularly significant in helping us identify principles of application that reflect how contemporary Jains strive to bring together their Jain identity on one hand and the competing scientific values and ethical sensibilities of their broader cultural and social contexts on the other. Examining these contemporary approaches through a historical perspective allowed us to indicate lines of continuity and discontinuity between earlier and contemporary debates and dilemmas.

We hope that our book will provide a foundation for future studies in the scarcely researched field of Jain bioethics. Particularly exciting areas of possible research include lay approaches to bioethical issues beyond Jain medical professionals and academics, contemporary mendicants and medicine, Jain bioethics in conversation with the views of other South Asian religious traditions, and in-depth comparative studies of Jain bioethical viewpoints and Western normative ethics on the various issues that we covered in the book. Other salient research topics might include the wide social and ecological arenas of human-animal-plant relations and emerging technologies. Our research shows that Jain positions on bioethical topics do not easily match any of the predominant normative ethics theories, but further cross-cultural work needs to be done in this area to explore where the Jain voice fits into the bioethical debates and what its potential contributions to contemporary discussions are. Our work also opens up questions about representation: What do we mean when we speak of a "Jain" approach, and who represents "Jain" (bio)ethics? Combining textual studies with fieldwork could be particularly fruitful for the future study of Jain bioethics in this regard.

Our intention was to show that Jainism can be in a meaningful conversation with contemporary bioethics. In the beginning of the book, we pointed out the roots of Western bioethics, which are—in the call for an expansive understanding of life and the notion of a moral subject—reminiscent, at least in certain respects, of Jainism (and were perhaps even influenced by it). Our book traces a long history of practical ideals and pragmatic accommodations that developed in following such a wide-ranging metaphysics of life and corresponding ethical guidelines. We highlighted the personal, professional, and public conflicts and commitments that continue to interconnect in the Jain encounters with the issues of birth, life, death, illness, health, liberation, and well-being. Ethical duties toward one's *jīva* and the approaches to one's body ensuing from those duties are not stricly individualized. Rather, these aspects of Jain practice are informed by broader communal concerns and, as such, provide a foundation for addressing bioethical issues in their personal and public dimensions.

We strove to write a book that was not prescriptive in character. Rather than developing a model of what Jain bioethics should look like, we outlined and analyzed the foundations and applications that are already present in the tradition. Bioethics is not an alien discipline to Jainism, and issues related to it continuously arise in clinical settings. We were interested in learning how Jains have navigated what we today understand as bioethical concerns and to what extent, and how, their responses have drawn from their philosophical-religious background. It is our hope that this work has done justice to the rich tradition of Jainism, the ever-emerging field of bioethics, and the multiplicity of insistent lives with whom we share this experience of existence.

# NOTES

## CHAPTER 1. WHY JAINISM AND BIOETHICS?

1. Paul Dundas notes that the term "Jain" in reference to a follower of a specific religious path was most likely employed as early as the first centuries of the Common Era (2002, 3–4). Padmanabh Jaini points out that the word "Jina" was used also by other renunciant groups to refer to their teachers, but probably came to be used exclusively for Jains from the ninth century on (2001/1979, 2, fn. 3). An earlier designation for Jain mendicants was *nirgrantha* (Pkt. *niggaṃṭha*; Pāli *nigaṇṭha*), meaning "without knots/bonds" or attachments. While Jains use this term to refer to their own mendicants in the canon, the term is also found in early Buddhist and Vedic/Hindu texts referring to a heretical group that follows Mahāvīra. On the basis of these textual references, Hermann Jacobi—in his introduction to the 1879 edition of the *Kalpa-sūtra* and in his 1880 article "Mahāvīra and his Predecessors"—challenged the prevalent idea that Jainism was a part of either Buddhism or Hinduism and argued that it is distinct from other Indian religious traditions (Flügel 2005, 2; Jacobi 1879, 1–6; Jacobi 1880).

2. Traditional dates for the birth of Mahāvīra are 599 BCE for the majority of Śvetambaras and 582 BCE for Digambaras. He died at the age of seventy-two, in 527 BCE for most Śvetāmbaras and 510 BCE for Digambaras. The historical dating for Mahāvīra varies slightly within the Jain tradition and among scholars who date these Jain figures in accordance with the revised later dating of the Buddha. The latter places Mahāvīra's death at around 425 BCE. See Dundas (2002, 24, 30–32) and Wiley (2009, 134–35).

3. Main Śvetāmbara sectarian traditions include Mūrtipūjaka, Sthānakavāsī, and Śvetāmbara Terāpanthī. The central issue of disagreement between them is the worship of images, which the latter two reject. Main Digambara sectarian traditions include Bīsapanthī and Digambara Terāpanthī, where the main issue of contention is the recognition of the authority of *bhaṭṭārakas*, sedentary mendicant leaders, which only the first group accepts. There are also the Tāraṇ Svāmī Panth, centered on the teachings of scholar-monk Tāraṇ

Svāmī, and Kānjī Svāmī Panth, a neo-Digambara tradition based on the teachings of the layman Kānjī Svāmī. Another popular lineage crossing sect lines is the Kavi Panth, which follows the teachings of the philosopher-mystic-layman Śrīmad Rājacandra (1867–1901). For a narrative summary of how these sectarian traditions developed in relation to one another, see Wiley (2009, 14–18) and Dundas (2002, 45–49, 246–71). For an examination of the broader Śrīmad Rājacandra movement, see Salter (2006).

4. WRD uses four sources to estimate global religions: (1) the World Christian Database, (2) censuses in which a religious question is asked, (3) censuses in which an ethnicity or language question is asked, and (4) other surveys and polls. A full description of each of these sources, as well as the wider methods of the WRD, can be found at https://worldreligiondatabase.org/wrd/doc/WRD_Methodology.pdf (accessed June 1, 2020). The WRD requires a subscription through a university or institution.

5. Some Jains feel that the Jain population reported in the official Census of India is undercounted as a result of hybrid Hindu-Jain identification, and community efforts to generate more accurate counts persist (Flügel 2005, 4–5; Jain and Jain 2019; Rashkow 2013). According to the 2011 Census of India, the Jain population has entered a phase of slowed growth since 1981, increasing by only 5.37 percent between 2001 and 2011, less than other minority communities in the country; the next census will be in 2021 (Bajaj 2016, 1–2). For an overview of Jain population trends between the nineteenth and twenty-first centuries, see Jain (2019).

6. This data set from the WRD can be found by selecting "All religions global totals" on the WRD home page. Clicking on the annual numeric figures will open a document with country totals. The Federation of Jain Associations in North America (JAINA) states that it currently represents over 150,000 Jains in North America (but does not provide a country breakdown; "JAINA in Action" n.d.). The estimate of one hundred thousand Jains in the United States is a frequently cited estimate in modern publications (Lee 2010, 487–88). Many of these figures lack data for support, so the WRD offers a somewhat more substantiated figure to corroborate these estimates.

7. Jainism was granted "minority religion" status in 2014 per Section 2(c) of the National Commission for Minorities (NCM) Act, 1992 (National Commission for Minorities 2014).

8. Jains who had completed at least twelve years of education: women, 55.8%; men, 57.6% (Ministry of Health and Family Welfare 2016, 61–62).

9. The economic contribution is difficult to track with national measures. Various Jain-authored sources state that Jains contribute 24 percent of Indian tax revenue and 62 percent of the national charity fund, but as of this writing, we could not verify these figures through governmental data ("Jains' Contribution" 2007). In 2015, Jains were awarded 7 percent of the national Padma Awards, the highest civilian honors in India for contributions in philanthropy, arts, and human service ("Jains Steal the Show" 2015).

10. While a comprehensive proposal was published in Jahr's 1927 article "Bio-Ethik: Eine Umschau über die ethischen Beziehungen des Menschen zu Tier und Pflanze" in the journal *Kozmos: Handweiser für Naturfreunde* (Jahr 1927), he also mentions the term in his 1926 article "Wissenschaft vom Leben und Sittenlehre (Alte Erkenntnisse in neuem Gewande)," published in *Die Mittelschule: Zeitschrift für das gesamte mittlere Schulwesen* (Jahr 1926).

11. It seems that Jahr found inspiration for formulating the term "Bio-Ethik" in Rudolf Eisler's introduction of "Bio-Psychik," a field exploring the souls of all living beings. He felt

that there was a logical progression between the two: "From Biopsychics it is only one step to *Bio-Ethics* [Bio-Ethik], i.e. the assumption of ethical responsibilities not only towards humans, but towards all living beings" (Jahr 2013, 17). This is particularly relevant for the present monograph, since Jain ethics is strongly rooted in the recognition of a wide-ranging presence of life (as will be shown in chapters 2 and 3).

12. He expanded on his ideas in the 1971 book *Bioethics: Bridge to the Future*.

13. Potter dedicated his first book on bioethics to Leopold (1887–1948), who he felt "anticipated the extension of ethics to Bioethics" (Potter 1971). In *A Sand County Almanac, and Sketches Here and There*, published in 1949, Leopold introduces the term *land ethic*, emphasizing the interdependence of the ecosystem and understanding humans as just one part of the community that forms the living organism of the land. In his book *Global Bioethics: Building on the Leopold Legacy* (1988), Potter describes Leopold as "the first bioethicist" (xiii; Ten Have 2012, 75).

14. The conception of bioethics as ethics oriented toward life sciences and healthcare was proposed by André Hellegers and R. Sargent Shriver not long after the publication of Potter's article. While the pioneers of the discipline had different visions with regard to what the term *bioethics* should denote, the understanding of bioethics as a discipline concerned with ethical issues that emerge with technological advancements in the fields of medicine and life sciences has been predominant.

15. See, for example, Ramsey (2002/1970), McCormick (1981), and Jakobovits (1975/1959).

16. Founded in 1971, the institute was initiated and sponsored by Shriver and the Kennedy family; Hellegers was the first director.

17. Established by Daniel Callahan and Willard Gaylin in 1969, initially as the Institute of Society, Ethics, and the Life Sciences.

18. (1) Brianne Donaldson served on the steering committee for the 2012 International Jain Bioethics Conference, August 24–25, 2012, in Claremont, California, which focused only on bioethics-related themes from Jainism and other global religious traditions (see Dilip Shah, "First Ever International Jain Bioethics Conference," Institute of Jainology, at www.jainology.org/jain-bioethics-conference/, accessed September 10, 2019). (2) The 2016 International Conference on Science and Jain Philosophy (January 8–10, 2016) at the Indian Institute of Technology Bombay, Mumbai, included some exploration of bioethics in terms of neuroscience, consciousness, soul, and karma, though the overall conference explored several other topics (summary available at http://jvbi.ac.in/pdf/menu/departments/bmirc/SUMMARY_OF_INTERNATIONAL_CONFERENCE_ON_SCIENCE_AND_JAIN_PHILOSOPHY.pdf, accessed January 20, 2020). (3) The 2017 National Seminar: Engaging Jainism with Modern Issues (February 24–26, 2017) at the Jain Vishva Bharati Institute, Ladnun, featured bioethics as a subtheme among six possible topics participants could address (summary available at "BMIRC National Seminar," *HereNow4U*, www.herenow4u.net/index.php?id=123357, accessed September 12, 2019).

19. The Gyan Sagar Science Foundation (GSSF) was started in 2009 by forty-one founding Jain scientists in India for the purposes of "bridging science and society" (see "Gyan Sagar," *HereNow4U*, www.herenow4u.net/index.php?id=110933, accessed September 12, 2019). In addition to hosting annual conferences, GSSF publishes a journal with relevant articles and also cosponsored the 18th Jaina Studies Workshop on Jainism and Science (2016) at the School of Oriental and African Studies (SOAS), University of London.

20. For two examples of such healthcare guidelines in the United Kingdom and the United States, see "Caring for the Jain Patient" and "Guidelines for Healthcare Providers."

## CHAPTER 2. LIFE, NONLIFE, AND KARMA

1. See, for example, BhS 5.9§247b: "The venerable Pārśva, the one to be accepted by the people, described the world as eternal, without a beginning or end, limited (i.e. of definite size), surrounded [by the non-world]. In the lower part it is expanded, in the middle it is tight, in the upper part it is wide: below it has a form of a pallet, in the middle [it is like] a narrow grip of an excellent thunderbolt weapon, in the upper part it is placed upwards in the shape of a *mṛd-aṅga* drum" (trans. Balcerowicz 2011, 96). TBh 3.6 compares this shape to an hourglass-shaped stand, which TṬ 3.6 explains as "a tool made of reed placed on which clothes are perfumed [with incense]" (trans. Balcerowicz 2011, 96, fn. 4).

2. It has been suggested that the cosmos has been visually represented in Jain art as a human being from around the sixteenth century on (Dundas 2002, 90; cf. Caillat and Kumar 1981). Some scholars have pointed to much earlier textual references that describe the cosmos as having the shape of a person with specific body parts, even a womb (Balcerowicz 2011).

3. Knowledge about the nature of the cosmos has been passed on through textual sources, visual representations, and popular stories, remaining a topic of interest among contemporary Jains (Del Bontà 2013, 47; Dundas 2002, 92; see also Aukland 2016, 220; Balbir 1990, 182).

4. Contemplating the nature of the cosmos is one of the twelve *anuprekṣās* (Dig.), or *bhāvanās* (Śv.), discussed in chapters 3 and 7.

5. Among modern Jains who strive to demonstrate their tradition's compatibility with science, the presence of heavenly beings and hell-beings in the Jain account of embodied living beings is not necessarily seen as an obstacle, but merely a premodern notion of multiple forms of life (Aukland 2016; Donaldson 2020).

6. TS$^{Dig}$ 3.35.

7. The middle world also contains luminous heavenly beings (*jyotiṣka-deva*—suns, moons, planets, constellations, and scattered stars), which continuously move in the human realms but are static beyond them. Semi-heavenly beings also exist in the lower world and in the area between the lower and the middle worlds.

8. Ohira dates this text between the sixth/fifth and first centuries BCE (1994, 1).

9. See also chapter 6.

10. All nine "reals" are mentioned already in the Śvetāmbara canon, but K.K. Dixit points out that rather than providing lists of "reals," canonical texts tend to refer to them in sets—for example, as living and nonliving entities (*jīva-ajīva*), bondage and liberation (*bandha-mokṣa*), nonmeritorious and meritorious types of karma (*puṇya-pāpa*), and so on. He suggests that presenting "reals" in the form of a list is Umāsvāti's response to the Nyāya-Vaiśeṣika list of the objects of valid knowledge (*prameya*), a clear comprehension of which is supposed to lead one to liberation (cf. den Boer 2020, 81–82). Dixit proposes that the fact that Umāsvāti presents "reals" as being causally connected, with karmic influx leading to bondage, and stoppage and removal of karma leading to liberation, he follows a similar causal formula in Buddhism, which identifies the cause of suffering (*duḥkha*) in craving

(*tṛṣṇā*) and proposes a way to liberation through its elimination (Dixit 1971, 5). While the "reals" already feature in canonical sources, Umāsvāti as one of the earliest systematizers of the Jain teachings chooses to present his whole doctrinal system and soteriological project through them, which was not characteristic of textual sources prior to him (Ohira 1982, 56). His intention is attested by the title of his work, which purports to explain the meaning of the "reals" (*tattva-artha*).

11. See US 28.14 and SthS 9§667.

12. For a list of nine "reals" in Digambara texts, see DS 28 and PañS 108.

13. For the triplet, see US 23.33. Perhaps inspired by the Buddhist four noble truths, Umāsvāti adds the word "right" (*samyak*) to them, which is the formulation that has come to be most frequently used (Ohira 1982, 56). "Three Jewels" are also called "Three Gems" or "Three Qualities" (*guṇa-traya*). In the Jain symbol, the three jewels are visually represented with three dots located above the fourfold *svastika*. See figure 3.

14. For a discussion of the difference between US's and TS's treatment of this topic, see den Boer 2002, 78–79. For an overview of different Jain articulations of the meaning of right worldview, see Williams (1963, 41).

15. See US 28.1–3.

16. It is important to note that the arrangement of reality into living and nonliving entities develops gradually within Jainism. The *Ācārāṅga-sūtra*, for example, does not mention the term "nonliving" (*ajīva*) and instead divides existing entities into those that have thought and those that do not (Dundas 2002, 93).

17. Because historically not all Jain mendicants have been educated, this topic has been a matter of concern within Jain communities. In an effort to promote the intellectual education of Jain mendicants (in this case the Tapā Gaccha of the Mūrtipūjaka community), Ācārya Oṃkārasūri stated at a mendicant conference in Ahmedabad, Gujarat, in 1988: "What must monks and nuns be taught? It is necessary for them to be given knowledge in a graduated manner. This way they can learn the scriptures, and become knowledgeable. To accomplish this we must think about devising a curriculum. It is also necessary to establish an institution for study so that they can learn in the proper manner. It is impossible for a soul desirous of liberation to maintain conduct without knowledge of Jain metaphysics" (Śeṭha 1988, 35, cited in Cort 2001b, 328).

18. See $TS^{Dig}$ 5.29.

19. Translating these terms as "soul" can be problematic in monotheist contexts of Judaism, Christianity, or Islam wherein the "soul" often represents a defining characteristic of human life that distinguishes it from soulless matter and other living beings (Donaldson 2016).

20. See Bronkhorst (2000) for an analysis of the development of the concept of *pudgala* and its possible connections with the Buddhist doctrines.

21. Digambaras generally accept the existence of a separate substance of time, whereas Śvetāmbaras are divided with regard to the issue, and some understand time as the modal modification of the other five kinds of substances rather than an independent substance (Bajželj 2017, 1238–41).

22. This implies that knowing one substance perfectly is, in some way, knowing all of reality perfectly. An early formulation of this idea appears in the ĀS 1.3.4.1. See Johnson (2014, 143) regarding whether this statement is descriptive or prescriptive.

23. See, for example, BhS 7.2§299b.

24. Also *nyāsa*.

25. Literally "the doctrine of maybe (*syāt*)."

26. Jain philosophers maintain not only that the world is multiplex, but that it is infinitely complex, every object being endowed with an infinite number of properties. This means that an infinite number of assertions can be made about a single object. Some assertions are seemingly incompatible, but Jains claim that none actually exclude one another, since all are only conditionally valid and based on distinct contextual parameters. While omniscient beings are the only ones that cognize the entire range of the properties of a single object, as discussed below, ordinary people cognize objects in a limited way—that is, from particular standpoints and viewpoints.

27. Jain texts do not explicitly state whether non-one-sidedness also holds for disembodied liberated *jīvas*, which we will discuss below (Bajželj 2018).

28. An exception to this equality is a category of living beings that Jain texts define as being devoid of the inner ability to attain liberation (*bhavyatva*), since the capacity of these *jīvas*' qualities is always limited (Jaini 2010a).

29. As detailed below, this does not mean that a *jīva* is completely disembodied.

30. Because the Jain cosmos is considered to be without a beginning or end, there is no time when *jīvas* were not bound by karmic matter. This means that *jīvas* were never pure before a "fall" into karmic bondage. Even though their inherent nature is perfect and not polluted, their manifestation as such is expressed primarily as a potentiality that *jīvas* can strive for (Jaini 2001/1979, 107).

31. Much like the cosmography discussed above, the Jain karmic doctrine gradually developed into a sophisticated and independent branch of learning (Dundas 2002, 99).

32. Ohira notes that while the term *karman* tends to mean "action" in the earliest portions of the Śvetāmbara canon, in the late first canonical stage the meaning seems to be a material substance like dust (*rajas*) (1994, 7–8; for her chronology of canonical stages, see 1–2).

33. TS$^{Śv}$ 5.32–35.

34. As Dundas points out, the idea that karmically bondable material aggregates are spread out throughout the entire cosmos is not present in the earliest Jain doctrine (2002, 97).

35. This is similar to comparing an embodied *jīva* to a large leaky boat fully submerged in water to illustrate the bondage between matter and *jīvas* (BhS 1.6§83b).

36. TS$^{Śv}$ 8.2–3.

37. See chapter 3 for the other factors of bondage and to see how all of them relate to the wider goal of nonviolence in Jainism and map onto the path of liberation through the fourteen stages (*guṇa-sthāna*).

38. See, for example, US 31.3.

39. See chapter 3. For an analysis of the concept of passions in early Jainism, particularly with regard to the emergence of *kaṣāyas* as a central doctrinal element, see Bruhn (1987).

40. Nemicandra explains that the activities of the *jīva* and passions affect different aspects of karmic bondages. Type bondage (*prakṛti-bandha*) and quantity bondage (*pradeśa-bandha*) result from activities, whereas duration bondage (*sthiti-bandha*) and intensity bondage (*anubhāga-bandha*) result from passions (DS 33). See SSi 8.3§736; Jaini (2001/1979, 113); and Wiley (2008, 44, fn. 5).

41. Ohira dates most of this Śvetāmbara canonical text between the sixth/fifth and fourth centuries BCE (1994, 1).

42. See Dundas's analysis of these similes (2002, 97–98).

43. Jain philosophers usually do not explicitly address the issue of the interaction between two essentially different substances, in this case the immaterial *jīva* and matter. Kundakunda, however, indicates that he is aware of the problem when he states: "When karmically bondable aggregates meet with the modifications (*pariṇati*) of the *jīva*, they attain the state of karma (*karma-bhāva*). They are not modified by the *jīva*" (PS 2.77). His commentator Amṛtacandrasūri expands on this and concludes that since the interaction is indirect (i.e., through modifications only), the self (*puruṣa*) is not the agent (*kartṛ*) of the karmic state of material aggregates (TD 2.77). Similarly, karmic aggregates do not directly affect the *jīva*. In Jaini's words, karmic matter is merely an efficient (*nimitta*; i.e., instrumental) rather than a material (*upādāna*) cause of karmic effects (Jaini 2001/1979, 117). See also the idea that earlier, karma was understood to be nonmaterial (Ohira 1980, 44–45; Wiley 2008, 51–52), the idea that *jīva* was understood to be material (Johnson 1995b, 45; cf. Dundas 1997, 509–10), and the idea that the current understanding of the *jīva* allows for some flexibility with regard to its exact nature (Jaini 1979/2001, 113–15). For the doctrine of *leśya*s, or colors of the *jīva*, see Wiley (2000b).

44. See also the idea that a portion of the merit generated in future worship is received by the donor (Cort 2003, 138).

45. For the Śvetāmbara Mūrtipujaka Jain sectarian tradition in relation to the other sects, see chapter 1, note 3.

46. This specific worship is related to the festival of Navpad Oḷī, which is observed mostly by women with a specific purpose of granting health and well-being to their families (Cort 2003, 142).

47. See Granoff (1992b) for Jain mortuary rituals performed on behalf of the dead, including praying for them.

48. Wiley points out that "although different 'molecules' of karmic matter are capable of producing different effects, there is apparently no definable physical quality by which one can determine which among the undifferentiated 'molecules' will form a specific variety (*prakṛti*) of karmic matter. Instead, karmic matter is discussed in more general terms" (Wiley 2003, 339).

49. See note 43 above. It should be noted that the type of karma that is drawn to the *jīva* is also related to the activity's degree of mental intention and intensity. For instance, telling a very elaborate, intentional lie for the sake of personal gain would draw more karma that will be bound for a longer time than uttering an exaggeration in a moment of excitement, though both attract karma. See chapter 3 for the concept of intention in Jainism as well as a more detailed analysis of the historical development of the concepts of activity and meritorious/nonmeritorious karma.

50. Dundas translates them as "harming" and "nonharming" (2002, 99).

51. Dundas notes that the division into eight kinds can be traced at least as far back as the *Bhagavatī-sūtra* (Dundas 2002, 99). See, for example, BhS 8.10§421b.

52. Also translated as "confusing karma" (Schubring 2000/1962, 180).

53. See note 28 above for an exception. For a definition of *omniscience*, see TBh 5.2.

54. Pūjyapāda defines activity (*yoga*) also as the vibration of the self (*ātman*) (SSi 6.1§610).

55. Jaini explains the latter with an example of illness preventing one from "giving free reign to a particular sensual impulse" (Jaini 2001/1979, 123), highlighting the complex dynamics between illness and the operation of the various karmic types.

56. TS$^{Śv}$ 2.37.

57. Apart from the four passions discussed above, conduct-deluding karma also produces nine subsidiary passions or emotions (*no-kaṣāya*), including laughter, pleasure and displeasure in sense activity, sorrow, fear, disgust, and sexual feelings/desires (Jaini 2001/1979, 118–21). While sexual feeling or desire (*veda*) is produced by conduct-deluding karma, biological sex (*liṅga*) is produced by name-determining karma, which will be discussed next. This points to the Jain distinction between the two (Sethi 2012, 71–74; Zwilling and Sweet 1996). See chapter 5.

58. Wiley translates this as "identity-producing karma" (1999, 114) and Schubring as "individuality or personality karma" (2000/1962, 181–82).

59. Wiley also translates it as "family karma" (1999, 114).

60. Schubring translates it as "the one to be perceived through the senses" (2000/1962, 180).

61. For a detailed account of nondestructive karmas, see Wiley (2000a).

62. The particular number 8,400,000 may have been an adaptation from a *śramaṇa* tradition known as the Ājīvikas, closely related to the early Jain community. The Ājīvika doctrine suggests that *every jīva* must pass through 8,400,000 great time periods (*mahākalpa*) before reaching liberation. The Jain tradition may have transformed this into the number of possible birth states (Balcerowicz 2016, 82–84; Jaini 2010ab, 130).

63. Glasenapp points out that ascetics can use this body to burn other living beings or objects (1942/1915, 12). Schubring explains this power as "radiation of either heat or coolness as an effect of either curse or blessing" (2000/1962, 139). Wiley notes that according to some Jain authors, after rigorous ascetic practices, certain heavenly beings, hell-beings, and five-sensed humans and animals can form a secondary fiery body, which can either stay in the body or travel out of it. The latter is subdivided into an auspicious (cooling) kind, which removes suffering, and an inauspicious (fiery) kind, which causes it (2000a, 145–47). See Wiley (2012, 163–64).

64. For example, it can assume a very small or an extremely large form, it can become very heavy or extremely light, and so on. Heavenly beings, hell-beings, and some one-sensed possess this body naturally, and humans can attain it through practices of purification (TS$^{Dig}$ 2.46–47 = TS$^{Śv}$ 2.47–48; Glasenapp 1942/1915, 12; Wiley 2012, 164–65, 191).

65. TS$^{Śv}$ 2.38–40.

66. TS$^{Śv}$ 2.43.

67. Once the longevity-determining karma is bound, the birth state is fixed and can no longer be changed. Many other aspects of the forthcoming embodiment that are influenced by the types of karma that are always arising and passing away, however, can still be modified, including the exact length of life, at least according to the Digambaras (Wiley 2003, 348–51).

68. TS$^{Śv}$ 8.13.

69. Nemicandra compares knowledge- and perception-obscuring karmas to a veil (*paṭa*) and a doorkeeper (*pratīhāra*), respectively, energy-obstructing karma to a treasurer (*bhaṇḍa-āgārika*), bliss-defiling karma to wine (*madya*), name-determining karma to

a painter (*citra*), longevity-determining karma to stock (*hali*), status-determining karma to a potter (*kulāla*), and feeling-determining karma to a sword (*asi*) (GKK 21; Glasenapp 1999/1925, 186). According to Jaini, the wine analogy highlights the idea that the attribute of bliss alone undergoes proper defilement, just as "drunkenness involves an actual alteration of one's internal chemistry" (Jaini 2001/1979, 117).

70. In fact, there developed a notion that a *jīva* has, in the course of its wanderings through the cycle of rebirths, attracted and cast off all karmic matter there is (SSi 2.10§275).

71. TS$^{Śv}$ 10.7.

72. These are sometimes also translated as "destinies."

73. See US 36.12, 36.79, 36.87, 36.101.

74. See J.L. Jaini's commentary to GJK 183.

75. Ohira dates much of this Śvetāmbara canonical text between the sixth/fifth and fourth centuries BCE (1994, 1).

76. The period of forty-eight minutes has considerable significance in the Jain tradition. Sometimes referred to as a *muhūrta*, this period represents one-thirtieth of a twenty-four-hour day. An *antar-muhūrta*, which is the term used in the text, is a period of less than forty-eight minutes.

77. We are mainly following Jacobi's translation of all of these classifications from the *Uttarādhyayana-sūtra*.

78. This unfortunate karmic turn was, according to the Jains, the fate of the leader of the Ājīvikas, Makkhali Gosāla.

79. Śvetāmbaras classify all living beings that undergo ordinary rebirths as *vyāvahārika*, or "specifiable." In relation to them, those beings who have known only the life of a *nigoda* are irregular and are thus designated as *avyāvahārika*, "unspecifiable." See Jaini (2010b, 128).

80. The *Bhagavatī-sūtra* states that the number of living beings does not increase or decrease but stays constant (BhS 5.8§244a).

81. This is interesting, particularly with regard to the belief that two-, three-, and four-sensed beings are capable of attaining rebirth in a human form but incapable of attaining liberation in that very human life, "rendering them inferior in this respect even to the *nitya-nigodas*" (Jaini 2003, 4). As noted above, fire-bodied and air-bodied beings are denied the possibility of rebirth in a human form, even though they represent higher birth forms than the *nitya-nigodas*. Jaini also notes the lack of stories that would describe earth- and water-bodied beings taking rebirth in a human form and attaining liberation (4).

82. According to Wiley, Digambara texts state that the bodies of Kevalins cannot act as hosts for gross-bodied *nigodas* (2000a, 229). *Nigodas*, further, cannot occupy the bodies of heavenly beings, hell-beings, and earth-, water-, fire-, and air-bodied beings (Jaini 2010b, 127).

83. For a distinction between *sātā/asātā* and *sukha/duḥkha*, see Wiley (2000a, 274).

84. For a more detailed analysis of the two aspects of sense cognition, see den Boer (2020, 148–50).

85. The *Tattvārtha-bhāṣya* 2.25 explains reflective awareness (*saṃpradhāraṇa-saṃjñā*) as reflection (*vicāraṇā*) on merits (*guṇa*) and demerits/defects (*doṣa*).

86. The *Bhagavatī-sūtra* states that this description applies also to two- to four-sensed beings (BhS 1.2§39a).

87. See note 85 above.

88. $TS^{Śv}$ 2.25.

89. For a discussion on how long this time period might be and on which beings can bind the two kinds of karma discussed here, see Wiley 2000a, 129–30.

90. $TS^{Śv}$ 2.32.

91. Ohira dates this Śvetāmbara canonical text in the first half of the fourth century CE (1994, 1).

92. For a further discussion on the violence of sex acts, see chapter 5.

93. For exceptions where a pregnancy is not a result of sex acts, see chapter 5.

94. $TS^{Śv}$ 2.34.

95. Life span is the only vitality that is a product not of the rising of the *nāma-karman* but of *āyu-karman* (GJK 131; Wiley 2000a, 187).

96. This means that besides having basic bodily and sensory functions, one-sensed beings that are capable of attaining complete development also develop a faculty of respiration. In the *Bhagavatī-sūtra*, Mahāvīra's student Gautama acknowledges that respiration is observed in two- through five-sensed beings. He points out, however, that respiration cannot be observed in the case of one-sensed beings and asks Mahāvīra whether these beings—despite our inability to observe it—breathe. Māhāvīra confirms that one-sensed beings possess respiration and, consequently, inhale and exhale (BhS 2.1§109). This dialogue presents another Jain caution against the assumption that if something does not look alive, it means that it is not alive.

97. See section above on "Ability to Develop a Body's Capacity."

98. In his comment on the *Gommaṭasāra-jīva-kāṇḍa* 119, Jaini explains that the difference between the *āhāra-paryāpti* and the *śarīra-paryāpti* is that "while the first helps in transforming the *āhāra vargaṇā* molecules into liquid and solid forms, the second effects the formation of the trunk, flesh, blood and bones etc." (1927, 84; Wiley 2000a, 128–29, fn. 27).

99. Ohira dates this Śvetāmbara canonical between the second half of the fourth century and the fifth century CE (1994, 2).

100. We here mainly follow the translation from Krümpelmann (2006, 8).

101. Umāsvāti compares a *jīva* to a lamplight in its ability to contract (*saṃhāra*) and expand (*visarga*) its space-points (*pradeśa*) (TS 5.16).

102. This shows the dependence of nondestructive types of karma on the destructive ones. See Jaini (2001/1979, 124, fn. 47).

103. The feeling-determining karma may sometimes be bound in larger quantities than other nondestructive karmas, which requires a special process of karmic thinning through which a *jīva* expands to the size of the cosmos and "shakes off" excessive karmic matter (Dundas 2002, 104; Jaini 2001/1979, 268–70; Schubring 2000/1962, 183–85).

104. $TS^{Śv}$ 10.3.

105. For a study of the *jīva*'s travel to the space of liberated beings, see Bajželj (2019).

106. Schubring suggests that this idea may have developed by observing the shrinking of the corpse (2000/1962, 329).

## CHAPTER 3. NONVIOLENCE AND THE FRAMEWORK OF JAIN ETHICS

1. In her analysis of words for violence in the early texts of the Śvetāmbara canon, Colette Caillat notes that the root *han-* seems to have had "a general meaning: it is liable to

express any form of aggression, of violence, torture . . . , including those which result in death" (1993, 219). While *hiṃs-* is a desiderative form, Caillat points out that forms derived from the roots *han-* and *hiṃs-* are occasionally exchanged and that words such as *hiṃsā* never reflect a desiderative meaning (207).

2. Mūrtipūjaka Jains accept all forty-five Āgamas; Sthānakavāsis and Terāpanthīs accept thirty-two (Wiley 2009, xix). The councils, arguably held at Pāṭaliputra (under Sthūlabhadra), at Mathurā (under Skandila), at Valabhī (under Nāgarjuna), and later at Valabhī (under Devarddhigaṇin Kṣemāśramaṇa), are typically dated in the fourth century BCE (first council) and from the fourth to sixth centuries CE (the other three councils). However, Royce Wiles cautions against acceptance of these dates and names without adequate historical support, as most scholars use quite late sources to determine this information (2006).

3. Suzuko Ohira dates these portions of the canon to the sixth/fifth to fourth centuries BCE (1994, 1). For more on how these early texts developed and how they relate to each other, see Dixit (1978, 2–3).

4. Dixit states that "at the most one can say that this treatment represents the earliest stage when Jaina speculation became acquainted with the concept of 5 *mahāvratas*" (1978, 7). He even suggests that all of these references to the five great vows may be later interpolations (19).

5. For an analysis of various words used for expressing violence in the early texts of the Śvetāmbara canon, see Caillat (1993).

6. For a few examples of these attachments and the harms they cause, see ĀS 1.2.2.2, 1.2.3.3–5, 1.2.4.1–3, 1.2.5.1; SKS 1.3.2.1–22, 1.7.4–9, 1.9.2–10.

7. Specifically, these early portions of the canon talk about six kinds of living beings (*jīva-nikāya*) that can be violated: earth-bodied, water-bodied, fire-bodied, wind-bodied, plant-bodied, and mobile beings (Ohira 1994, 5; see chapter 2).

8. See also the related *labh-*, with a prefix *ā-*, which means to kill or sacrifice, and to take hold of, touch, or handle (Monier-Williams 1899, 153; Johnson 1995a, 38; Whitney 1885, 136, 145–46).

9. See, for example, ĀS 1.3.1.3, where suffering (*duḥkha*) is defined as "born of *ārambha* (*ārambha-ja*)."

10. Kristi Wiley expresses doubt "that a reconstruction of an early version of Jain karma theory can be made on the basis of what is found and what is absent in these sources," particularly considering the detailed expositions of karma in later sources that are believed to be based on the no-longer-extant Aṅga, called *Dṛṣṭivāda*, itself thought to be based on the no-longer-extant earliest portions of the canon, the Pūrvas (Wiley 2016, 78).

11. Hermann Jacobi's decision to use the word *allow* in his translation opens up interesting questions of whether initially Jain mendicants were taught to prevent violence rather than merely refrain from approving of it. We discuss this issue in more detail later in this chapter. Cf. Jacobi's translation of ĀS 1.2.5.3 and SKS 1.1.1.3, where he uses the word *consent* instead.

12. This formula is repeated throughout the early canon. See, for example, ĀS 1.1.2.6, 1.1.3.8, 1.1.4.7, 1.1.5.7, 1.1.6.6, 1.1.7.7.

13. In his translation, Jacobi glosses the word as a *prāyaścitta* (1884, 48, fn. 2). For a detailed discussion of Jain atonements, see Caillat (1975).

14. Discussing the specific section of the *Uttarādhyayana-sūtra* mentioned above, Dixit states: "Certainly, in the course of time it became a common practice for monks to wander

about in the form of a unit functioning under the headship of an *ācārya* assisted by a staff made up of *upādhyāya* etc. This replaced the old practice of a young student staying with his preceptor just for the duration of his education. . . . [F]or this final practice [of wandering about in a unit] must be the result as soon as disciples make it a point not to take leave of their preceptor even when their education was over" (1978, 24–25). Dixit also points out the *Uttarādhyayana-sūtra* 32.4–5 as a possible intermediary stage between the two mendicant lifestyles. These two verses encourage mendicants to seek companions equal or superior to themselves, but if they cannot find any, it is suggested that they should wander alone (24).

15. Ohira states that earlier even the existence of a heavenly realm (*deva-loka*) was rejected (1994, 6).

16. The *Uttarādhyayana-sūtra* belongs to a group of texts called the Mūla-sūtras, or "Root Texts," that every novice had to master upon entering mendicancy. It is believed to be the last sermon of Mahāvīra.

17. See chapter 1 for an explanation of the cycles of time, in accordance with which liberation is possible only in particular periods in our part of the cosmos.

18. Like the *Uttarādhyayana-sūtra*, the *Daśavaikālika-sūtra* also belongs to the instructional Mūla-sūtras for novice mendicants. Shortly after its composition, it replaced the *Ācārāṅga-sūtra* in the mendicant curriculum and is today perhaps the most important Jain book on mendicant conduct.

19. Controlling the body, speech, and mind is mentioned already in the *Sūtrakṛtāṅga-sūtra* I (1.2.1.22). Ohira suggests that the notion of the triplet of bodily, verbal, and mental activities was borrowed from Buddhism (1994, 9).

20. The third term that developed from the original *karman*, Ohira explains, was *kriyā*, which came to designate "evil action" that a practitioner should avoid (1992, 19). See Donaldson (2021) for an analysis of the term *kriyā*.

21. Padmanabh Jaini states that historically, "Jainas have not been blind to the importance of resisting injustice and aggression" (2001/1979, 171). He particularly points out the example of self-defense for the purpose of which violent acts came to be permitted. For the Jain approaches to self-defense (*virodhī-hiṃsā*), see Dundas (2007b, 44), Jaini (2004), and chapter 6 in relation to antibiotic use.

22. Ohira dates a large portion of this Śvetāmbara canonical text to the first century BCE/first century CE to third century CE (1994, 1).

23. Petit describes how the two parts of the *Gommaṭasāra*—*Jīva-kāṇḍa* and *Karma-kāṇḍa*—address unique aspects of the fourteen stages (2015, 110).

24. Glasenapp notes that the *Karmagranthas* include carelessness under nonrestraint (1942/1915, 62, fn. 1).

25. See Glasenapp (1942/1915, 62–63) and Petit (2015, 99–100) for a detailed list of these. Every primary cause also has a number of secondary subcauses (*uttara-hetu*), which together add up to fifty-seven (Glasenapp 1942/1915, 62).

26. According to Jaini, this is an initial confrontation with the "knot" (*granthi*) of the gross passions and deluding karmas. The term *yathā-pravṛtta-karaṇa* normally refers to the *jīva*'s "ineradicable tendency towards spiritual growth," he notes, and points out that the fact that it is used in this context indicates how important the event of becoming aware of the "knot" and the first resistance to one's karmic entrapment is for the *jīva*'s development (2001/1979, 143–44).

27. The second rung, called *sāsvādana* ("taste of right belief") (SSN 13.8 and GJK 9, trans. Petit), describes a momentary instant when gross (*ananta-anubandhī*) passions reassert themselves (Jaini 2001/1979, 145). Cort equates this stage with adherents of other traditions who possess more wrong understanding than right (2001a, 25). This stage can only be reached during a fall back to the first rung from a higher level (Jaini 2001/1979, 272; Tatia 1951, 276–77), exemplifying the advancements and regressions upon the ladder toward liberation. The third rung, called *samyag-mithyātva* or *miśra* ("mixed") (GJK 9 and SSN 13.8, trans. Petit), is also a brief intermediate stage. This is a stage of indifference, in which passions are not yet fully reasserted, but the insight is not clear anymore (Cort 2001a, 26; Jaini 2001/1979, 145).

28. For other new characteristics that arise with the experience of the fourth rung, see Jaini (2001/1979, 151–56) and Williams (1963, 42–46).

29. Robert Williams remarks that *anukampā* refers to both the internal attitude as well as the actions stemming from it: "In its material aspect this virtue takes the form of practical steps to remedy suffering where one has the power and in its non-material aspect it expresses itself in tenderness of the heart" (1963, 42).

30. TS$^{Dig}$ 6.12.

31. TS$^{Dig}$ 7.11.

32. Ācārya Suśīlkumār was the second Jain monk to come to the United States. Citrabhānu (1922–2019), who left his life as a Śvetāmbara Mūrtipūjaka mendicant after twenty-nine years, came to the United States in 1971, starting the Jain Meditation International Center for non-Jains interested in nonviolence and self-realization and helping establish the Federation of Jain Associations in North America (JAINA) (Shah 2017b, 109–18).

33. Signe Kirde notes that the *pratimā* ladder is also called *ekādaśa-sthāna* and *śrāvaka-pada* (2011, 11). According to Petit, *pratimā*, meaning "image" or "statue," likely refers to the statues of the Jinas in the motionless position of *kāyotsarga*, "standing with their arms at their sides," which are to be emulated by the followers (2015, 106; see also Williams 1963, 172). For a summary chart of the *pratimās*, see Jaini (2001/1979, 186) and Petit (n.d.).

34. Several scholars have noted that very few laypersons take these vows under the formal direction of a mendicant as prescribed in early texts devoted to the practices of lay life (Dundas 2002, 189–91; Jaini 2001/1979, 160; Laidlaw 1995, 173–75).

35. See also the "Four Refuges" (*catuḥ-śaraṇa*) (Jaini 2001/1979, 164).

36. For the variations in the Digambara and Śvetāmbara understanding of the *mūla-guṇas*, see Williams (1963, 50–55).

37. TS$^{Dig}$ 6.4–6.

38. TS$^{Śv}$ 8.10.

39. The *sāmāyika-pratimā* also includes *pūjā* such as worshipping the Jinas or other temple rituals, of which mendicants do only the former.

40. Describing the (un)boiled water concerns, Cort notes that "by boiling water, one prevents the birth of infinite invisible organisms, and therefore actually prevents much *hiṃsā*. The small amount of *hiṃsā* that one causes from boiling water is much less than that which results from drinking unboiled water with all its microorganisms" (2001a, 131). Laidlaw additionally explains that a layperson who boils the water takes the karmic harm of killing organisms upon him or herself: "One goes through the division of labour: the person who boils the water and so does the killing may not be the person who drinks it. This indeed

is routinely the case, as [mendicants] never boil water themselves. They are forbidden to use fire with just the same severity as they are forbidden to use unboiled water and their water is boiled in advance by lay people" and usually, he adds, by senior women (1995, 155–56).

41. For other foods in this category, see Williams (1963, 176–77).

42. Although the concept of carelessness has various meanings throughout the canon (Donaldson 2019c), by the time of the *Tattvārtha-sūtra*, the term takes on a technical meaning, designated as one of the five causes of bondage (TS 8.1) that must be overcome to progress toward further stages of karmic removal. The *Samayasāra-nāṭaka* lists five types of carelessness (SSN 13.79), while the *Gommaṭasāra-jīva-kāṇḍa* lists eighty possible combinations of carelessness (GJK 32–44).

43. In addition to the *saṃjvalana* passions, Glasenapp suggests that sleep also induces carelessness, and gestures toward other causes as well (1942/1915, 82).

44. For a deeper analysis of *anuprekṣā*, see the introduction in Upadhye (1960).

45. These obligatory practices were detailed in the earliest portions of the *Āvaśyaka-sūtra* (second to third centuries CE).

46. The *Tattvārtha-sūtra* states that fourteen hardships are experienced in *guṇa-sthānas* 10–12. Only eleven hardships are experienced by the Jinas in *guṇa-sthānas* 13–14, although, since passions and deluding karmas are no longer operative at these two stages, the hardships occur without inciting any response (TS 9.10–11).

47. Jaini describes the nature of omniscience in this stage (2001/1979, 266–67).

48. $TS^{Śv}$ 6.23. Jaini states that one of the sixteen forms of action that are conducive to producing these Jina-related karmas is "service to sick mendicants," which is his explanation of *vaiyāvṛttya-karaṇa*, listed as "service to the teacher and other mendicants" under the "internal ascetic practices" earlier in this chapter. In fact, he writes, service to the sick is regarded as one of the three most important of the sixteen kinds of action (2001/1979, 260; derived from TS 6.23).

49. Tatia states that the fourteenth rung "lasts only for the period of time required to pronounce five short syllables at the ordinary speed. . . . At the end of this period the soul attains *unembodied emancipation*" (1951, 279; emphasis added). See SSN 13.8 and Glasenapp (1942/1915, 91–92).

50. $TS^{Śv}$ 7.20.

51. $TS^{Śv}$ 7.21.

52. $TS^{Śv}$ 7.22.

53. $TS^{Śv}$ 7.23.

54. $TS^{Śv}$ 7.24.

55. In the medieval period, Amṛtacandrasūri offers a near duplication of this list in his *Puruṣārtha-siddhyupāya* (PSU 190).

56. Ohira dates this text to the fourth century CE (1994, 1).

57. These are listed in the *Sāgāra-dharmāmṛta* by the Digambara author Āśādhara (Williams 1963, 117).

58. For example, the Śvetāmbara *Śrāddha-vidhi* by Ratnaśekhara (sixteenth century CE) and the Digambara *Traivarṇika-ācāra* by Somasena (seventeenth century CE).

## CHAPTER 4. JAINISM'S EVOLVING VIEW OF MEDICINE

1. Drawing from *Niśītha-bhāṣya*, Willem Bollée notes that the difference between *vyādhi* and *roga* is that while "the former is lethal in a short time, the latter is a slow killer"

(2003–2004, 162; see also Stuart 2014, 77). Further, *roga*, according to Madhu Sen, can be cured only through a slow healing process (1975, 182). Examples of *vyādhi* include fever, asthma, cough, internal heat, diarrhea, and others; examples of *roga* include tremor, bent back, diabetes, deafness, blindness, and others. Mental illness, discussed next, is considered *roga* (Bollée 2003–2004, 174; see also Sen 1975, 183). Two other common terms for illness are *ātaṅka* and *āmaya*, and Sen notes that, like *vyādhi, ātaṅka* was understood to be a serious illness from which one could die in a very short period of time (1975, 182–83).

2. While the life spans of humans in the "lands of enjoyment" can thus not be shortened by factors such as illness, life spans in the "lands of action" can be (see chapters 2 and 7).

3. For *prāṇas*, see chapter 2.

4. They both agree that this type of karma is also associated with injury (*vadha*) (TS 9.16; TVā 8.8.2).

5. Śvetāmbaras seem to connect *upaghāta-nāma-karman* with an irregular bodily formation, such as an additional finger or a protruding tooth, that is not deadly but can prove to be painful or embarrassing (Wiley 2000a, 171–72). For a list of irregularities in bodily stature as they relate to a subtype of name-determining karma called *saṃsthāna-nāma-karman*, see Glasenapp (1942/1915, 14–15).

6. Ugrāditya discusses specific illnesses arising from the disturbances of the three humors in chaps. 8–19 of his *Kalyāṇa-kāraka* (KK).

7. Monier Monier-Williams translates *rasa* as "a constituent fluid or essential juice of the body, serum, (esp.) the primary juice called chyle (formed from the food and changed by the bile into blood)" (1899, 869). *Rasa* also represents female fluid, which is a vital component needed in the conception of a child (see chapter 5).

8. See Varṇī (2012/1970, vol. 1, 471).

9. See Bollée (2003–2004, 166) for blood as a cause of an eye disease in addition to the three humors.

10. For an example of blood disturbance due to the three humors, see Bollée (2003–2004, 169).

11. Meulenbeld points out that blood is also defined both as a humor, which is a secondary bodily constituent according to the division noted above, and as a primary bodily constituent (*dhātu*) (KK 3.61; Meulenbeld 2000, vol. IIB, 175).

12. In his commentary to the *Sthānāṅga-sūtra*, Abhayadevasūri explains that in the case of the first three kinds, the main cause of illness (*nidāna*) is that factor alone, whereas the last one is a combination (*saṃyoga*) of either two or three of them (Jambūvijaya 2003, 452–53). N.L. Jain suggests that this fourfold system is different from the āyurvedic system of the three humors and points out that, by contrast, the *Bhagavatī-ārādhanā* and *Kalyāṇa-kāraka* both follow the āyurvedic system (1996, 533). For a discussion of how certain humors affect predispositions and lifestyle preferences of mendicants and how these should be accommodated in the community, see Stuart (2014, 77–78).

13. See Stuart (2014, 73). For other examples of an illness arising from improper food, see JK 5 and Granoff (1998a, 244).

14. Cf. ĀS 1.8.4.1, which states that Mahāvīra refused to take medicine. See also Dixit (1978, 5, 13), Granoff (1998a, 241–42), and Wujastyk (1984).

15. See, for example, Abhayadevasūri's commentary, as noted in Deleu (1996/1970, 219). See also chapter 6.

16. The idea behind this is that their ascetic practices have provided them with extraordinary healing powers (Granoff 1998a, 245; Wiley 2012, 159–60, 174–75). For ascetics

providing religious healing, including treatment of leprosy, bringing the dead to life, and producing missing limbs, in exchange for religious conversion, see Granoff (1989, 198–99, 204–7, 214).

17. For deities healing injuries and illnesses, see Granoff (1989, 210–11) and Granoff (1998a, 221, 239–41, 244–46). For deities and ascetics imbuing objects and children with healing properties, see Granoff (1989, 210–11, 213).

18. Some religious hymns are believed to have been composed with the specific purpose of healing, such as Mānatuṅga's *Bhaktāmara-stotra*, which was created with the intention of ending a plague in the city of Takṣaśilā (Granoff 1998a, 219). For another example of a religious healing of a plague, see Granoff (1998c, 124).

19. Related to these different variations of improper eating is also eating at night as a cause of illness (Bollée 2003–2004, 164; see chapter 3).

20. "Excessive sensuous pleasures" are considered a cause of mental illness, which we will return to below.

21. For various cases of illnesses where lifestyle choices are related to the three humors, see Bollée (2003–2004). Granoff, further, mentions an account according to which Abhayadevasūri suffered from a *blood imbalance* due to his "overzealous fasting and studying" (1998a, 219, 239–40).

22. The Jain approaches to the prevention of illness will be further explored in chapter 6.

23. For an example of leprosy resulting from theft and dishonesty, see Granoff (1998a, 248).

24. Granoff notes that the illnesses most frequently cured are those that were brought on by evil heavenly beings (1998a, 224, 230).

25. See SthS 2.1.75, which states the same. For an example of a possession caused by a human being, see Granoff (1998a, 234).

26. Stuart suggests a connection between deluding karmas and bodily humors: "One might say that the deluding karmas are a particularly Jain way of understanding disturbed bodily *doṣas*—or perhaps more accurately, what the Jains perceive as their underlying cause" (2014, 88).

27. See also Bollée (2003–2004, 176).

28. He does not provide the source but is perhaps at least partially drawing from the *Bhagavatī-sūtra* 3.7§197b. Jain also mentions *udvega-graha* as a "psychological/emotional disease."

29. Suzuko Ohira dates this Śvetāmbara canonical text to the fourth century CE (1994, 1).

30. For more on possession and Jainism, see Aukland (2010, 2013), Gordeeva (2015), Humphrey and Laidlaw (1994), Kelting (2001, 104), and Vallely (2002a, 115–39; 2011).

31. TS$^{\text{Śv}}$ 8.11.

32. Likewise, Anne Vallely states that "possession results in the diversion or shifting of *agency* from the self to the alien other" (2002a, 128).

33. Deo identifies the acceptance of medicine particularly within the postcanonical commentaries on the Cheda-sūtras and the Mūla-sūtras (1954–1955, 437–38); Stuart examines three postcanonical commentaries: *Niśītha-bhāṣya*, *Vyavahāra-bhāṣya*, and *Bṛhatkalpa-bhāṣya*.

34. For an explanation of the *Ācārāṅga* I and the *Sūtrakṛtāṅga* I, see chapter 3.

35. We are using the standard translations of the Jain understanding of various illnesses.

36. Approving of others receiving or providing medical care is not mentioned in the passage.

37. As in chapter 3, we here follow the canonical chronology proposed by Ohira (1994).

38. For a reference to a hospital (*cikitsā-śālā*) with a variety of staff, see JK 13.

39. For *bhūtikarma*, see Mitra (1939, 175). The *Sthānāṅga-sūtra* states that *bhūtikarma* leads to the accrual of *abhiyogatva* types of karma that result in rebirth as a subordinate *abhigoyika* heavenly being (SthS 4.568).

40. Ohira dates this text to the fourth century CE (1994, 1).

41. See also Jain (1947, 179).

42. The *Niśītha-sūtra* is one of the Cheda-sūtras, or texts on mendicant discipline.

43. Drawing from later canonical sources, Jagdish Chandra Jain notes that "meat and wine were freely prescribed as diet by physicians" (1947, 180). See also Deo (1954–1955, 177, fn. 237, 210).

44. Drawing from the *Vyavahāra-sūtra*, Stuart notes that "service" in this period means "attending to a person's daily needs and, in cases of sickness, caring for him or her" (2014, 76).

45. Granoff identifies this obligatory duty to help the sick as beginning in the *Bṛhatkalpa-sūtra* and continuing through the postcanonical commentaries. Cf. Granoff (2017, 35–37), where extraordinary circumstances, under which patients may be abandoned, are listed; among others, these are plague, being under a threat of a ruler, or in times of unrest. Nevertheless, it is made clear that such practice is far from ideal, and it is indicated that truly great mendicants will never leave the sick behind, even when in danger.

46. Stuart describes this commentary, composed by Śvetāmbara monk Saṅghadāsa, as representing "by far the richest and lengthiest discussions on medicine in Jain mendicant life" (2014, 77).

47. See Granoff (2017, 36–37) for an interpretation of caring for the sick as restraint (*saṃyama*) and austerity (*tapas*).

48. Granoff notes that the *Bhagavatī-sūtra* deems one who provides care for the ill as doing reverence to the Jina by following the "Three Jewels" of right worldview, knowledge, and conduct (2014, 236).

49. Cf. Stuart (2014, 76–77).

50. For allowance of non-Jain food in case of illness, see, for example, Deo (1954–1955, 417–18). For instruction on differentiating between major and minor illnesses of varying intensity, see Stuart (2014, 77).

51. It should be noted that a class of semi-renunciant Śvetāmbara mendicants, called *yati*s, who dwelt in one place, were known for, among other things, their expertise in āyurvedic medicine (Wiley 2009, 240). They provided their services for money. Medical knowledge and services of *yati*s and *bhaṭṭāraka*s, their approximate Digambara equivalent, is an important topic in need of further research.

52. For more on the various extraordinary healing powers, see Granoff (1998a), Granoff (1998c), and Wiley (2012).

53. For a Digambara example, see Granoff (1998a, 236–38).

54. See Wiley (2000a: chap. 1) for an introduction to the various lands of the Jain cosmos. Additionally, as Wiley explains, it seems that birth in the *bhoga-bhūmi*s ("lands

of enjoyment") often takes place when circumstances would normally warrant rebirth in heaven but a slightly less desirable birth as a human in the *bhoga-bhūmis* is attained instead (60).

55. Meulenbeld explains: "After a maṅgala addressed to the first Tīrthaṅkara, Ṛṣabha, the book opens with the Jain version of the descent (*avatāra*) of āyurveda (1.2–10): the medical science was revealed by Ādinātha (= Ṛṣabha) with the goddess Sarasvatī as an intermediary, to the first cakravartin, Bharata, and others, when mankind became oppressed by disease in the present avasarpiṇī; subsequently every Tīrthaṅkara proclaimed this science, until it was acquired by the gaṇadharas, śrutakevalins and other holy men, who transmitted it to their pupils" (2002, vol. IIA, 151).

56. For Jain alchemy, see Balbir (1992).

## CHAPTER 5. POTENTIALS OF (RE)BIRTH

1. The National Health Portal of India offers a hospital directory database at www.nhp.gov.in/directoryservices/hospitals. The number of Jain-sponsored hospitals was calculated by searching this directory using the keywords "Jain," "Jaina," "Mahavir" (including alternate spellings), and "Parshva(natha)" (including alternate spellings), arriving at a total of 213 facilities, though there are certain hospitals with Jain affiliations that were overlooked in this count. Additionally, there are other medical programs associated with Jain endeavors—such as the health clinics of Veeryatan, started by Ācārya Candanā (Wiley 2009, 65), or the Anekant Community Center in Southern California—that were not explicitly included.

2. Personal email correspondence with Sanmati Thole, president of the Jain Medical Doctors Association of India, January 19, 2018. Additional organizations include Jain Doctors' Federation in Mumbai and National Jain Doctors' Association, although we were not able to get definitive membership data from these two groups. Jain physicians can also be found by searching the Indian Medical Directory.

3. See chapter 1 for demographic details and sources.

4. Personal email correspondence with Manoj Jain, December 21, 2017.

5. The introductory video is available online at www.youtube.com/watch?v=Tw9joiNJDkU&list=UUgZi8PYp1Mfa6p8dfgwCSiQ&index=3&t=0s.

6. Some data totals may not equal 100 percent, for two primary reasons: (1) we only round fractions up over 0.5 and, thus, lesser fractions will sometimes constitute a missing percentage; or (2) a rare participant error (such as selecting all options) required removing their response from the set for accuracy.

7. Some participants ($n = 21$) optionally listed their MD specializations, which included internal medicine and surgery (6), anesthesiology (3), family medicine (3), pathology (2), urology, psychiatry, emergency medicine, neonatology, pediatrics, gastroenterology, and cardiology. "Other" ($n = 3$) included doctor of physical therapy, pharmaceutical development, and three-year bachelor's degree.

8. For an analysis of Jain temple education, or *pāṭhaśālā*, in the United States, see Donaldson (2019a, 2019b).

9. As discussed in chapters 2 and 3, only liberation represents the end of (re)births. In line with this, early mendicant manuals assert that wise persons should avoid conception and birth the same as they would evade the passions, delusion, and suffering (ĀS 1.3.4.4; see also US 32.7).

10. $TS^{Śv}$ 2.32–36.

11. It should be noted that Śvetāmbara Terāpanthīs do not celebrate the event of conception, while the Śvetāmbara Mūrtipūjaka Kharatara Gaccha sect sometimes celebrates a sixth auspicious event, the transfer of embryo, which will be described below (Wiley 2009, 115–16). See also Cort (2010, 23–24).

12. Peter Harvey asserts that about half of the pre-Mahāyāna schools, including Theravāda, did not share the idea of an intermediate existence between death and rebirth (*antarā-bhava*) (2013/1990, 71).

13. Kundakunda describes a moment as the time needed for the smallest material particle to move across one space unit (PS 2.47).

14. $TS^{Śv}$ 2.26–30. For greater detail on the transitional period between births, see chapter 2 and Wiley (2000a, 153–63).

15. The *Sthānāṅga-sūtra* 5.2.103 describes five ways in which a woman can conceive without having had intercourse: (1) if she is sitting and draws in semen; (2) if a piece of cloth containing semen enters her vagina; (3) if she puts semen into her vagina herself; (4) if somebody else does it; and (5) if semen enters her while she is taking a bath. N.L. Jain, however, states, "The canons do not seem to give confirmed examples of such uncopulated births except in the case of mother of Keśīkumāra in the second category" (1996, 547). Drawing from the *Vṛtti*, Surendra Bothra in his translation of the *Sthānāṅga-sūtra* explains: "Keshi Kumar's mother had put a bunch of hair in her vagina either for pacifying itching or to stop flow of blood. That bunch of hair was soiled with semen and as a consequence she became pregnant" (Bothra 2004, 146, see under SthS). For human beings born through agglutination (which is not the result of sex acts and takes place in open space), see chapter 2.

16. For a deeper account of substances involved in conception, see Das (2003).

17. Pūjyapāda describes the womb/belly (*udara*) of the mother as a mixed place of birth (*miśra-yoni*), since blood and semen are not conscious (*acitta*), but they are mixed (*miśraṇa*) with the vitality or self (*ātman*) of the mother that has consciousness (*cittavat*) (SSi 2.32§324) (Tatia 2011, 53; Wiley 2000a, 136). See also SthS 3.1.100.

18. Kristi Wiley points to the *Yaśodhara-caritra* where it is said that a *jīva* can enter a womb for up to seven days after a sex act, such that a *jīva* of a male goat who previously engaged in intercourse with a female goat can enter this same female goat's womb after it dies as a male goat (2000a, 190–91; see Granoff 1993, 122). This indicates that it is technically possible to be one's own parent. Such complicated interlinking of lives is common in Jain narratives and, as Dundas states, "seem[s], at an ideal level, to have been intended to destabilise any fixed sense of social and familial identity and so ease the individual's path into a spiritual journey in which such ties eventually have to be abandoned" (Dundas 2002, 101; see chapter 3).

19. For other reasons why a woman cannot conceive, see SthS 5.2.104.

20. We discuss the implications of this for the understanding of sex as a violent act later in this chapter.

21. Various terms that Jains use for the "third sex" include *napuṃsaka* (lit. "not-a-male"), *tṛtīya* ("third"), *trairāśika* ("third heap"), *klība* (sexually defective man), and *paṇḍaka* (perhaps meaning "impotent" or "sterile") (Zwilling and Sweet 1996, 363–64).

22. *Taṇḍula-vaicārika* states that the *jīva* is transmuted into an embryo after it has had food for the first time at the union of the maternal *ojas* and the paternal semen (p. 5, 1–3). Caillat suggests that while the *Vṛtti* explains *ojas* as menstrual blood (*ārtavaṃ śoṇitam*), it

may be possible to interpret it as that which is carried by menstrual blood, thus being able to feed the embryo (Caillat 2019, 5, fn. 20).

23. Defective parental fluids can lead to dysfunctions in the embryo. For an example of an embryo disfigurement caused by a defect in parents, see Bollée (2003–2004, 167).

24. The *Taṇḍula-vaicārika* states that an embryo stays in the material womb for about 277½ days, that is, 8,325 *muhūrtas* (Caillat 2018, 4). The *Bhagavatī-sūtra* states that a human pregnancy can last anywhere from less than a *muhūrta* to twelve years (BhS 2.5§133a).

25. Wiley explains that sense faculties accompany *jīvas* even without the principal body (2000a, 177). Nascent embryos are said to possess the fiery and karmic bodies, not the gross physical, transformational, and translocational bodies (BhS 1.7§86b).

26. For more on *dohada*, see Bauer (1998, 220–21, 219–69; 2003) and Jain (1996, 543–44).

27. Mahāvīra's mother is said to see an elephant, a bull, a lion, the goddess Śrī, a garland, the moon, the sun, a flag, a vase, a lotus lake, the ocean, a heavenly abode, a heap of jewels, and a flame (KS 2.3–4). The dreams vary slightly across texts and within the Digambara tradition (Jaini 2001/1979, 7).

28. Conception in a womb of a Brahmin woman is not considered accidental. It is linked to one of Mahāvīra's previous lives as Marīci, the heretical grandson of Ṛṣabha, the first Jina of our time and place. Since Marīci felt pride about the prestige of his family and his destiny of becoming a future Jina, which his grandfather had predicted, he attracted low-birth karma. The coming to fruition of this karma resulted in his conception in the Brahmin caste, which Jains considered to be lower than the warrior caste (Appleton 2012, 6–7). For other hypotheses on the significance of the Brahmin womb in this story, see Bauer (1998, 96–108).

29. Bauer describes Hariṇegamesī as a deity associated with successful birth, miscarriage, burglary, and plague in the wider Indian context (1998, 56–58).

30. Bauer mentions a retelling of this story on a videotape entitled *Tirthankar Bhagwan Shri Mahavir: Audio Visual on the Life of Lord Mahavir* (Institute of Jainology, London) that presents Triśalā's original embryo—"the nameless child of no notable destiny"—as female (1998, 132–33). He also claims, somewhat controversially, that the transfer could be viewed as an abortion (500) or miscarriage for Devānandā (66).

31. Robert Zydenbos argues that the embryo transfer is an example of Jain authors integrating Hindu figures such as Indra into their own narratives (2000, 93). Other scholars have cautioned against any simple accounts of cultural absorption, since *bhakti* traditions were present in the earliest strata of Jain literature, and Jains also imbued these figures with their own Jain ideals (Cort 1987, 249–50; Qvarnström 2000, 119–21).

32. De Clercq draws from the ninth-century *Mahāpurāṇa* of Jinasena and Guṇabhadra and the twelfth-century *Triṣaṣṭiśalākāpuruṣa-caritra* of Hemacandra, which offer elaborate tales of the Jinas' life stories.

33. The deep mutual connection between Jinas and their mothers seems to hold even in the case of Mahāvīra and his initial Brahmin mother. When Mahāvīra later meets Devānandā, he knows she is his first mother, and milk flows in Devānandā's breast out of a two-directional love for her original son (BhS 9.33§458a).

34. It should also be pointed out that Jain texts recognize the possibility of the child's spiritual learning in the womb, where the mother's role during her child's gestation may be

particularly important. For instance, if a child *in utero* hears spiritual stories from a learned teacher—ostensibly exposed to such a teacher by a mother—and gains a love for religion and beneficial karma, it can be reborn in heaven in case it dies in the womb (BhS 1.7§86b). Similarly, an embryo can attract unmeritorious karma. There is an unusual account of an embryo who has fully developed senses and mind and by extraordinary powers (transformational body) participates in a war from a distance, dies in the womb, and is reborn as a hell-being (BhS 1.7§86b).

35. In the *Sūtra-prābhṛta* (Pkt. *Sutta-pāhuḍa*) 7, Kundakunda, further, describes the innate violence of the female body, stating: "In the genital organs of women, in between their breasts, in their navels, and in the armpits, it is said (in the scriptures that) there are very subtle living beings" which leads to a constant violation of the vow of nonviolence. This assertion plays a role in the debates regarding the spiritual liberation of women (Jaini 1991a, 35, 142–43).

36. See BhS 2.5§133b, which states that the number of lives produced through a sex act ranges from a minimum of one, two, or three to a maximum of nine hundred thousand. As noted in chapter 2, this idea relates to the "undevelopable" humans (*aparyāpta*) who exist briefly without a womb (see GJK 118–28; Wiley 2000a, 136–41).

37. Bauer suggests that the queen's attempt at abortion could be viewed as a form of self-defense, though one that produces consequences throughout the mother's life as she cares for a son with severe illness (1998, 247–48).

38. Suzuko Ohira dates this Śvetāmbara canonical text between the latter half of the fourth and the fifth century CE (1994, 2).

39. Medical abortion involves drugs such as mifepristone followed by misoprostol, methotrexate followed by misoprostol, and misoprostol alone.

40. Medical abortion is available only in certain countries such as the United States, Canada, France, China, Turkey, and Tunisia (Ngo et al. 2011).

41. See Wiley (2000a, 132) and Vallely (2020, 562–64) for a more detailed description of the rarity of birth as a (womb-born) human.

42. See Dundas (2002a, 276) for details of the degeneration during the fifth and sixth spoke.

43. See "Jain Declaration on the Climate Crisis" (2019) as well as Chapple (2002). The volume by Chapple was produced as part of a series of conferences on religious traditions and ecology that took place at Harvard University during 1996–98.

44. In a survey of Jain students and teachers in US temple education (*pāṭhaśālā*), one of the most cited issues respondents desired to discuss more was intermarriage (Donaldson 2019b).

45. See Donaldson (2019b), wherein Jain *pāṭhaśālā* students note an interest in discussing birth control in temple education class.

46. This history of IVF begins in the late 1800s with animal models in Europe. The first successful human procedure was completed by Patrick Steptoe and Robert Edwards when baby Louise Brown was born in the United Kingdom in 1978.

47. See also note 15 above, where various ways in which a woman can conceive without having had intercourse are listed. Bothra comments that "a woman conceives when semen molecules enter her vagina irrespective of the fact that it is accidental or by artificial means. In modern times the process of artificial insemination has also been developed on the same basis" (2004, 146).

48. Sethi also describes commonalities between Jain nuns and laywomen, such as "male dominance, vulnerability to sexual and physical violence and so on" (2012, 39). Sethi describes how renunciation is still portrayed as an essential male pursuit, in spite of the recognition that women are equal participants in the Jain community and vision (64).

49. See also chapter 2.

50. For a more technical description of how karma impacts rebirth, see Wiley (2000a).

51. Dowry, or the financial burden of a woman's family, is contrasted with "brideprice," which is the cost a husband's family will pay for the marriage (Anderson 2007).

52. In Hinduism, a son is also required to complete specific Vedic funerary rites (*śrāddha*) when his parents die (Chidester 2002, 78–79).

53. For a description of the *puṃsavana* ritual, its variations, and textual sources, see Stork (1992, 92–93).

54. Anecdotally, in casual conversations over the years with Jain women, at least three have expressed relief at having an institutional excuse not to go to temple during their monthly menstruation, when the shedding of the uterine lining is considered to result in harm to numerous living beings (see chapter 2). Each of these women was extremely involved in temple life and also had professional careers and families, making me (Brianne) wonder if some Jain women view this prohibition both through the lens of karma and as a needed social break, though I have never followed up on this question formally. Additionally, at a conference session on women in Jainism held at Claremont School of Theology (August 23–24, 2013), several Jain men described the prohibition as a positive rest for women, suggesting a modern reinterpretation worth future investigation. For contemporary discussion among lay Jains, see also "Menstruation" (2020).

55. See Kelting (n.d.), "Candanbālā."

56. For a more detailed analysis of these types of karma, see chapter 2 and Wiley (2000a).

## CHAPTER 6. WAGES OF LIFE

1. Robert Williams provides the Śvetāmbara list in a hierarchy of desirability: trade, practice of medicine, agriculture, artisanal crafts, animal husbandry, service of a ruler, and begging. The Digambara list (excluding medicine) is trade, clerical occupations, agriculture, artisanal crafts, and military occupations (1963, 122).

2. Jain here seems to be employing a modern interpretation of non-one-sidedness as tolerance of alternative views (cf. chapter 2). For a historical overview of the changes in the Jain understanding of non-one-sidedness, see Barbato (2017).

3. $TS^{Śv}$ 7.21.

4. See Donaldson (2020) for an account of Jain views on Darwinian evolution.

5. See chapter 7 regarding end-of-life care.

6. See Donaldson's two-part analysis of US Jains navigating their identity through temple education (2019a, 2019b).

7. The meaning of *sūkṣma* here seems to be different from the technical meaning of the term as defining bodies that cannot be harmed (see chapter 2). Here, it indicates the minuteness of life-forms rather than their indestructability.

8. Alternative translations: "animalcules" (Schubring), "organisms" (Lalwani), and "micro-beings" (Bothra).

9. Alternative translations: "[organic] dust [as found in cracks]" (Schubring), "ants" (Lalwani), and "micro-dwellings" (Bothra).

10. We follow Schubring's translation. Alternative translations: "moss" (Lalwani) and "micro-fungi" (Bothra).

11. Alternative translations: "[indistinguishable] plants" (Schubring), "greenery" (Lalwani), and "micro-vegetation" (Bothra).

12. Sikdar defines "cell" using a term of embryonic development—*arbuda*—noted in the *Taṇḍula-vaicārika*, which refers to the stage of being a "long round mass," described in chapter 5 (Sikdar 1975, 12, fn. 44).

13. For more on the development of *virodhī-hiṃsā* as an acceptable mode of self-defense, see Dundas (2007b, 44) and Jaini (2004).

14. For more on *pratikramaṇa* in relation to animals, plants, and people, see Donaldson (2016).

15. TS$^{Dig}$ 7.25 (= TS$^{Śv}$ 7.20) lists *chavi-ccheda*, or "piercing/cutting the skin," as one of the transgressions of the minor vow of nonviolence (see also YŚ 3.90). As Williams notes, "the word *chavi* is . . . variously interpreted as 'body' or 'skin'" (1963, 68).

16. For dead bodies as breeding grounds of *nigoda*s, see Jaini (2001/1979, 169) and Williams (1963, 54, 65).

17. For a discussion on the payment for treatment in such cases, see Shāntā (1997, 564). It is also important to note that Ladnun has a care center (Seva Kendra) for elderly and ill Terāpanthī nuns (565).

18. Shāntā adds: "The Terāpanthīs are on the whole strict and little in favor of surgical operations; in certain cases a *sādhvī* may, after an operation, receive a new *dīkṣā* [initiation]" (1997, 563, fn. 7).

19. Vallely (2011) describes two other laywomen experiencing possession; the first attributed the possession to a goddess neglected by her ancestors in need of propitiation, and the second who battled her *bhūta*s at a temple associated with the powerful presence of the sixth Jina.

20. Survey question: "What percentage of your patients are lay Jains?" ($n$ = 42): 0–5% (60%), 5–20% (14%), 20–40% (0%), 40–60% (2%), 60–80% (0%), 80–100% (0%), 100% of patients are Jain (0%), None of my patients are Jain (0%), I am not aware how many are Jain (10%), Not applicable (12%), Other (2%).

21. Suzuko Ohira dates this Śvetāmbara canonical text to the fourth century CE (1994, 1).

22. See chapter 2 for responsibility for one's own karma and karmic mobility.

23. In 2015, Shaleen and Shilpi Shah opened the first no-kill animal sanctuary outside India based on Jain ideals (www.luvinarms.org). See Dilip V. Shah (2017a), "My Visit to an Animal Sanctuary."

24. See Donaldson (2016, 37–42).

25. Jain food commitments have generated conflict in India when Jains used political channels to influence national food policy. In 2014, Jain monks engaged in a public fast to demand that the Jain pilgrimage city of Palitana ban all animal slaughter and meat sales, leading to conflicts with the city's Muslim inhabitants. In 2015, the government banned animal slaughter in Mumbai during the Jain festival of Paryuṣana, a conflict currently being adjudicated by the city's high court (Bhalerao 2018).

26. For more on vitalities, see chapter 2.

27. Nuanced debates on the topic are rare, but they do exist. See the Hastings Center collaborative resources (Gilbert et al. 2012). The Center for Alternatives to Animal Testing at Johns Hopkins University and the Wyss Institute for Biologically Inspired Engineering at Harvard also research nonanimal alternatives.

## CHAPTER 7. CALCULATIONS OF DEATH

1. For other places that had a similar status to Śravaṇa Beḷgoḷa, see Dhaky (1980, 8, fn. 49) and Granoff (1992b, 183, fn. 4, 188). See also Caillat (1977, 54, 64, fn. 88).

2. Jains were not alone in this belief. Franklin Edgerton traces the emergence of similar ideas in Hindu and Buddhist textual traditions—such as the value of meditating on Kṛṣṇa or the five Buddhist precepts at the hour of death (1926–1927, 222–26; see also Jaini 2001/1979, 227–28). The Jain vows—and related austerities such as fasting, limited movement, cultivating equanimity for attachments and aversions, among many other practices—function as preparation for meeting death with a serene state of mind.

3. Kristi Wiley notes three times when karma has an opportunity to be bound, according to the Śvetāmbara texts, starting with the moment when one-third of the current longevity-determining karma remains, followed by its next remaining one-third, and the remaining one-third after that. If the binding does not occur during any of these times, it may happen during the final *antar-muhūrta* (less than forty-eight minutes) of one's life (2003, 341, cf. 343). In line with this, Helmuth von Glasenapp, referencing the *Loka-prakāśa* by Vinayavijaya (seventeenth century), states that the "*āyus* of the new existence is always bound during the life immediately preceding it, especially in the 3rd, 9th, or 27th part or within the last 48 minutes of it" (1942/1915, 11). Conversely, Wiley points out that Digambara sources describe eight such times when longevity-determining karma may be bound: the first forty-eight minutes of the remaining one-third of a life span, the first forty-eight minutes of the next remaining one-third, and so on eight times. If it is not bound during any of these times, Digambaras, similarly to the Śvetāmbaras, maintain that it must be bound within the final forty-eight minutes of one's life (2003, 342, cf. 343).

4. For a discussion of factors that impel people to become Jain mendicants, see Cort (2001b), Dundas (2002, 153–55), Sethi (2012, 87–130), and Shāntā (1997, 445–48).

5. For an example of an animal being ceremonially cremated after it had fasted unto death, see Granoff (1992, 191–92).

6. For the early Jain approaches to the dead bodies of mendicants, see Flügel (2010, 44; 2018, 122) and Wiley (2002a, 321–22, fn. 53).

7. For Jain relic worship, see Flügel (2010; 2018, 120–25, 129) and Granoff (1992b, 184, fn. 5, 189).

8. For another description of contemporary Jain lay funerary customs, particularly with regard to food, see Mahias (1985, 229–34).

9. In the funeral guidelines for the community, published in the US, Tansukh J. Salgia advises that in the case of stillbirth, the child be buried rather than cremated (2004, 6).

10. For a description of seventeen types of death most commonly listed in Jain texts, see Settar (2017/1990, 8–16).

11. Human beings in our part of the cosmos whose longevity-determining karma was not subject to reduction were those who were undergoing their last life before liberation,

Jinas, Cakravartins, Vāsudevas, and so on (Wiley 2000a, 50). Wiley also emphasizes: "*Āyu karma* that is being experienced in one's current life (*bhujamāna āyu* or *ihabhava āyu*) cannot be experienced at a slower rate. Therefore, the life span of one's current life cannot be extended under any circumstances" (2003, 340, fn. 1; see also chapter 2, note 67).

12. Living beings that always die "naturally," without external efficient causes, include heavenly beings, hell-beings, and humans residing in the "lands of enjoyment," whose life span is measured in uncountable years (see chapter 2).

13. Cf. the historical practice of self-immolation by some Jain women up to the nineteenth century (Dundas 2002a, 179, fn. 69).

14. The seventh lecture in the *Ācārāṅga-sūtra* is considered lost. Consequently, the lecture on "Liberation" (*vimokṣa*) that describes the approach of death is typically lecture eight, though Jacobi does not follow this convention.

15. Some texts mention a fourth wise death, called *bāla-paṇḍita-maraṇa*, referring to the death of those who could not renounce the householding life even in the face of death. Such persons would aim to limit the passions and assume the minor vows (Wiley 2000a, 319). Luitgard Soni describes this death as "the death of laypeople with *samyak-cāritra*" (2014, 6).

16. See US 36.249–54, Deo (1954–55, 201–2), and Wiley (2002a, 315–16) for an alternative meaning of *sallekhanā* as an extensive series of fasts that functions as a preparation for the final fast unto death and that can last up to twelve years.

17. Suzuko Ohira dates these canonical texts from the second half of the fourth to the fifth century CE (Ohira 1994, 1).

18. $TS^{\acute{S}v}$ 7.17.

19. The twelve vows include the five *aṇu-vrata*s, three *guṇa-vrata*s, and four *śikṣa-vrata*s (see chapter 3).

20. Later texts provide rare examples of mendicants and laity killing themselves by means other than fasting unto death in order to maintain individual dedication to religious practice or protect the reputation of the Jain community. These kinds of death, Soni remarks, are "accepted under certain very precarious circumstances when keeping the right path is likely to become impossible" (2014, 10). Soni recounts two stories from the *Bṛhat-kathā-kośa* to illustrate these exceptional deaths. One narrates how King Dharmasiṃha allows himself to be eaten by vultures rather than be forced to abandon his mendicant path for palace life. Likewise, in the other story, the Jain teacher Yativṛṣabha cuts open his own belly as restitution for a false Jain ascetic who killed the local king in order to protect the Jain community; this act of sacrifice gains Yativṛṣabha *samādhi-maraṇa* and access to heaven (2014, 9–11).

21. Other texts offer slightly different accounts of this process; see Williams (1963, 167–69).

22. $TS^{\acute{S}v}$ 9.34.

23. TC 4.1.157, 4.2.187, 4.3.33, 4.4.90, 4.5.70, 6.3.6, 6.4.5, 6.5.8, 10.1.106.

24. See Appleton (2015, 26–29) for accounts of the importance of a pure and serene mind among animals at the moment of their death.

25. Jaini locates this story in the *Uttara-purāṇa* 86.207–8 (2010d, 266, fn. 21), while De Clercq locates it in the *Mahā-purāṇa* 74.120–219 and the *Triṣaṣṭiśalākāpuruṣa-caritra* TC 10.1.182 (2013, 149, fn. 22).

26. Depending on the state, POLST forms go by other acronyms such as MOST, MOLST, POST, or TPOPP; www.polst.org.

27. A POLST or DNR form can be respected only if medical professionals know they exist. Patients nearing the end of life are encouraged to inform their families, doctors, care teams, and assisted-living staff about these documents, have them on file, and post them visibly on bright paper in relevant living spaces.

28. For more on antibiotic use in the Jain tradition, see chapter 6.

29. See William Dalrymple's story about a young Jain nun who decides to fast to death (2009).

# REFERENCES

## PRIMARY SOURCES


AA [Banārsīdās, *Avasthā-aṣṭaka*]. Portions of the text are translated in Jérôme Petit, "Banārasīdās Climbing the Jain Stages of Perfection." In *Puṣpikā: Tracing Ancient India through Texts and Traditions: Contributions to Current Research in Indology, Vol. 3*, edited by Robert Leach and Jessie Pons, 96–117. Oxford: Oxbow Books, 2015.

ĀA [Guṇabhadra, *Ātmānuśāsana*]. *Atmanushasana (Discourse to the Soul) by Shri Guna-Bhadra Acharya*. The Sacred Books of the Jainas, vol. 7. Edited and translated by Rai Bahadur J.L. Jaini. Lucknow, India: Central Jaina Publishing House, 1928.

AD [*Antakṛd-daśāḥ*, Pkt. *Aṃtagaḍa-dasāo*]. *The Antagaḍa-dasāo and Aṇuttarovavāiya-dasāo*. Translated by L.D. Barnett. London: Royal Asiatic Society, 1907.

ĀS [*Ācārāṅga-sūtra*, Pkt. *Āyāraṃga-sutta*]. (1) *The Âyâraṃga Sutta of the Çvetâmbara Jains*. Part I—Text. Edited by Hermann Jacobi. London: Henry Frowde for the Pali Text Society, 1882. (2) *Gaina Sûtras, Part 1, The Âkârâṅga Sûtra. The Kalpa Sûtra*. The Sacred Books of the East, vol. 22. Translated by Hermann Jacobi. Oxford: Clarendon Press, 1884.

BhĀ [Śivārya (Śivakoṭi), *Bhagavatī-ārādhanā*, Pkt. *Bhagavaī-ārāhaṇa*]. *Mūlārādhanā (Aparanāma Bhagavatī Ārādhanā)*. Sholapur, India: Svāmī Devendrakīrti, 1935. Portions of the text are translated in Luitgard Soni, "Jaina Modes of Dying in Ārādhanā Texts." *International Journal of Jaina Studies* 10 (2), 2014: 1–14.

BhS [*Bhagavatī-sūtra/Vyākhyāprajñapti-sūtra*, Pkt. *Bhagavaī-sutta/Viyāhapaṇṇatti-sutta*]. (1) *Bhagavatī Sūtra*. Four volumes. Translated by K.C. Lalwani 1999–2007/1973–1985. Calcutta: Jain Bhawan. (2) *Viyāhapannatti (Bhagavaī): The Fifth Anga of the Jaina Canon*. Lala Sundar Lal Jain Research Series, vol. 10.

Introduction, Critical Analysis, Commentary, and Indexes by Jozef Deleu. Delhi: Motilal Banarsidass, 1996/1970. Originally published in 1970 in Brugge, Belgium, by "De Tempel." The numbering in the in-text references follows Deleu.

ChU [*Chāndogya-upaniṣad*]. *The Early Upaniṣads: Annotated Text and Translation.* Translated and edited by Patrick Olivelle. New York: Oxford University Press, 1998, 166–287.

DS [Nemicandra, *Davva-saṃgaha*] *Dravyasaṃgraha*. Translated by Nalini Balbir. Mumbai: Hindi Granth Karyalay, 2010.

DVS [*Daśavaikālika-sūtra*, Pkt. *Dasaveyāliya-sutta*]. (1) *The Dasaveyāliya Sutta: Introduction, Text and Variants.* Edited by Ernst Leumann. Translated by Walther Schubring. Ahmedabad, India: The Managers of Sheth Anandji Kalianji, 1932. Reprinted in Walther Schubring, *Kleine Schriften*, 109–248. Wiesbaden: Franz Steiner Verlag, 1977. (2) *Ārya Sayyambhava's Daśavaikālika Sūtra (Dasaveyalia Sutta).* Translated by Kastur Chand Lalwani. Delhi: Motilal Banarsidass, 1973. (3) Illustrated *Dashavaikalik Sutra: The Basic Compendium of Shraman Conduct.* Translated by Surendra Bothara. Delhi: Padma Prakashan, 1997. The numbering in the in-text references follows Leumann.

GJK [Nemicandra, *Gommaṭasāra-jīva-kāṇḍa*]. *Gommatsara Jiva-Kanda (The Soul).* The Sacred Books of the Jainas, vol. 5. Edited and translated by Rai Bahadur J.L. Jaini. Lucknow, India: Central Jaina Publishing House, 1927.

GKK [Nemicandra, *Gommaṭasāra-karma-kāṇḍa*]. *Gommatsara Karma-Kanda (Part 1).* The Sacred Books of the Jainas, vol. 6. Edited and translated by J.L. Jaini. Lucknow, India: Central Jaina Publishing House, 1927.

JK [*Jñātṛdharma-kathā*, Pkt. *Nāyādhamma-kahāo*]. *Illustrated Jñātā Dharma Kathāṅga Sūtra.* Two volumes. Translated by Surendra Bothara. Delhi: Padma Prakashan, 1996–1997.

KG [Devendrasūri, *Karma-grantha*] *Catvāraḥ Karmagranthāḥ with Svopajña-vṛtti.* Edited by Muni Chaturavijayaji. Bhavnagar, India: Śrī Jain Ātmānanda Sabhā, 1934.

KK [Ugrāditya, *Kalyāṇa-Karāka*] *The Kalyāṇa-karākam of Ugrādityacharya.* Edited by Vardhaman Parshwanath Shastri. Sholapur, India: Seth Govindji Raoji Doshi, Sakharam Nemchand Granthamala, 1940.

KS [Bhadrabahu, *Kalpa-sūtra*, Pkt. *Kappa-sutta*] (1) *The Kalpa Sûtra of Bhadrabâhu.* Edited by Hermann Jacobi. Leipzig: F.A. Brockhaus, 1879. (2) *Gaina Sûtras, Part 1, The Âkârâṅga Sûtra. The Kalpa Sûtra.* The Sacred Books of the East, vol. 22. Translated by Hermann Jacobi. Oxford: Clarendon Press, 1884.

MS [*Manu-smṛti*]. (1) *Manu's Code of Law: A Critical Edition and Translation of the Mānava-Dharmaśāstra.* Edited and translated by Patric Olivelle. Oxford: Oxford University Press, 2005. (2) *The Laws of Manu.* Translated by Wendy Doniger and Brian K. Smith. New York: Penguin Books, 1991. The numbering in the in-text references follows Olivelle.

NS [*Niryāvalī-sūtra*, Pkt. *Nirayāvaliyāo*]. *The Nirayāvaliyāo: The Last Five Upangas of the Jain Canon.* Edited and translated by A.S. Gopani and V.J. Chokshi. Ahmedabad, India: Gurjar Grantha Ratna Karyalaya, 1934.

NSā [Kundakunda, *Niyama-sāra*, Pkt. *Ṇiyama-sāra*] *Niyamsara (The Perfect Law)*. The Sacred Books of the Jainas, vol. 9. Translated by Uggar Sain. Lucknow, India: Central Jaina Publishing House, 1931.

PP [Umāsvāti, *Praśamarati-prakaraṇa*] *Ācārya Umāsvāti Vācaka's Praśamarati-prakaraṇa*. L.D. Series 107. Edited and translated by Yajneshwar S. Shastri. Ahmedabad, India: L.D. Institute of Indology, 1989.

PS [Kundakunda, *Pravacana-sāra*, Pkt. *Pavayaṇa-sāra*] (1) *Śrī Kundakundācārya's Pravacanasāra (Pavayaṇasāra): A Pro-canonical Text of the Jainas, The Prakrit Text Critically Edited with the Sanskrit Commentaries of Amṛtacandra and Jayasena and a Hindī Commentary of Pāṇḍe Hemarāja, with an English Translation of the Text, a Topical Index and the Text with Various Readings, and with an Exhaustive Essay on the Life, Date and Works of Kundakunda and on the Linguistic and Philosophical Aspects of Pravacanasāra by A.N. Upadhye*. Second edition. Edited and translated by A.N. Upadhye. Bombay: The Parama-Śruta-Prabhāvaka Maṇḍala, 1935. (2) *The Pravacana-sāra of Kunda-kunda Ācārya Together with the Commentary, Tattva-dīpikā, by Amṛtacandra Sūri*. Translated by Barend Faddegon. Edited with an Introduction by F.W. Thomas. Cambridge: Cambridge University Press, 2014/1935.

PSU [Amṛtacandrasūri, *Puruṣārtha-siddhyupāya*] *Purushartha-Siddhyupaya (Jaina-Pravachana-Rahasya-Kosha)*. Edited and translated by Ajit Prasada. The Sacred Books of the Jainas, vol. 4. Lucknow, India: Central Jaina Publishing House, 1933.

RŚr [Samantabhadra, *Ratnakaraṇḍa-śrāvakācāra*]. (1) *Samantabhadra's Ratnakaraṇḍaka-Śrāvakācāra*. Translated by Willem Bollée. Śravaṇabelagola: National Institute of Prakrit Studies and Research, 2010. (2) *The Ratna-Karanda-Sravakachara (or the Householder's Dharma) of Sri Samanta Bhadra Acharya*. The Library of Jaina Literature, vol. 9. Translated by Champat Rai Jain. Arrah, India: Central Jaina Publishing House, 1917.

ŚĀ [Vasunandin, *Śrāvaka-ācāra*]. Portions of the text are translated by Signe Kirde in "Vasunandin's Śrāvakācāra (57–205): English Translation with Critical Notes," PhD diss., University of Tübingen, 2011.

SKS [*Sūtrakṛtāṅga-sūtra*, Pkt. *Sūyagaḍaṃga-sutta*]. *Gaina Sûtras, Part 2, The Uttarâdhyayana Sûtra. The Sûtrakritâṅga Sûtra*. The Sacred Books of the East, vol. 45. Translated by Hermann Jacobi. Oxford: Clarendon Press, 1895.

SP [*Saṃstāraka-prakīrṇaka*, Pkt. *Saṃthāraga-paiṇṇayaṃ*]. *Santhārgapaiṇṇayaṁ (Saṁstāraka-Prakīrṇaka)*. Edited by D.S. Baya. Udaipur, India: Āgama Ahiṃsā Samatā Evaṁ Prākṛta Saṁsthāna, 2003.

SS [Kundakunda, *Samaya-sāra*]. (1) *Samayasāra (The Soul-Essence)*. The Sacred Books of the Jainas, vol. 8. Translated by Rai Bahadur J.L. Jaini. Lucknow, India: Central Jaina Publishing House, 1930. (2) *Ācārya Kundakunda's Samayasāra*. Translated by A. Chakravarti. New Delhi: Bharatiya Jnanpith, 2008.

SSi [Pūjyapāda Devanandin, *Sarvārtha-siddhi*, includes the Digambara recension of the *Tattvārtha-sūtra* = $TS^{Dig}$] (1) *Ācārya Pūjyapāda's Sarvārthasiddhi [The Commentary on Āchārya Griddhapiccha's Tattvārtha-sūtra]*. Seventh edition. Edited and translated into Hindi by Phoolchandra Shastri. New Delhi: Bharatiya

Jnanpith, 1997. (2) *Reality: English Translation of Shri Pujyapada's Sarvarthasiddhi*. Translated by S.A. Jain. Calcutta: Vira Sasana Sangha, 1960.

SSN [Banārsīdās, *Samayasāra-nāṭaka*]. Portions of the text are translated in Jérôme Petit, "Banārasīdās Climbing the Jain Stages of Perfection." In *Puṣpikā: Tracing Ancient India through Texts and Traditions: Contributions to Current Research in Indology, Vol. 3*, edited by Robert Leach and Jessie Pons, 96–117. Oxford: Oxbow Books, 2015.

SthS [*Sthānāṅga-sūtra*, Pkt. *Ṭhāṇaṃga-sutta*]. *Illustrated Sthananga Sutra*. Two volumes. Translated by Surendra Bothra. Delhi: Padma Prakashan, 2004. In-text citations follow the numbering in this translation.

TBh See TS.

TC [Hemacandra, *Triṣaṣṭiśalākāpuruṣa-caritra*] *Triṣaṣṭiśalākāpuruṣacaritra or The Lives of Sixty-Three Illustrious Persons*, vols. 1 and 2. Gaekwad's Oriental Series, vols. 51 and 77. Translated by Helen M. Johnson. Baroda: Oriental Institute, 1931 and 1937.

TD See PS.

TS [Umāsvāti, *Tattvārtha-sūtra*]. When there is no difference between the Śvetāmbara ($TS^{Śv}$) and the Digambara ($TS^{Dig}$) recension of the text, we refer to it as TS.

$TS^{Dig}$ See SSi.

$TS^{Śv}$ [Umāsvāti, *Tattvārtha-sūtra* with Śvetāmbara commentaries, includes the Śvetāmbara recension of *Tattvārtha-sūtra* = $TS^{Śv}$] (1) *Tattvārthādhigamasūtra (A Treatise on the Fundamental Principles of Jainism) by His Holiness Śrī Umāsvāti Vāchaka, Together with His Connective Verses Commented upon by Śrī Devaguptasūri & Śrī Siddhasenagaṇi and His Own Gloss Elucidated by Śrī Siddhasenagaṇi*. Two volumes. Edited by H.R. Kapadia. Sheth Devchand Lalbhai Jain Pustakoddhar Fund Series Nos. 67 and 76. Bombay: Jivanchand Sakerchand Javeri, 1926 (Part I: Chapters 1–5), 1930 (Part II, Chapters: 6–10). (2) *Tattvārthādhigama by Umāsvāti Being in the Original Sanskrit with the Bhāṣya by the Author Himself*. Edited by K.P. Mody. Bibliotheca Indica New Series 1044, 1079, 1118. Calcutta: Asiatic Society of Bengal, 1903, 1904, 1905.

TṬ See $TS^{Śv}$ 1.

TV [*Taṇḍula-vaicārika*, Pkt. *Tandula-veyāliya*]. *Tandulaveyāliya: Ein Paṇṇaya des Jaina Siddhānta*. Edited by Walther Schubring. Mainz: Verlag der Akademie der Wissenschaften und der Literatur (in Kommission bei Franz Steiner Verlag, Wiesbaden), 1969.

TVā [Akalaṅka, *Tattvārtha-vārttika* (*Rāja-vārttika*)]. *Tattvārtha-vārttika [Rāja-vārttika] of Śrī Akalaṅkadeva*. Two volumes. Edited and translated into Hindi by M.K. Jain. New Delhi: Bharatiya Jnanpith, 2008 (Part I: Chapters 1–4; 8th ed.), 2013 (Part II: Chapters 5–10; 9th edition).

US [*Uttarādhyayana-sūtra*, Pkt. *Uttarajjhayaṇa-sutta*]. *Gaina Sûtras, Part 2, The Uttarâdhyayana Sûtra. The Sûtrakritâṅga Sûtra*. The Sacred Books of the East, vol. 45. Translated by Hermann Jacobi. Oxford: Clarendon Press, 1895.

YŚ [Hemacandra, *Yoga-śāstra*]. *The Yogaśāstra of Hemacandra: A Twelfth Century Handbook on Śvetāmbara Jainism*. Translated by Olle Qvarnström. Cambridge, MA: Harvard University Press, 2002.

## SECONDARY SOURCES

Abrevaya, Jason. 2009. "Are There Missing Girls in the United States? Evidence from Birth Data." *American Economic Journal: Applied Economics* 1 (2): 1–34.

"A Definition of Irreversible Coma: A Report of the Ad Hoc Committee of the Harvard Medical School to Examine the Definition of Brain Death." 1968. *Journal of the American Medical Association* 205 (6): 337–40.

Aiken, Abigail R.A., Irena Digol, James Trussell, and Rebecca Gomperts. 2017. "Self Reported Outcomes and Adverse Events after Medical Abortion through Online Telemedicine: Population Based Study in the Republic of Ireland and Northern Ireland." *British Medical Journal* 357: j2011.

Aleccia, Jonel. 2017. "Legalizing Aid in Dying Doesn't Mean Patients Have Access to It." *NPR.org*, January 25. Accessed December 24, 2020: npr.org/sections/health-shots/2017/01/25/511456109/legalizing-aid-in-dying-doesn't-mean-patients-have-access-to-it.

Alsdorf, Ludwig. 2010/1961. "Contributions to the History of Vegetarianism and Cow-Veneration in India." Translated by Bal Patil. Revised by Nichola Hayton. In *The History of Vegetarianism and Cow-Veneration in India*, edited by Willem Bollée, 1–89. New York: Routledge. Originally published in German in 1961 in Mainz, Germany, by Verlag der Akademie der Wissenschaften und der Literatur.

Anderson, Siwan. 2007. "The Economics of Dowry and Brideprice." *Journal of Economic Perspectives* 21 (4): 151–74.

"Animal Protection Index." n.d. World Animal Protection. Accessed on September 1, 2018: https://api.worldanimalprotection.org/.

Appleton, Naomi. 2011. "Heir to One's Karma: Multi-life Personal Genealogies in Early Buddhist and Jain Narratives." *Religions of South Asia* 5 (1–2): 227–44.

———. 2012. "The Multi-life Stories of Gautama Buddha and Vardhamāna Mahāvīra." *Buddhist Studies Review* 29 (1): 5–16.

———. 2014. *Narrating Karma and Rebirth: Buddhist and Jain Multi-life Stories*. New York: Cambridge University Press.

Aramesh, Kiarash. 2009. "The Ownership of Human Body: An Islamic Perspective." *Journal of Medical Ethics and History of Medicine* 2: 1–4.

"ART Success Rates." 2016. Centers for Disease Control and Prevention. Last modified May 16, 2018. Accessed May 13, 2019: www.cdc.gov/art/artdata/index.html.

"Assisted Reproduction." 2004. In *Reproduction and Responsibility: The Regulation of New Biotechnologies*. The President's Council on Bioethics. Accessed January 25, 2018: https://bioethicsarchive.georgetown.edu/pcbe/reports/reproductionandresponsibility/fulldoc.html.

Aukland, Knut. 2010. *The Cult of Nākoḍā Bhairava: Deity Worship and Possession in Jainism*. MA thesis, University of Oslo.

———. 2013. "Understanding Possession in Jainism: A Study of Oracular Possession in Nakoda." *Modern Asian Studies* 47 (1): 109–34.

———. 2016. "The Scientization and Academization of Jainism." *Journal of the American Academy of Religion* 84 (1): 192–233.

Babb, Lawrence A. 1996. *Absent Lord: Ascetics and Kings in a Jain Ritual Culture*. Berkeley: University of California Press.

Bagheri, A. 2007. "Individual Choice in the Definition of Death." *Journal of Medical Ethics* 33 (3): 146–49.

Bajaj, J.K. 2016. "Declining Share of Jains in the Population of India [Census 2011]." Center for Policy Studies, India. Accessed May 11, 2019: www.cpsindia.org/dl/Blogs/Blog10.pdf.

Bajželj, Ana. 2017. "Time (Jainism)." In *Encyclopedia of Indian Religions: Buddhism and Jainism*, edited by K.T.S. Sarao and Jeffery D. Long, 1238–41. Dordrecht, The Netherlands: Springer.

———. 2018. "Kundakunda on the Modal Modification of Omniscient *Jīvas*." In *Jaina Studies: Select Papers Presented in the 'Jaina Studies' Section at the 16th World Sanskrit Conference, Bangkok, Thailand & the 14th World Sanskrit Conference, Kyoto, Japan*, edited by Nalini Balbir and Peter Flügel, 97–110. New Delhi: DK.

———. 2019. "Like a Castor Seed: Jaina Philosophers on the Nature of Liberation." *Journal of Hindu Studies* 12 (1): 28–48.

———. 2020. "Clay Pots, Golden Rings, and Clean Upper Garments: Causality in Jaina Philosophy." In *Framing Intellectual and Lived Spaces in Early South Asia*, edited by Lucas den Boer and Elizabeth Cecil, 197–223. Berlin: De Gruyter.

Balbir, Nalini. n.d. "Five 'Fundamental Vows.'" *Jainpedia: The Jain Universe Online*. Accessed May 11, 2019: www.jainpedia.org/themes/principles/vows/five-fundamental-vows.html.

———. 1990. "Recent Developments in a Jaina Tīrtha: Hastinapur (U.P.)—A Preliminary Report." In *The History of Sacred Places in India as Reflected in Traditional Literature: Papers on Pilgrimage in South Asia*, edited by Hans Bakker, 177–91. Leiden, The Netherlands: Brill.

———. 1992. "La fascination jaina pour l'alchimie." *Journal of the European Āyurvedic Society* 2: 134–50.

———. 1993. *Āvaśyaka-Studien: Introduction générale et traductions*. Alt- und Neu-Indische Studien, vol. 45: 1. Stuttgart, Germany: Franz Steiner Verlag.

———. 1994a. "An Investigation of Textual Sources on the *samavasaraṇa* ("The Holy Assembly of the Jina")." In *Festschrift Klaus Bruhn*, edited by Nalini Balbir and Joachim K. Bautze, 67–104. Reinbek, Germany: Verlag für Orientalistische Fachpublikationen.

———. 1994b. "Women in Jainism." In *Religion and Women*, edited by Arvind Sharma, 121–38. Albany, NY: SUNY Press.

———. 2015. "Lay Atonements: Investigation into the Śvetāmbara Textual Tradition." In *Jaina Scriptures and Philosophy*, edited by Peter Flügel and Olle Qvarnström, 68–129. New York: Routledge.

Balcerowicz, Piotr. 2001. "The Logical Structure of the *Naya* Method of the Jainas." *Journal of Indian Philosophy* 29: 379–403.

———. 2003. "Some Remarks on the *Naya* Method." In *Essays in Jaina Philosophy and Religion*, edited by Piotr Balcerowicz, 37–68. Delhi: Motilal Banarsidass.

———. 2011. "The Body and the Cosmos in Jaina Mythology and Art." In *Art, Myths and Visual Culture of South Asia*, edited by Piotr Balcerowicz in collaboration with Jerzy Malinowski, 95–151. Delhi: Manohar.

———. 2016. *Early Asceticism in India: Ājīvikism and Jainism*. New York: Routledge.

Banks, Marcus J. 1991. "Orthodoxy and Dissent: Varieties of Religious Belief among Immigrant Gujarati Jains in Britain." In *The Assembly of Listeners: Jains in Society*, edited by Michael Carrithers and Caroline Humphrey, 241–59. New York: Cambridge University Press.

Barbato, Melanie. 2017. *Jain Approaches to Plurality: Identity as Dialogue*. Leiden, The Netherlands: Brill Rodopi.

Bauer, Jerome H. 1998. "Karma and Control: The Prodigious and the Auspicious in the Śvetāmbara Canonical Mythology." PhD diss., University of Pennsylvania.

———. 2003. "Dohada (Pregnancy Cravings)." In *South Asian Folklore: An Encyclopedia*, edited by Margaret A. Mills, Peter J. Claus, and Sarah Diamond, 163. New York: Routledge.

Baya, D.S. 2006. *Jainism: The Creed for All Times*. Jaipur, India: Prakrit Bharati Academy.

Beard, T. Randolph, and Rigmar Osterkamp. 2014. "The Organ Crisis: A Disaster of Our Own Making." *European Journal of Health Economics* 15: 1–5.

Beauchamp, Tom L. 2007. "History and Theory in 'Applied Ethics.'" *Kennedy Institute of Ethics Journal* 17 (1): 55–64.

Beauchamp, Tom L., and James F. Childress. 2001. *Principles of Biomedical Ethics*. Oxford: Oxford University Press.

Bendorf, Aric, Ian H. Kerridge, and Cameron Stewart. 2013. "Intimacy or Utility? Organ Donation and the Choice between Palliation and Ventilation." *Critical Care* 17: article 316.

Bentham, Jeremy. 2007/1789. *An Introduction to the Principles of Morals and Legislation*. Mineola, NY: Dover.

Bernat, James L., Bernard Gert, and R. Peter Mogielnicki. 1993. "Patient Refusal of Hydration and Nutrition: An Alternative to Physician-Assisted Suicide or Voluntary Active Euthanasia." *Archives of Internal Medicine* 153 (24): 2723–31.

Bhalerao, Sanjana. 2018. "Mumbai Abattoirs Shut, No Sale of Meat in Civic Markets on Thursday Due to Jain Festival." *Hindustan Times*, September 13. Accessed August 30, 2019: www.hindustantimes.com/mumbai-news/mumbai-abattoirs-shut-no-sale-of-meat-in-civic-markets-on-thursday-due-to-jain-festival/story-Lh564GJarxiiPh9Zz8zTxO.html.

Bhansali, Ayush. 2018. "Ahimsa in a Pro-Choice World." *Young Minds*, October 22. Accessed August 2, 2020: https://youngminds.yja.org/ahimsa-in-a-pro-choice-world-ab5e563e2fa4.

Bhargava, Dayanand. 1968. *Jaina Ethics*. Delhi: Motilal Banarsidass.

Bhatnagar, R.P. 1984. *Jaina Āyurveda kā Itihāsa*. Udaipur, India: Surya Prakashan Sansthan.

Bhattacharyya, Swasti. 2006. *Magical Progeny, Modern Technology: A Hindu Bioethics of Assisted Reproductive Technology*. Albany, NY: SUNY Press.

Bobra, D.K. 2008. "Bio Medical Ethics in Jainism." *HereNow4U*. Last modified July 30, 2015. Accessed June 25, 2018: www.herenow4u.net/index.php?id=66653.

Bollée, Willem B. 2003–2004. "Notes on Diseases in the Canon of the Śvetāmbara Jains." *Studia Asiatica. International Journal for Asian Studies* 4–5: 161–92.

Bothra (Bothara), Surendra, trans. 2004. *Illustrated Sthananga Sutra*, vol. 2. Delhi: Padma Prakashan.

———. 2004/1987. *Ahimsā: The Science of Peace (As Developed by Jain Thinkers)*. Jaipur, India: Prakrit Bharati Academy.

Braun, Whitny. 2008. "Sallekhana: The Ethicality and Legality of Religious Suicide by Starvation in the Jain Religious Community." *Medicine and Law* 27 (4): 913–24.

Brekke, Torkel. 2005. *Religious Motivation and the Origins of Buddhism: A Social-Psychological Exploration of the Origins of a World Religion*. London: RoutledgeCurzon.

Brockopp, Jonathan E. 2003. "Taking Life and Saving Life: The Islamic Context." In *Islamic Ethics of Life: Abortion, War, and Euthanasia*, edited by Jonathan E. Brockopp, 1–24. Columbia: University of South Carolina Press.

Brody, Baruch. 2010. "Ethical Issues in Clinical Trials in Developing Countries." In *Biomedical Ethics*, 7th ed., edited by David DeGrazia, Thomas A. Mappes, and Jeffrey Brand-Ballard, 248–87. New York: McGraw-Hill.

Bronkhorst, Johannes. 2000. "Abhidharma and Jainism." In *Abhidharma and Indian Thought: Essays in Honors of Professor Doctor Junsho Kato on His Sixtieth Birthday*, edited by Committee for the Felicitation of Professor Doctor Junsho Kato's Sixtieth Birthday, Nagoya, 598–81 (13–30). Tokyo: Shuju-sha.

Brown, W. Norman. 1941. *Manuscript Illustrations of the Uttarādhyayana Sūtra*. New Haven, CT: American Oriental Society.

Bruhn, Klaus. 1987. "Soteriology in Early Jainism." In *Hinduismus und Buddhismus: Festschrift für Ulrich Schneider*, edited by Harry Falk, 60–86. Freiburg: Hedwig Falk.

Caillat, Colette. 1974a. "Sur les doctrines médicales dans le *Tandulaveyāliya* [*Taṇḍula-vaicārika*]: 1. Enseignements d'embryologie." *Indologica Taurinensia* 2: 45–55.

———. 1974b. "Sur les doctrines médicales du *Tandulaveyāliya* [*Taṇḍula-vaicārika*]: 2. Enseignements d'anatomie." *Adyar Library Bulletin* 38 (Mahāvīra Jayaṇti Volume): 102–14.

———. 1975. *Atonements in the Ancient Ritual of the Jaina Monks*. L.D. Series 49. Ahmedabad, India: L.D. Institute of Indology.

———. 1977. "Fasting unto Death According to the Jaina Tradition." *Acta Orientalia* 38: 43–66.

———. 1993. "Words for Violence in the 'Seniors' of the Jaina Canon." In *Jain Studies in Honour of Jozef Deleu*, edited by Rudy Smet and Kenji Watanabe, 207–36. Tokyo: Hon-No-Tomosha.

———. 2018. "On the Medical Doctrines in the *Tandulaveyāliya*: 1. Teachings of Embryology." Translated by Brianne Donaldson. *International Journal of Jaina Studies (Online)* 14 (1): 1–14.

———. 2019. "On the Medical Doctrines in the *Tandulaveyāliya*: 2. Teachings of Anatomy." Translated by Brianne Donaldson. *International Journal of Jaina Studies (Online)* 15 (1): 1–12.

Caillat, Colette, and Ravi Kumar. 1981. *The Jain Cosmology*. Translated by R. Norman. Basel, Switzerland: Harmony Books.

Carbone, Larry. 2004. *What Animals Want: Expertise and Advocacy in Laboratory Animal Welfare Policy*. Oxford: Oxford University Press.

Cardon, Andrew D., Matthew R. Bailey, and B. Taylor Bennett. 2012. "The Animal Welfare Act: From Enactment to Enforcement." *Journal of the American Association for Laboratory Animal Science* 51 (3): 301–305.

"Caring for the Jain Patient." n.d. *Ashford and St. Peter's Hospitals*. Accessed May 11, 2019: www.ashfordstpeters.info/images/other/PAS08.pdf.

Chandanaji, Acharya, and Vastupal Parikh. 2009. *Walk with Me—The Story of Mahavir: A Remarkable Revolutionary*. Toronto: Peace Publications.

Chapple, Christopher K. 1993. *Nonviolence to Animals, Earth, and Self in Asian Traditions*. Albany, NY: SUNY Press.

———, ed. 2002. *Jainism and Ecology: Nonviolence in the Web of Life*. Cambridge, MA: Harvard University Press for the Center for the Study of World Religions, Harvard Divinity School.

———. 2006. "Inherent Value without Nostalgia: Animals and the Jaina Tradition." In *A Communion of Subjects: Animals in Religion, Science, and Ethics*, edited by Paul Waldau and Kimberley Patton, 241–49. New York: Columbia University Press.

———. 2010. "Eternal Life, Death, and Dying in Jainism." In *Religion, Death, and Dying, Vol. 3: Bereavement and Death Rituals*, edited by Lucy Bregman, 198–211. Santa Barbara, CA: Praeger Perspectives.

———. 2013. "Ethics of Synthetic Life: A Jaina Perspective." *Worldviews: Global Religions, Culture, and Ecology* 17 (1): 77–88.

———. 2016a. "Aid to Dying: What Jainism—One of India's Oldest Religions—Teaches Us." *The Conversation*, June 10, 2016. Accessed June 12, 2019: https://theconversation.com/aid-to-dying-what-jainism-one-of-indias-oldest-religions-teaches-us-60828.

———, ed. 2016b. *Yoga in Jainism*. New York: Routledge.

Charitrapragya, Samani. 2004. "Mahāvīra, Anekāntavāda and the World Today." In *Ahiṁsā, Anekānta and Jainism*, edited by Tara Sethia, 75–84. Delhi: Motilal Banarsidass.

Chhapia, Hemali. 2015. "In 7 Years, Mumbai Suburb Sees 400 Santharas." *Times of India*, August 16. Accessed November 5, 2018: https://timesofindia.indiatimes.com/city/mumbai/In-7-years-Mumbai-suburb-sees-400-Santharas/articleshow/48498345.cms.

Chidester, David. 2002. *Patterns of Transcendence: Religion, Death, and Dying*, 2nd ed. Belmont, CA: Wadsworth/Thomson Learning.

Childress, James F. 1990. "The Place of Autonomy in Bioethics." *The Hastings Center Report* 20 (1): 12–17.

Clardy, Jon, Michael A. Fischbach, and Cameron R. Currie. 2009. "The Natural History of Antibiotics." *Current Biology* 19 (11): R437–41.

"Controversies in the Determination of Death." 2009. The President's Council on Bioethics. Accessed January 25, 2018: https://bioethicsarchive.georgetown.edu/pcbe/reports/death/chapter1.html.

Cort, John E. 1987. "Medieval Jaina Goddess Traditions." *Numen* 34 (2): 235–55.

———. 1993. "An Overview of the Jaina Purāṇas." In *Purāṇa Perrennis: Reciprocity and Transformation in Hindu and Jaina Texts*, edited by Wendy Doniger, 185–206. Albany, NY: SUNY Press.

———. 2000. "'Intellectual Ahiṃsā' Revisited: Jain Tolerance and Intolerance of Others." *Philosophy East and West* 50 (3): 324–47.

———. 2001a. *Jains in the World: Religious Values and Ideology in India*. Oxford: Oxford University Press.

———. 2001b. "The Intellectual Formation of a Jain Monk: A Śvetāmbara Monastic Curriculum." *Journal of Indian Philosophy* 29 (3): 327–49.

———. 2002a. "Bhakti in the Early Jain Tradition: Understanding Devotional Religion in South Asia. *History of Religions* 42 (1): 59–86.

———. 2002b. "Green Jainism? Notes and Queries toward a Possible Jain Environmental Ethic." In *Jainism and Ecology: Nonviolence in the Web of Life*, edited by Christopher K. Chapple, 63–94. Cambridge, MA: Harvard University Press for the Center for the Study of World Religions, Harvard Divinity School.

———. 2003. "Doing for Others: Merit Transfer and Karma Mobility in Jainism." In *Jainism and Early Buddhism: Essays in Honor of Padmanabh S. Jaini, Part 1*, edited by Olle Qvarnström, 129–49. Fremont, CA: Asian Humanities Press.

———. 2009. "The Cosmic Man and the Human Condition." In *Victorious Ones: Jain Images of Perfection*, edited by Phyllis Granoff, 35–47. Rubin Museum of Art, New York, in association with Mapin Publishing, Ahmedabad, India.

———. 2010. *Framing the Jina: Narratives of Icons and Idols in Jain History*. Oxford: Oxford University Press.

Coward, Harold G., Julius J. Lipner, and Katherine K. Young, eds. 1989. *Hindu Ethics: Purity, Abortion, and Euthanasia*. Albany, NY: SUNY Press.

Crawford, S. Cromwell. 1995. *Dilemmas of Life and Death: Hindu Ethics in North American Context*. Albany, NY: SUNY Press.

———. 2003. *Hindu Bioethics for the Twenty-first Century*. Albany, NY: SUNY Press.

Culver, Charles, and Bernard Gert. 2006. "The Definition and Criterion of Death." In *Biomedical Ethics*, 6th ed., edited by Thomas Mappes and David DeGrazia, 312–19. New York: McGraw-Hill.

Dalrymple, William. 2009. *Nine Lives: In Search of the Sacred in Modern India*. London: Bloomsbury.

Das, Rahul Peter. 2003. *The Origin of the Life of a Human Being: Conception and the Female According to Ancient Indian Medical and Sexological Literature*. Delhi: Motilal Banarsidass.

Dash, Bhagwan, and R.N. Basu. 1968. "Methods for Sterilization and Contraception in Ancient and Medieval India." *Indian Journal of History of Science* 3 (1): 9–24.

Davis, Dena S. 1990. "Old and Thin." *Second Opinion* 15: 26–32.

Dean, Signe. 2017. "9 Amazing Things We've Achieved in 2017 with Help from CRISPR." *Science Alert*, July 21. Accessed June 30, 2018: www.sciencealert.com/9-amazing-things-we-have-already-achieved-this-year-with-help-from-crispr.

Debroy, Sumitra. 2013. "In Mumbai, 85% Eyes, 95% Skin Donated by Gujaratis, Jains." *Times of India*, March 31. Accessed June 2, 2018: https://timesofindia.indiatimes.com/india/In-Mumbai-85-eyes-95-skin-donated-by-Gujaratis-Jains/articleshow/19299085.cms.

De Clercq, Eva. 2009. "The Great Men of Jainism in Utero: A Survey." In *Imagining the Fetus: The Unborn in Myth, Religion, and Culture*, edited by Vanessa R. Sasson and Jane Marie Law, 33–54. Oxford: Oxford University Press.

———. 2013. "Karman and Compassion: Animals in the Jain Universal History." *Religions of South Asia* 7 (1–3): 141–57.

"Defining Death: Medical, Legal and Ethical Issues in the Determination of Death." 1981. President's Commission for the Study of Ethical Problems in Medicine and Biomedical and Behavioral Research. July. Accessed February 2021: repository.library.georgetown.edu/bitstream/handle/10822/559345/defining_death.pdf?sequence=1&isAllowed=y.

DeGrazia, David. 2010. "On the Ethics of Animal Research." In *Biomedical Ethics*, 7th ed., edited by David DeGrazia, Thomas A. Mappes, and Jeffrey Brand-Ballard, 305–13. New York: McGraw-Hill.

DeGrazia, David, Thomas A. Mappes, and Jeffrey Brand-Ballard. 2010. *Biomedical Ethics*, 7th ed. New York: McGraw-Hill.

Del Bontà, Robert J. 2013. "Saṃgrahaṇī-Sūtra Illustrations." *Jaina Studies: Newsletter of the Centre of Jaina Studies* (SOAS, University of London) 8: 47–50.

Deleu, Jozef. 1996/1970. *Viyāhapannatti (Bhagavaī): The Fifth Anga of the Jaina Canon.* Lala Sundar Lal Jain Research Series, vol. 10. Introduction, Critical Analysis, Commentary, and Indexes. Delhi: Motilal Banarsidass. Originally published in 1970 in Brugge, Belgium, by "De Tempel."

den Boer, Lucas. 2020. "Early Jaina Epistemology: A Study of the Philosophical Chapters of the *Tattvārthādhigama* with an English Translation of the *Tattvārthādhigamabhāṣya* I, II.8–25, and V." PhD diss., Leiden University.

Deo, S.B. 1954–1955. "The History of Jaina Monachism (from Inscriptions and Literature)." *Bulletin of the Deccan College Research Institute* 16 (1–4): 1–608.

Deshpande, Madhav M. 2008. "Sanskrit in the South Asian Sociolinguistic Context." In *Language in South Asia*, edited by Braj B. Kachru, Yamuna Kachru, and S.N. Sridhar, 177–88. Cambridge: Cambridge University Press.

Dhaky, M.A. 1980. "Ūrjayatgiri and Jina Ariṣṭanemi." *Journal of the Indian Society of Oriental Art*, New Series 11: 1–33.

Dhanki, Bhavik. 2017. "Is a Jain Monk Allowed to Take Antibiotic Medication?" *Quora*, July 21, 2017. Accessed November 29, 2018: www.quora.com/Is-a-Jain-monk-allowed-to-take-antibiotic-medication.

Dhanwate, Anant Dattatray. 2014. "Brainstem Death: A Comprehensive Review in Indian Perspective." *Indian Journal of Critical Care Medicine* 18 (9): 569–605.

Dhar, Deepali, and John His-en Ho. 2009. "Stem Cell Research Policies around the World." *Yale Journal of Biology and Medicine* 82 (3): 113–15.

Diamond-Smith, Nadia, Nancy Luke, and Stephen McGarvey. 2008. "'Too Many Girls, Too Much Dowry': Son Preference and Daughter Aversion in Rural Tamil Nadu, India." *Culture, Health and Sexuality* 10 (7): 697–708.

Dixit, K.K. 1971. *Jaina Ontology*. L.D. Series 31. Ahmedabad, India: L.D. Institute of Indology.

———. 1978. *Early Jainism*. L.D. Series 64. Ahmedabad, India: L.D. Institute of Indology.

Donaldson, Brianne. 2015. *Creaturely Cosmologies: Why Metaphysics Matters for Animal and Planetary Liberation*. Lanham, MD: Lexington Books.

———. 2016. "From Ancient Vegetarianism to Contemporary Advocacy: When Religious Folks Decide That Animals Are No Longer Edible." *Religious Studies and Theology* 35 (2): 143–60.

———. 2017. "Ṇamōkāra Mantra." *Encyclopedia of Indian Religions: Buddhism and Jainism*, edited by K.T.S. Sarao and Jeffery D. Long, 805–806. New York, Springer.

———. 2019a. "Transmitting Jainism in U.S. Pāṭhaśālā Temple Education Part 1: Implicit Goals, Curriculum as 'Text,' and Authority of Teachers, Family, and Self." *Transnational Asia* 2 (1): 1–45.

———. 2019b. "Transmitting Jainism in U.S. Pāṭhaśālā Temple Education Part 2: Navigating Non-Jain Contexts, Cultivating Jain-Specific Practices and Social Connections, Analyzing Truth Claims, and Future Directions." *Transnational Asia* 2 (1): 1–41.

———. 2019c. "Bioethics and Jainism: From *Ahiṃsā* to an Applied Ethics of Carefulness." *Religions:* Special Issue *"New Directions in Jaina Studies"* 10 (4), 243.

———. 2020. "Jainism and Darwin: Evolution beyond Orthodoxy." *Asian Religious Responses to Darwinism: Evolutionary Theories in Middle Eastern, South Asian, and East Asian Cultural Contexts*, edited by C. Mackenzie Brown, 185–208. Cham, Switzerland: Springer.

———. 2021 (Forthcoming). "The Hunter, the Bow, and the Arrow: The Development of Intentional Harm as *Kriyā* in the Early Jaina Canon." In *(Non) Violence in Jaina Philosophy, Literature and Art*, edited by Peter Flügel. New Delhi: Dev Publishers.

Doniger, Wendy. 2009. *The Hindus: An Alternative History*. New York: Penguin Press.

Doshi, Sachin. 2018. "What to Do When Your Parents Don't Understand Your Mental Health." *Young Minds*, May 22. Accessed August 12, 2020: https://youngminds.yja.org/what-to-do-when-your-parents-dont-understand-your-mental-health-3acd9fa32dda.

Doudna, Jennifer. 2015. "Perspective: Embryo Editing Needs Scrutiny." *Nature* 528 (S6). Accessed June 12: www.nature.com/articles/528S6a.

Dundas, Paul. 1996. "Jain Attitudes towards the Sanskrit Language." In *Ideology and Status of Sanskrit: Contributions to the History of the Sanskrit Language*, edited by Jan E.M. Houben, 137–56. Leiden, The Netherlands: E.J. Brill.

———. 1997. "The Laicisation of the Bondless Doctrine: A New Study of the Development of Early Jainism." Book review of W.J. Johnson's *Harmless Souls. Journal of Indian Philosophy* 25 (5): 495–516.

———. 2000. "The Meat at the Wedding Feasts: Kṛṣṇa, Vegetarianism and a Jain Dispute." In *Jain Doctrine and Practice: Academic Perspectives*, edited by Joseph T. O'Connell, 95–112. Toronto: University of Toronto, Centre for South Asian Studies.

———. 2002a. *The Jains*, 2nd ed. New York: Routledge.

———. 2002b. "The Limits of a Jain Environmental Ethic." In *Jainism and Ecology: Nonviolence in the Web of Life*, edited by Christopher K. Chapple, 95–117. Cambridge, MA: Harvard University Press for the Center for the Study of World Religions, Harvard Divinity School.

———. 2007a. *History, Scripture and Controversy in a Medieval Jain Sect*. New York: Routledge.

———. 2007b. "The Non-violence of Violence: Jain Perspectives on Warfare, Asceticism, and Worship." In *Religion and Violence in South Asia: Theory and Practice*, edited by John R. Hinnells and Richard King, 39–58. New York: Routledge.

———. 2011. "A Digambara Jain Saṃskāra in the Early Seventeenth Century: Lay Funerary Ritual According to Somasenabhaṭṭāraka's *Traivarṇikācāra*." *Indo-Iranian Journal* 54 (2): 99–147.

Edgerton, Franklin. 1926–1927. "The Hour of Death: Its Importance for Man's Future Fate in Hindu and Western Religions." *Annals of the Bhandarkar Oriental Research Institute* 8: 219–49.

Embury-Dennis, Tom. 2018. "Terminally-Ill Children Become Youngest Ever to Be Euthanised, Aged Nine and 11." *The Independent*, August 7. Accessed June 2, 2018: www.independent.co.uk/news/world/europe/children-euthanasia-belgium-youngest-killed-terminally-ill-cfcee-a8481311.html.

Eplett, Layla. 2015. "Rite to Die: Sallekhana and End of Life." *Scientific American Blog*, September 29. Accessed June 2, 2018: https://blogs.scientificamerican.com/food-matters/rite-to-die-sallekhana-and-end-of-life/.

Evans, Brett. 2013. "A Perspective on *Panjarapoles* (Animal Shelters) of India." *HereNow4U*. Last modified July 30, 2015. Accessed August 1, 2018: www.herenow4u.net/index.php?id=95254.

Fackler, Martin. 2007. "Risk Taking Is in His Genes." *New York Times*, December 11. Accessed March 2, 2018: www.nytimes.com/2007/12/11/science/11prof.html.

"Fair Benefits for Research in Developing Countries." 2002. Participants in the 2001 Conference on Ethical Aspects of Research in Developing Countries. *Science* 298 (5601): 2133–34.

"Farm Animal Statistics: Slaughter Totals." 2013. The Humane Society of the United States, June 27. Accessed December 28, 2020: https://perma.cc/M9XR-ZT2M.

Farrugia, A., J. Penrod, and J.M. Bult. 2015. "The Ethics of Paid Plasma Donation: A Plea for Patient Centeredness." *HEC Forum: An Interdisciplinary Journal on Hospitals' Ethical and Legal Issues* 27 (4): 417–29.

"Female Infanticide Worldwide: The Case for Action by the UN Human Rights Council." 2016. Asian Centre for Human Rights. Accessed June 12, 2019: www.global-sisterhood-network.org/gsn/downloads/FemaleFoeticideWorldwide.pdf.

Filliozat, Jean. 1967. "L'abandon de la vie par le sage et les suicides du criminel et du héros dans la tradition indienne." *Arts Asiatiques* 15: 65–88.

Fitzpatrick, Emily F., Alexandra L.C. Martiniuk, Heather D'Antoine, June Oscar, Maureen Carter, and Elizabeth J. Elliott. 2016. "Seeking Consent for Research with Indigenous Communities: A Systematic Review." *BMC Medical Ethics* 17: 65.

Flügel, Peter. 2005. "The Invention of Jainism: A Short History of Jaina Studies." *International Journal of Jaina Studies* 1 (1): 1–14.

———. 2006. "Demographic Trends in Jaina Monasticism." In *Studies in Jaina History and Culture: Disputes and Dialogues*, edited by Peter Flügel, 312–98. New York: Routledge.

———. 2010. "The Jaina Cult of Relic Stūpas." *Numen* 57 (3): 389–504.

———. 2018. "Jaina Afterlife Beliefs and Funerary Practices." In *The Routledge Companion to Death and Dying*, edited by Christopher M. Moreman, 119–32. New York: Routledge.

Fohr, Sherry. 2006. "Restrictions and Protection: Female Jain Renouncers." In *Studies in Jaina History and Culture: Disputes and Dialogues*, edited by Peter Flügel, 157–80. New York: Routledge.

Folkert, Kendall W. 1993. *Scripture and Community: Collected Essays on the Jains*. Edited by John E. Cort. Atlanta, GA: Scholars Press.

Galib, A.C. Kar, M.M. Rao, and Ala Narayan. 2008. "Concepts of Contraception in Ancient India and Status in Present Scenario." *Journal of Indian Institute of History of Medicine* 38: 79–88.

Ganzini, Linda, Elizabeth R. Goy, and Steven K. Dobscha. 2008. "Prevalence of Depression and Anxiety in Patients Requesting Physicians' Aid in Dying: Cross Sectional Study." *The BMJ* 337 (7676): a1682.

Ganzini, Linda, Elizabeth R. Goy, Lois L. Miller, Theresa A. Harvath, Ann Jackson, and Molly A. Delorit. 2003. "Nurses' Experiences with Hospice Patients Who Refuse Food and Fluids to Hasten Death." *New England Journal of Medicine* 349 (4): 359–65.

Gardiner, D., S. Shemie, A. Manara, and H. Opdam. 2012. "International Perspective on the Diagnosis of Death." *British Journal of Anaesthesia* 108 (1): i14–i27.

Ghatnekar, Ravindra G., and B.P. Nanal. 1979. "The Pharmacological Concepts, Materia Medica, Medicinal Preparations etc. with Special Reference to Kalyana-karakam of Ugraditya." *Studies in History of Medicine* 3 (2): 93–99.

Gilbert, Susan, Gregory E. Kaebnick, and Thomas H. Murray, eds. 2012. *Animal Research Ethics: Evolving Views and Practices, Hastings Center Special Report* 42 (6): S1–S40.

Glantz, Leonard H., George J. Annas, Michael A. Grodin, and Wendy K. Mariner. 2010. "Research in Developing Countries: Taking Benefit Seriously." In *Biomedical Ethics*, 7th ed., edited by David DeGrazia, Thomas A. Mappes, and Jeffrey Brand-Ballard, 278–83. New York: McGraw-Hill.

Glasenapp, Helmuth von. 1942/1915. *The Doctrine of Karman in Jain Philosophy*. Translated by G. Barry Gifford. Edited by Hiralal R. Kapadia. Bombay: Bai Vijibai Jivanlal Panalal Charity Fund. Originally published in German in 1915 in Leipzig, Germany, by Otto Harrassowitz.

———. 1999/1925. *Jainism: An Indian Religion of Salvation*. Lala Sundar Lal Jain Research Series, vol. 14. Translated by Shridhar B. Shrotri. Delhi: Motilal Banarsidass. Originally published in German in 1925 in Berlin, Germany, by Alf Häger.

"Global Processed Meat Market Will Reach $1,567.00 Billion by 2022." 2017. *Intrado: Globe News Wire*, February 8. Accessed November 22, 2017: https://globenewswire.com/news-release/2017/02/08/915112/0/en/Global-Processed-Meat-Market-will-reach-1-567-00-Billion-by-2022-Zion-Market-Research.html.

Goldim, José Roberto. 2009. "Revisiting the Beginning of Bioethics: The Contribution of Fritz Jahr (1927)." *Perspectives in Biology and Medicine* 52 (3): 377–80.

Gordeeva, Aleksandra. 2015. "Jainism." In *Spirit Possession around the World: Possession, Communion, and Demon Expulsion across Cultures*, edited by Joseph P. Laycock, 173–78. Santa Barbara, CA: ABC-CLIO.

Granoff, Phyllis. 1989. "Religious Biography and Clan History among the Śvetāṃbara Jains in North India." *East and West* 39 (1): 195–215.

———. 1992a. "The Violence of Non-violence: A Study of Some Jain Responses to Non-Jain Religious Practices." *Journal of the International Association of Buddhist Studies* 15 (1): 1–43.

———. 1992b. "Worship as Commemoration: Pilgrimage, Death and Dying in Medieval Jainism." *Bulletin d'Etudes Sanskrites et Indiennes* 10: 181–202.

———, ed. 1993. *The Clever Adulteress and Other Stories: A Treasury of Jaina Literature*. Delhi: Motilal Banarsidass.

———. 1995. "Jain Stories Inspiring Renunciation." In *Religions of India in Practice*, edited by Donald S. Lopez Jr., 412–17. Princeton, NJ: Princeton University Press.

———. 1998a. "Cures and Karma: Healing and Being Healed in Jain Religious Literature." In *Self, Soul and Body in Religious Experience*, edited by Albert I. Baumgarten with Jan Assmann and Guy G. Stroumsa, 218–55. Studies in the History of Religions (*Numen* Book Series), vol. 78. Leiden, The Netherlands: E.J. Brill.

———. 1998b. "Cures and Karma II: Some Miraculous Healings in the Indian Buddhist Story Tradition." *Bulletin de l'Ecole Française d'Extrême-Orient* 85: 285–304.

———. 1998c. "The Jina Bleeds: Threats to the Faith and Rescue of the Faithful in Medieval Jain Stories." In *Images, Miracles, and Authority in Asian Religious Traditions*, edited by Richard H. Davis, 121–39. Boulder, CO: Westview Press.

———. 2000. "Being in the Minority: Medieval Jain Reactions to Other Religious Groups." In *Jain Doctrine and Practice: Academic Perspectives*, edited by Joseph T. O'Connell, 136–64. Toronto: University of Toronto, Centre for South Asian Studies.

———. 2014. "Between Monk and Layman: *Paścātkṛta* and the Care of the Sick in Jain Monastic Rules." In *Buddhist and Jaina Studies: Proceedings of the Conference in Lumbini, February 2013*, edited by Jayandra Soni, Michael Pahlke, and Christoph Cüppers, 229–51. Lumbini, Nepal: Lumbini International Research Institute.

———. 2017. "Patience and Patients: Jain Rules for Tending the Sick." *eJournal of Indian Medicine* 9: 23–38.

Greenberg, Gary. 2014. "Lights Out: A New Reckoning for Brain Death." *The New Yorker*, January 15. Accessed April 22, 2018: www.newyorker.com/tech/annals-of-technology /lights-out-a-new-reckoning-for-brain-death.

"Guidelines for Healthcare Providers Interacting with Patients of the Jain Religion and Their Families." 2002. Metropolitan Chicago Healthcare Council. Accessed December 1, 2017: www.kyha.com/assets/docs/PreparednessDocs/cg-jain.pdf.

Guinn, David E., ed. 2006. *Handbook of Bioethics and Religion*. New York: Oxford University Press.

Harvey, Peter. 2000. *An Introduction to Buddhist Ethics: Foundations, Values and Issues*. New York: Cambridge University Press.

———. 2013/1990. *An Introduction to Buddhism: Teachings, History and Practices*, 2nd ed. New York: Cambridge University Press.

Hegewald, Julia. 2019. *Jaina Temple Architecture in India: The Development of a Distinct Language in Space and Ritual*. Mumbai: Hindi Granth Karyalay.

Hosseinbor, Mohsen, Seyed Mojtaba, Yassini Ardekani, Saeed Bakhshani, and Somayeh Bakhshani. 2014. "Emotional and Social Loneliness in Individuals with and without Substance Dependence Disorder." *International Journal of High Risk Behaviors & Addiction* 3 (3): e22688.

"How Vaccines Work." n.d. *The History of Vaccines: An Educational Resource by the College of Physicians of Philadelphia*. Accessed August 27, 2018: https://ftp.historyofvaccines.org /index.php/content/how-vaccines-work.

Humphrey, Caroline, and James Laidlaw. 1994. *The Archetypal Actions of Ritual: A Theory of Ritual Illustrated by the Jain Rite of Worship*. Oxford: Clarendon Press.

"International Guidelines for the Determination of Death—Phase 1." 2012. World Health Organization. May 30–31. Accessed June 2, 2018: www.who.int/patientsafety/montreal -forum-report.pdf.

Iyer, Sriya. 2002. *Demography and Religion in India*. Oxford: Oxford University Press.

Jacob, Tony George. 2013. "History of Teaching Anatomy in India: From Ancient to Modern Times." *Anatomical Sciences Education* 6 (5): 351–58.

Jacobi, Hermann. 1880. "On Mahāvīra and His Predecessors." *Indian Antiquary* 9: 158–63.

Jakobovits, Immanuel. 1975/1959. *Jewish Medical Ethics: A Comparative and Historical Study of the Jewish Religious Attitude to Medicine and Its Practice*. New York: Bloch.

Jaggi, O.P. 1981. *Āyurveda: Indian System of Medicine*. History of Science, Technology and Medicine in India, vol. 4. Delhi: Atma Ram & Sons.

Jahr, Fritz. 1926. "Wissenschaft vom Leben und Sittenlehre (Alte Erkenntnisse in neuem Gewande)." *Die Mittelschule: Zeitschrift für das gesamte mittlere Schulwesen* 40: 604–5.

———. 1927. "Bio-Ethik: Eine Umschau über die ethischen Beziehungen des Menschen zu Tier und Pflanze." *Kosmos: Handweiser für Naturfreunde* 24 (1): 2–4.

———. 2013. *Essays in Bioethics 1924–1948*, edited and translated by Irene M. Miller and Hans-Martin Sass. Vienna: LIT Verlag.

Jain, Champat Rai. 1934. *Jainism and World Problems: Essays and Addresses, Part II*. Bijnor, India: The Jaina Parishad.

"Jain Declaration on the Climate Crisis." 2019. *JAINA*, October 17. Accessed July 3, 2020: https://cdn.ymaws.com/www.jaina.org/resource/resmgr/jaindeclarationonclimatechange/Update_Jain_Declaration_on_C.pdf.

Jain, Jagdish Chandra. 1947. *Life in Ancient India as Depicted in the Jain Canons (with Commentaries): An Administrative, Economic, Social and Geographical Survey of Ancient India Based on the Jain Canons*. Bombay: New Book Company.

Jain, Jyoti Prasad. 1950. "Ugrāditya's Kalyāṇakāraka and Ramagiri." *Proceedings of the Indian History Congress* 13: 127–33.

Jain, Manish, Anmol Mathur, Santhosh Kumar, Prabu Duraiswamy, and Suhas Kulkarni. 2009. "Oral Hygiene and Periodontal Status among Terapanthi Svetambar Jain Monks in India." *Brazilian Oral Research* 23 (4): 370–76.

Jain, N.L. 1996. *Scientific Contents in the Prākṛta Canons*. Varanasi, India: Pārśvanātha Vidyāpīṭha.

Jain, Parshv. 2017. "Is a Jain Monk Allowed to Take Antibiotic Medication?" *Quora*, July 16, 2017. Accessed July 2, 2019: www.quora.com/Is-a-Jain-monk-allowed-to-take-antibiotic-medication.

Jain, Prakash C., ed. 2019. *Studies in Jain Population and Demography*. Jaipur, India: Rawat Publications.

Jain, Prem Suman. 2015. "A Rare Manuscript of the Bhagavatī Āradhanā." In *Jaina Scriptures and Philosophy*, edited by Peter Flügel and Olle Qvarnström, 21–33. London: Routledge.

Jain, Ravindra. 2016. "Does Jainism Allow the Usage of Antibiotics?" *Quora*, December 13, 2016. Accessed November 29, 2018: www.quora.com/Does-Jainism-allow-the-usage-of-antibiotics.

Jain, Rekha N. 1991. *Contributions of Jainism to Ayurveda*. Pune, India: Chakor Publications.

Jain, S.M. 2003. *Pristine Jainism (Beyond Rituals and Superstitions)*. Parshwanath Vidyapeeth Series, No. 143. Varanasi, India: Parshwanath Vidyapeeth.

Jain, Shalin. 2012. "Divided Identities: The Jain Sects in Medieval India." *Proceedings of the Indian History Congress* 73: 450–60.

———. 2017. *Identity, Community and the State: The Jains under the Mughals*. Delhi: Primus Books.

Jain, Shugan C., and Prakash C. Jain. 2019. "Under-enumeration of Jain Population: Evidence from Two Delhi Surveys." In *Studies in Jain Population and Demography*, edited by Prakash C. Jain, 222–41. Jaipur, India: Rawat Publications.

Jain, Sulekh C. 2016. *An Ahimsa Crisis: You Decide*. Jaipur, India: Prakrit Bharati Academy.

Jain, Sulekh C., and Yashwant K. Malaiya. 2011. "Can Jainism Survive in 21st Century?" *HereNow4U*. Last modified March 3, 2017. Accessed August 12, 2018: www.herenow4u.net/index.php?id=82539.

Jain, Yogendra. 2007. *Jain Way of Life: A Guide to Compassionate, Healthy and Happy Living*. [Place of publication not identified]: JAINA (Federation of Jain Associations of North America).

"JAINA in Action." n.d. JAINA: Federation of Jain Associations in North America. Accessed January 12, 2020: www.jaina.org/page/jaina_in_action.

"JAINA President's Message." 2017. *Jain Digest* 5 (May). Accessed January 14, 2019: https://c.ymcdn.com/sites/jaina.site-ym.com/resource/resmgr/e-jain_digest/E_Digest_May_2017.pdf.

Jaini, J.L., ed. and trans. 1920. *Tattvarthadhigama Sutra (A Treatise on the Essential Principles of Jainism)*. The Sacred Books of the Jainas, vol. 2. Arrah, India: Central Jaina Publishing House.

Jaini, Padmanabh S. 1990. "Ahimsa: A Jain Way of Personal Discipline." The 1990 Inaugural Roop Lal Jain Lecture. Toronto: Centre for South Asian Studies, University of Toronto.

———. 1991a. *Gender and Salvation: Jaina Debates on the Spiritual Liberation of Women*. Berkeley: University of California Press.

———. 1991b. "Is There a Popular Jainism?" In *The Assembly of Listeners: Jains in Society*, edited by Michael Carrithers and Caroline Humphrey, 187–99. New York: Cambridge University Press.

———. 2001a. "Saṃskāra-Duḥkhatā and the Jaina Concept of Suffering." In *Collected Papers on Buddhist Studies*, edited by Padmanabh S. Jaini, 133–38. Delhi: Motilal Banarsidass.

———. 2001b. "Śramaṇas: Their Conflict with Brāhmaṇical Society." In *Collected Papers on Buddhist Studies*, edited by Padmanabh S. Jaini, 47–96. Delhi: Motilal Banarsidass.

———. 2001/1979. *The Jaina Path of Purification*. Delhi: Motilal Banarsidass.

———. 2002. "Ecology, Economics, and Development in Jainism." *Jainism and Ecology: Nonviolence in the Web of Life*, edited by Christopher K. Chapple, 141–56. Cambridge, MA: Harvard University Press for the Center for the Study of World Religions, Harvard Divinity School.

———. 2003. "From *Nigoda* to *Mokṣa:* The Story of Marudevī." In *Jainism and Early Buddhism: Essays in Honor of Padmanabh S. Jaini, Part 1*, edited by Olle Qvarnström, 1–27. Fremont, CA: Asian Humanities Press.

———. 2004. "Ahiṃsā and 'Just War' in Jainism." In *Ahiṁsā, Anekānta and Jainism*, edited by Tara Sethia, 47–61. Delhi: Motilal Banarsidass.

———. 2010a. "Bhavyatva and Abhavyatva: A Jaina Doctrine of 'Predestination.'" In *Collected Papers on Jaina Studies*, edited by Padmanabh S. Jaini, 95–109. Delhi: Motilal Banarsidass.

———. 2010b. "*Karma* and the Problem of Rebirth in Jainism." In *Collected Papers on Jaina Studies*, edited by Padmanabh S. Jaini, 121–45. Delhi: Motilal Banarsidass.

———. 2010c. "Jaina Debates on the Spiritual Liberation of Women." In *Collected Papers on Jaina Studies*, edited by Padmanabh S. Jaini, 163–97. Delhi: Motilal Banarsidass. See also Jaini (1991) for extended analysis of this topic.

———. 2010d. "Indian Perspectives on the Spirituality of Animals." In *Collected Papers on Jaina Studies*, edited by Padmanabh S. Jaini, 253–66. Delhi: Motilal Banarsidass.

———. 2010e. "Fear of Food: Jaina Attitudes on Eating." In *Collected Papers on Jaina Studies*, edited by Padmanabh S. Jaini, 281–96. Delhi: Motilal Banarsidass.

"Jainism View on Having a Pet." 2019. *Jainism: Know It, Understand It & Internalize It* (blog), October 10. Accessed July 2, 2020: https://jainism-says.blogspot.com/2019/10/jainism-view-on-having-pet.html.

"Jains' Contribution to Exchequer 'Astounding.'" 2007. *The Hindu*, August 20. Last modified September 29, 2016. Accessed July 12, 2018: www.thehindu.com/todays-paper/tp-national/tp-tamilnadu/Jainsrsquo-contribution-to-exchequer-ldquoastoundingrdquo/article14819359.ece.

"Jains Hold Rally against Abortion." 2008. *The Hindu*, October 3. Last modified October 9, 2016. Accessed November 11, 2018: www.thehindu.com/todays-paper/tp-national/tp-andhrapradesh/Jains-hold-rally-against-abortion/article15315927.ece.

"Jains Steal the Show with 7 Padmas." 2015. *Times of India*, April 9, 2015. Accessed September 3, 2019: https://timesofindia.indiatimes.com/india/Jains-steal-the-show-with-7-Padmas/articleshow/46856659.cms.

Jambūvijaya, Muni, ed. 2003. *Sthānāṅgasūtra, Part 2, with the Commentary by Ācārya Śrī Abhayadev-Sūri Mahārāja*. Jaina Agama Series, no. 19 (2). Mumbai, Śrī Mahāvīra Jaina Vidyālaya.

Jansen, Lynn A. 2015. "Voluntary Stopping of Eating and Drinking (VSED), Physician-Assisted Suicide (PAS), or Neither in the Last Stage of Life? PAS: No; VSED: It Depends." *Annals of Family Medicine* 13 (5): 410–11.

Jansen, Lynn A., and Daniel P. Sulmasy. 2002. "Sedation, Alimentation, Hydration, and Equivocation: Careful Conversation about Care at the End of Life." *Annals of Internal Medicine* 136 (11): 845–49.

Jarvis Thomson, Judith. 2010. "A Defense of Abortion." In *Biomedical Ethics*, 7th ed., edited by David DeGrazia, Thomas A. Mappes, and Jeffrey Brand-Ballard, 479–87. New York: McGraw-Hill.

John Paul II. 1995. "Evangelium Vitae." The Vatican. Accessed May 2, 2019: https://w2.vatican.va/content/john-paul-ii/en/encyclicals/documents/hf_jp-ii_enc_25031995_evangelium-vitae.html.

Johnson, Todd M., and Brian J. Grim, eds. 2020. *World Religion Database*. Leiden, The Netherlands: Brill.

Johnson, William J. 1995a. *Harmless Souls: Karmic Bondage and Religious Change in Early Jainism with Special Reference to Umāsvāti and Kundakunda*. Delhi: Motilal Banarsidass.

———. 1995b. "The Religious Function of Jaina Philosophy: *Anekāntavāda* Reconsidered." *Religion* 25: 41–50.

———. 2014. "Jainism: From Ontology to Taxonomy in the Jaina Colonisation of the Universe." In *Categorisation in Indian Philosophy: Thinking inside the Box*, edited by Jessica Frazier, 133–45. Burlington, VT: Ashgate.

Jonsen, Albert R., Mark Siegler, and William J. Winslade. 2015. *Clinical Ethics: A Practical Approach to Ethical Decisions in Clinical Medicine*, 8th ed. New York: McGraw-Hill Education.

Kachhara, Narayan L. 2005. *Jaina Doctrine of Karma: The Religious and Scientific Dimensions*. Udaipur, India: Dharam Darshan Sewa Samstan.

———. 2014. *Scientific Explorations of Jain Doctrines (in 2 Parts), Part 1*. Delhi: Motilal Banarsidass.

Kachhara, Narayan Lal, Sohan Raj Tater, and Samani Unnat Prajna. 2017. "Karma, Living System, Genes and Human Performance." In *Scientific Perspectives of Jainism*, edited by Samani Chaitanya Prajna, Narendra Bhandari, and Narayan Lal Kachhara, 115–49. Ladnun, India: Jain Vishva Bharati Institute.

Kamptz, Kurt von. 1929. "Über die vom Sterbefasten handelnden älteren Paiṇṇa des Jaina-Kanons." PhD diss., University of Hamburg.

Kang, Xiangjin, Wenyin He, Yuling Huang, Qian Yu, Yaoyong Chen, Xingcheng Gao, Xiaofang Sun, and Yong Fan. 2016. "Introducing Precise Genetic Modification into

Human 3PN Embryos by CRISPR/Cas-mediated Genome Editing." *Journal of Assisted Reproduction and Genetics* 33 (5): 581–88.

Kapadia, H.R. 2010/1933. "Prohibition of Flesh-Eating in Jainism." In *The History of Vegetarianism and Cow-Veneration in India*, edited by Willem Bollée, 163–71. New York: Routledge. Originally published in 1933 in the *Review of Philosophy and Religion* 4: 232–39.

Katiyar, Arun. 1993. "Jain Research Centre in Gujarat Still Preaches That Earth Is Flat." *India Today*, March 31. Last modified August 13, 2013. Accessed June 12, 2019: www.indiatoday.in/magazine/offtrack/story/19930331-jain-research-centre-in-gujarat-still-preaches-that-earth-is-flat-810892-1993-03-31.

Kelting, M. Whitney. n.d. [a]. "Sulasā." *Jainpedia*. Accessed June 15, 2020: www.jainpedia.org/themes/people/women-in-the-jain-tradition/sulasa.html.

———. n.d. [b]. "Candanbālā." *Jainpedia*. Accessed August 2, 2019: www.jainpedia.org/themes/people/women-in-the-jain-tradition/candanbala.html.

———. 2001. *Singing to the Jinas: Jain Laywomen, Maṇḍaḷ Singing, and the Negotiations of Jain Devotion*. New York: Oxford University Press.

———. 2009. *Heroic Wives: Rituals, Stories, and the Virtues of Jain Wifehood*. New York: Oxford University Press.

Keown, Damien. 1995. *Buddhism and Bioethics*. New York: St. Martin's Press.

Kirde, Signe. 2011. "Vasunandin's *Śrāvakâcāra* (57–205): English Translation with Critical Notes." PhD diss., University of Tübingen.

Klaus, Daniela, and Arun Tipandjan. 2015. "Son Preference in India: Shedding Light on the North-South Gradient." *Comparative Population Studies* 40 (1): 77–102.

Koller, John M. 2000. "Syādvadā as the Epistemological Key to the Jaina Middle Way Metaphysics of Anekāntavāda." *Philosophy East and West* 50 (3): 400–407.

Kritzer, Robert. 2009. "Life in the Womb: Conception and Gestation in Buddhist Scripture and Classical Indian Medical Literature." In *Imagining the Fetus: The Unborn in Myth, Religion, and Culture*, edited by Vanessa Sasson and Jane Marie Law, 73–89. Oxford: Oxford University Press.

Krümpelmann, Kornelius. "The Sthānāṅgasūtra: An Encyclopaedic Text of the Śvetāmbara Canon." *International Journal of Jaina Studies* 2 (2): 1–13.

Kulkarni, Aniket D., Denise J. Jamieson, Howard W. Jones, Dmitry M. Kissin, Maria F. Gallo, Maurizio Macaluso, and Eli Y. Adashi. 2013. "Fertility Treatments and Multiple Births in the United States." *New England Journal of Medicine* 369 (23): 2218–25.

Laale, H. Willer. 1996. "Embryology and Abortion in Indian Antiquity: A Brief Survey." *Indian Journal of History of Science* 31 (3): 233–58.

Laidlaw, James. 1995. *Riches and Renunciation: Religion, Economy, and Society among the Jains*. Oxford: Clarendon Press.

Lalwani, Ganesh. 1997. *Jainism in India*. Jaipur, India: Prakrit Bharati Academy.

Ledford, Heidi. 2017. "CRISPR Fixes Disease Gene in Viable Human Embryos: Gene-editing Experiment Pushes Scientific and Ethical Boundaries." *Nature*. Accessed April 26, 2018: www.nature.com/news/crispr-fixes-disease-gene-in-viable-human-embryos-1.22382.

Lee, Jonathan H.X. 2010. "Jain Temples." In *Encyclopedia of Asian American Folklore and Folklife*, edited by Jonathan H.X. Lee and Kathleen M. Nadeau, 487–88. Santa Barbara, CA: ABC-CLIO.

Lewis, Ariane, James L. Bernat, Sandralee Blosser, J. Bonnie, Leon G. Epstein, John Hutchins, et al. 2018. "An Interdisciplinary Response to Contemporary Concerns about Brain Death Determination." *Neurology* 90 (9): 423–26.

Lipner, Julius J. 1989. "The Classical Hindu View on Abortion and the Moral Status of the Unborn." In *Hindu Ethics: Purity, Abortion, and Euthanasia*, edited by Harold G. Coward, Julius J. Lipner, Katherine K. Young, 41–69. Albany, NY: SUNY Press.

"Livestock Slaughter Annual [USDA] Summary." 2018. United States Department of Agriculture: Economics, Statistics and Market Information system. Accessed January 12, 2019: https://downloads.usda.library.cornell.edu/usda-esmis/files/r207tp32d/8336h934w/hq37vx004/lsslan19.pdf.

Loar, Russ. 1996. "Doctor Is Devoted to Religion That Inspired Gandhi." *Los Angeles Times*, June 24. Accessed January 25, 2018: http://articles.latimes.com/1996-06-24/local/me-17998_1_jain-religion.

Long, Jeffery D. 2009. *Jainism: An Introduction*. London: I.B. Tauris.

Löser, Peter, Jacqueline Schirm, Anke Guhr, Anna W. Wobus, and Andreas Kurtz. 2010. "Human Embryonic Stem Cell Lines and Their Use in International Research." *Stem Cells* 28 (2): 240–46.

Ma, Hong, Nuria Marti-Gutierrez, Sang-Wook Park, Jun Wu, Yeonmi Lee, Keiichiro Suzuki, et al. 2017. "Correction of a Pathogenic Gene Mutation in Human Embryos." *Nature* 548 (7668): 413–19.

Maayan, Inbar and Sean Cohmer. 2012. "John Bertrand Gurdon (1933–)." *The Embryo Project Encyclopedia*, October 11. Accessed January 21, 2018: https://embryo.asu.edu/pages/john-bertrand-gurdon-1933.

Mackler, Aaron L. 2003. *Introduction to Jewish and Catholic Bioethics: A Comparative Analysis*. Washington, DC: Georgetown University Press.

Maes, Claire. 2019. "Gāhāvaï *and* Gihattha: The Householder in the Early Jain Sources." In *Gṛhastha: The Householder in Ancient Indian Religious Culture*, edited by Patrick Olivelle, 75–91. New York: Oxford University Press.

Mahapatra, Dhananjay. 2015. "Supreme Court Permits Jain Community to Practice Santhara." *Times of India*, September 1. Accessed December 12, 2017: https://timesofindia.indiatimes.com/india/Supreme-Court-permits-Jain-community-to-practice-Santhara/articleshow/48751751.cms.

Mahāprajña, Ācārya. 2001. *Lord Mahavira's Scripture of Health*. Translated by Sarla Jag Mohan. Ladnun, India: Jain Vishva Bharati.

———. 2008. *The Happy and Harmonious Family*. Translated by Mukhya Niyojika Sadhvi Vishrut Vibha. Ladnun, India: Jain Vishva Bharati.

Mahias, Marie-Claude. 1985. *Délivrance et convivialité: Le systéme culinaire des Jaina*. Paris: Éditions de la Maison des sciences de l'homme.

Marks, Joel. 2012. "Accept No Substitutes: The Ethics of Alternatives." In *Animal Research Ethics: Evolving Views and Practices*, edited by Susan Gilbert, Gregory E. Kaebnick, and Thomas H. Murray. The Hastings Center Special Report. Accessed June 1, 2018: http://animalresearch.thehastingscenter.org/report/accept-no-substitutes-the-ethics-of-alternatives/.

Marquis, Don. 2010. "Why Abortion Is Immoral." In *Biomedical Ethics*, 7th ed., edited by David DeGrazia, Thomas A. Mappes, and Jeffrey Brand-Ballard, 475–79. New York: McGraw-Hill.

Matilal, Bimal K. 1981. *The Central Philosophy of Jainism (Anekānta-Vāda)*. L.D. Series 79. Ahmedabad, India: L.D. Institute of Indology.

McCarthy, Julie. 2015. "Fasting to the Death: Is It a Religious Rite or Suicide?" *NPR*, September 2. Accessed June 12, 2017: www.npr.org/sections/goatsandsoda/2015/09/02/436820789/fasting-to-the-death-is-it-a-religious-rite-or-suicide.

McCormick, Richard A. 1981. *How Brave a New World? Dilemmas in Bioethics*. Garden City, NY: Doubleday.

McMahan, Jeff. 2006. "An Alternative to Brain Death." *Journal of Law, Medicine, and Ethics* 34 (1): 44–48.

Mehta, Dhvani. 2018. "Jainism and Mental Health: How My Renewed Faith Made Me Stronger." *Young Minds*, February 1. Accessed August 12, 2020: https://youngminds.yja.org/jainism-and-mental-health-how-my-renewed-faith-made-me-stronger-8d584cfd1ecd.

Mehta, Mitul. 2015. "What Is Jainism's View on Embryonic Stem Cell Research?" *Quora*, October 3. Accessed January 11, 2018: www.quora.com/What-is-Jainisms-view-on-embryonic-stem-cell-research.

"Menstruation—Religious and Social Stigma." 2020. *Jainism: Know It, Understand It & Internalize It* (blog), November 25. Accessed December 23, 2020: https://jainism-says.blogspot.com/2020/11/menstruation-religious-and-social-stigma.html.

Meulenbeld, G. Jan. 1999–2002. *A History of Indian Medical Literature*. Five volumes. Groningen Oriental Studies, vol. 15. Groningen: Egbert Forsten.

Miles, John A., Jr. 1976. "Jain and Judaeo-Christian Respect for Life." *Journal of the American Academy of Religion* 44 (3): 453–57.

Ministry of Finance. 2018. "Gender and Son Meta-Preference: Is Development Itself an Antidote?" In *Ministry of Finance Economic Survey 2017–18*. Government of India, Ministry of Finance. Accessed January 8, 2018: https://issuu.com/utkarsh25/docs/102–118_chapter_07_english_vol_01_2.

Ministry of Health and Family Welfare. 2016. *National Family Health Survey (NFHS-4), 2015–16*. Government of India, Ministry of Health and Family Welfare. Mumbai: International Institute for Population Sciences. Accessed June 1, 2018: https://dhsprogram.com/pubs/pdf/FR339/FR339.pdf.

Mitra, Kalipada. 1939. "Magic and Miracle in Jaina Literature." *Indian Historical Quarterly* 15 (2): 175–82.

Monier-Williams, Monier. 1899. *A Sanskrit-English Dictionary: Etymologically and Philologically Arranged with Special Reference to Cognate Indo-European Languages*. Oxford: Clarendon Press.

Muzur, Amir, and Hans-Martin Sass. 2012. *Fritz Jahr and the Foundations of Global Bioethics: The Future of Integrative Bioethics*. Zürich/Berlin: LIT Verlag.

Muzur, Amir, and I. Rinčić. 2015. "Two Kinds of Globality: A Comparison of Fritz Jahr and Van Rensselaer Potter's Bioethics." *Global Bioethics* 26 (1): 23–27.

National Commission for Minorities. 2014. "Ministry of Minority Affairs Notification." Government of India, Ministry of Minority Affairs. January 27. Accessed May 29, 2020: http://ncm.nic.in/homepage/JainInclusion_Gazette.php.

Ngo, Thoai D., Min Hae Park, Haleema Shakur, and Caroline Free. 2011. "Comparative Effectiveness, Safety and Acceptability of Medical Abortion at Home and in a Clinic: A Systematic Review." *Bulletin of the World Health Organization* 89: 360–70.

"No Abortion—Jain Daily Pravacan." 2018. *YouTube*, February 18. Accessed July 29, 2018: www.youtube.com/watch?v=MzkM4du4GKU&t=5s.

Normile, Dennis. 2019. "Chinese Scientist Who Produced Genetically Altered Babies Sentenced to 3 Years in Jail." *Science*, December 30. Accessed July 30, 2020: www.sciencemag.org/news/2019/12/chinese-scientist-who-produced-genetically-altered-babies-sentenced-3-years-jail.

Notzer, Netta, David Zisenwine, Libi Oz, and Yoel Rak. 2006. "Overcoming the Tension Between Scientific and Religious Views in Teaching Anatomical Dissection: The Israeli Experience." *Clinical Anatomy* 19 (5): 442–47.

Ohira, Suzuko. 1975–76. "Jaina Concept of Siddhas." *Sambodhi* 4 (3–4): 17–21.

———. 1980. "Problems of the Purva." *Jain Journal* 15 (2): 41–55.

———. 1982. *A Study of Tattvārthasūtra with Bhāṣya with Special Reference to Authorship and Date*. L.D. Series 86. Ahmedabad, India: L.D. Institute of Indology.

———. 1994. *A Study of the Bhagavatīsūtra: A Chronological Analysis*. Prakrit Text Series, vol. 28. Ahmedabad, India: Prakrit Text Society.

Olivelle, Patrick. 2002. "*Abhakṣya* and *Abhojya:* An Exploration in Dietary Language." *Journal of the American Oriental Society* 122: 345–54.

———. 2017. "The Medical Profession in Ancient India: Its Social, Religious, and Legal Status." *eJournal of Indian Medicine* 9: 1–21.

Oliver, Michael, Alexander Woywodt, Aimun Ahmed, and Imran Saif. 2011. "Organ Donation, Transplantation and Religion." *Nephrology Dialysis Transplantation* 26 (2): 437–44.

Oram, John, and Paul Murphy. 2011. "Diagnosis of Death." *Continuing Education in Anaesthesia, Critical Care & Pain* 11 (3): 77–81.

Orentlicher, David. 2010. "The Supreme Court and Physician-Assisted Suicide: Rejected Assisted Suicide by Embracing Euthanasia." In *Biomedical Ethics*, 7th ed., edited by David DeGrazia, Thomas A. Mappes, and Jeffrey Brand-Ballard, 414–18. New York: McGraw-Hill.

Palmer, Barton W., and Alexandrea L. Harmell. 2016. "Assessment of Healthcare Decision-Making Capacity." *Archives of Clinical Neuropsychology* 31 (6): 530–40. Accessed August 2, 2010: https://doi.org/10.1093/arclin/acw051.

Pande, Rohini, and Anju Malhotra. 2006. "Son Preference and Daughter Neglect: What Happens to Living Girls?" *International Center for Research on Women (ICRW)*. Accessed June 2, 2018: www.icrw.org/wp-content/uploads/2016/10/Son-Preference-and-Daughter-Neglect-in-India.pdf.

"Passive Euthanasia Legalised: Jain Monk Hails SC Verdict, Catholic Bishop Calls It 'Painful.'" 2018. *DNA*, March 10. Accessed January 18, 2019: www.dnaindia.com/india/report-passive-euthanasia-legalised-jain-monk-hails-sc-verdict-catholic-bishop-calls-it-painful-2592473.

Patel, Vibhuti. 2014. "Sex Determination and Sex Pre-Selection Tests in India." In *Global Bioethics and Human Rights: Contemporary Issues*, edited by Wanda Teays, John-Steward Gordon, and Alison Dundes Renteln, 242–47. Lanham, MD: Rowman & Littlefield.

Patil, D.N., Darshan Babu N., Umapati C. Baragi, Pampanna Gouda H., and Patil N.J. 2015. "Kalyanakarakam: A Gem of Ayurveda." *Ayushdhara* 2 (3): 141–49.

Petit, Jérôme. 2015. "Banārasīdās Climbing the Jain Stages of Perfection." In *Puṣpikā: Tracing Ancient India through Texts and Traditions: Contributions to Current Research in Indology, Vol. 3*, edited by Robert Leach and Jessie Pons, 96–117. Oxford: Oxbow Books.

———. n.d. "Scales of Perfection." *Jainpedia*. Accessed April 3, 2019: www.jainpedia.org/themes/principles/jain-beliefs/karma/scales-of-perfection/mediashow/print.html.

Philbrick, Samuel. 2011. "Shinya Yamanaka (1962–)." *The Embryo Project Encyclopedia*. April 7. Accessed July 5, 2019: https://embryo.asu.edu/pages/shinya-yamanaka-1962.

Plofker, Kim. 2009. "The Mathematics of the Jain Cosmos." In *Victorious Ones: Jain Images of Perfection*, edited by Phyllis Granoff, 65–69. Rubin Museum of Art, New York, in association with Mapin Publishing, Ahmedabad, India.

Potter, Van Rensselaer. 1970. "Bioethics, the Science of Survival." *Perspectives in Biology and Medicine* 14 (1): 127–53.

———. 1971. *Bioethics: Bridge to the Future*. Englewood Cliffs, NJ: Prentice-Hall.

———. 1988. *Global Bioethics: Building on the Leopold Legacy*. East Lansing: Michigan State University Press.

Prasada, Ajit, ed. and trans. 1933. *Purushartha-siddhyupaya (Jaina-Pravachana-Rahasya-Kosha)*. The Sacred Books of the Jainas, vol. 4. Lucknow, India: Central Jaina Publishing House.

Quill, Timothy E., Bernard Lo, and Dan W. Brock. 1997. "Palliative Options of Last Resort: A Comparison of Voluntarily Stopping Eating and Drinking, Terminal Sedation, Physician-Assisted Suicide, and Voluntary Active Euthanasia." *JAMA* 278 (23): 2099–104.

Quill, Timothy E., and Ira R. Byock. 2000. "Responding to Intractable Terminal Suffering: The Role of Terminal Sedation and Voluntary Refusal of Food and Fluids." *Annals of Internal Medicine* 132 (5): 408–14.

Qvarnström, Olle. 2000. "Stability and Adaptability: A Jain Strategy for Survival and Growth." In *Jain Doctrine and Practice: Academic Perspectives*, edited by Joseph T. O'Connell, 113–35. Toronto: University of Toronto, Centre for South Asian Studies.

Rady, Mohamed Y., and Joseph L. Verheijde. 2012. "Distress from Voluntary Refusal of Food and Fluids to Hasten Death: What Is the Role of Continuous Deep Sedation?" *Journal of Medical Ethics* 38 (8): 510–12.

Ramsey, Paul. 2002/1970. *The Patient as Person: Explorations in Medical Ethics*, 2nd ed. New Haven, CT: Yale University Press.

Rankin, Aidan. 2018. *Jainism and Environmental Philosophy: Karma and the Web of Life*. New York: Routledge.

———. 2019. *Jainism and Environmental Politics*. New York: Routledge.

Rankin, Aidan, and Atul K. Shah. 2008. "Social Cohesion: A Jain Perspective." *Diverse Ethics*, August. Accessed September 15, 2018: www.diverseethics.com/files/resources/social-cohesion-reso/social-cohesion-lowres.pdf.

Rao, S.K. Ramachandra. 1985. *Encyclopaedia of Indian Medicine, Vol. 1: Historical Perspective*. Bombay: Popular Prakashan on behalf of Dr. V. Parameshvara Charitable Trust, Bangalore.

Rashkow, Ezra. 2013. "The Jain Endangerment Discourse." *Economic and Political Weekly* 48 (49): 24–27.

Reddy, D.V. Subba. 1960. "'Kalyana Karaka,' A Sanskrit Medical Treatise of the IX Century." *Indian Journal of the History of Medicine* 5 (1): 21–32.

Renou, Louis. 1953. *Religions of Ancient India*. London: University of London, The Athlone Press.

Renou, Louis, and Marie-Simone Renou. 1951. "Une secte religieuse dans l'Inde contemporaine." *Études* 268: 343–51.

"Revenue of the Worldwide Pharmaceutical Market from 2001 to 2016 (in Billion U.S. dollars)." 2017. *Statista*, December. Accessed January 26, 2019: www.statista.com/statistics/263102/pharmaceutical-market-worldwide-revenue-since-2001/.

Robertson, John A. 2012. "Preconception Gender Selection." In *Arguing about Bioethics*, edited by Stephen Holland, 83–92. New York: Routledge.

Robitaille, Marie-Claire. 2013. "Determinants of Stated Son Preference in India: Are Men and Women Different?" *Journal of Development Studies* 49 (5): 657–69.

Roy, Mira. 1966. "Methods of Sterilization and Sex-Determination in the *Atharva-veda* and the *Bṛhad-āraṇyakopaniṣad*." *Indian Journal of History of Science* 1 (2): 91–97.

Sade, Robert M. 2011. "Brain Death, Cardiac Death, and the Dead Donor Rule." *Journal of the South Carolina Medical Association* 107 (4): 146–49.

Salgia, J. Tansukh, comp. 2004. "Jain Funeral Practices & Observances: Practical Guidelines for the Community." Published by the author, Columbus, OH.

Salter, Emma. 2006. "Rethinking Religious Authority: A Perspective on the Followers of Śrīmad Rājacandra." In *Studies in Jaina History and Culture: Disputes and Dialogues*, edited by Peter Flügel, 241–62. New York: Routledge.

Sandel, Michael J. 2012. "The Case against Perfection: What's Wrong with Designer Children, Bionic Athletes, and Genetic Engineering?" In *Arguing about Bioethics*, edited by Stephen Holland, 93–104. New York: Routledge.

Sangave, Vilas Adinath. 1959. *Jaina Community: A Social Survey*. Bombay: Shri G.R. Bhatkal, at and for the Popular Book Depot.

———. 1997. *Jaina Religion and Community*. Long Beach, CA: Long Beach Publications.

———. 2001. *Aspects of Jaina Religion*. New Delhi: Bharatiya Jnanpith.

Sanghvi, Sukhlal. 2000/1974. *Pt. Sukhlalji's Commentary on Tattvārtha Sūtra of Vācaka Umāsvāti*. L.D. Series 44. Translated by K.K. Dixit. Ahmedabad, India: L.D. Institute of Indology.

Sanglikar, Mahaveer. 2016. "Do Jains Take Anti-Biotic Medication? Does It Not Go against Their Philosophy?" *Quora*, August 7. Accessed June 1, 2018: www.quora.com/Do-Jains-take-anti-biotic-medication-Does-it-not-go-against-their-philosophy.

Sarma, Deepak. 2013. "Jain Bioethics: Pontiff Charukeerthi Bhattaraka Sri Swamiji [interview]." *YouTube*, April 5. Accessed March 15, 2018: www.youtube.com/watch?v=-h-5tTX9R14.

Sass, Hans-Martin. 2007. "Fritz Jahr's 1927 Concept of Bioethics." *Kennedy Institute of Ethics Journal* 17 (4): 279–95.

———. 2014. "Bioethik–Bioethics." *Archiv für Begriffsgeschichte* 56: 221–28.

"SC Stays Rajasthan [High Court] Verdict Declaring Santhara Illegal." 2015. *The Hindu*, August 31. Last modified March 29, 2016. Accessed December 12, 2018: www.thehindu.com/news/national/sc-stays-rajasthan-hc-verdict-declaring-santhara-illegal/article7599349.ece.

Scharfe, Harmut. 1999. "The Doctrine of the Three Humors in Traditional Indian Medicine and the Alleged Antiquity of Tamil Siddha Medicine." *Journal of the American Oriental Society* 119 (4): 609–29.

Schenker, Joseph G. 2008. "The Beginning of Human Life: Status of Embryo. Perspectives in Halakha (Jewish Religious Law)." *Journal of Assisted Reproduction and Genetics* 25 (6): 271–76.

Schmidt, Hanns-Peter. 2010/1968. "The Origin of *Ahiṃsā*." In *The History of Vegetarianism and Cow-Veneration in India*, edited by Willem Bollée, 94–127. New York: Routledge. Originally published in 1968 in Mélanges d'Indianisme à la Mémoire de Louis Renou, 625–55. Publications de l'Institut de Civilisation indienne 28. Paris: Editions E. de Boccard.

Scholz, Sabine. 2012. "'The Jain Way of Life': Modern Re-use and Reinterpretation of Ancient Jain Concepts." In *Re-use: The Art and Politics of Integration and Anxiety*, edited by Julia A.B. Hegewald and Subrata K. Mitra, 273–87. Los Angeles: Sage.

Schubring, Walther. 2000/1962. *The Doctrine of the Jainas: Described after the Old Sources*. Lala Sundarlal Jain Research Series, vol. 15. Translated from the revised German edition by Wolfgang Beurlen. With three indices enlarged and added by Willem Bollée and Jayandra Soni. Delhi: Motilal Banarsidass. Translated from the original German version *Die Lehre der Jainas nach den alten Quellen dargestellt* published in Leipzig, Germany, by De Gruyter in 1935.

Sen, Amartya. 2005. *The Argumentative Indian: Writings on Indian Culture, History and Identity*. London: Penguin Books.

Sen, Madhu. 1975. *A Cultural Study of the Niśītha Cūrṇi*. Parshvanath Vidyashram Series, vol. 21. Amritsar, India: Sohanlal Jaindharma Pracharak Samiti.

Sethi, Manisha. 2009. "Chastity and Desire: Representing Women in Jainism." *South Asian History and Culture* 1 (1): 42–59.

———. 2012. *Escaping the World: Women Renouncers among Jains*. New Delhi: Routledge.

———. 2019. "Ritual Death in a Secular State: The Jain Practice of Sallekhana." *South Asian History and Culture* 10 (2): 136–51.

Sethia, Tara, ed. 2004. *Ahiṃsā, Anekānta and Jainism*. Delhi: Motilal Banarsidass.

Settar, S. 2016/1989. *Inviting Death: Historical Experiments on Sepulchral Hill*, revised ed. Delhi: Primus Books.

———. 2017/1990. *Pursuing Death: Philosophy and Practice of Voluntary Termination of Life*, revised ed. Delhi: Primus Books.

"Sex Ratio of India and Madhya Pradesh 1901–2011." 2011. *Gender Composition: Census India*. Accessed May 11, 2019: http://censusindia.gov.in/2011-prov-results/data_files/mp/06Gender%20Composition.pdf.

Shaefer, H. Luke, and Analidis Ochoa. 2018. "How Blood-Plasma Companies Target the Poorest Americans." *The Atlantic*, March 15. Accessed July 6, 2018: www.theatlantic.com/business/archive/2018/03/plasma-donations/555599/.

Shah, Amit. 2017. "Mental Health in South Asian & Jain Communities." *Young Minds*, May 2. Accessed August 12, 2020: https://youngminds.yja.org/mental-health-in-south-asian-jain-communities-65e098609657.

Shah, Atul K., and Aidan Rankin. 2017. *Jainism and Ethical Finance: A Timeless Business Model*. New York: Routledge.

Shah, Dilip V. 2017a. "My Visit to an Animal Sanctuary." *Gurudev Chitrabhanuji. Pramodaji Chitrabhanu. Jainism/Ahimsa/Nonviolence*, January 5. Accessed June 7, 2017: https://gurudevchitrabhanu.org/articles/animal-sanctuary-jain-philosophy/.

———. 2017b. *Chitrabhanu: Man of the Millennium*. Independently published.

Shah, Divyen K. 2014. "Health and Disease in Jaina Canonical Scriptures: A Modern Medical Perspective." *Jaina Studies: Newsletter of the Centre of Jaina Studies* 9: 31–33.

Shah, Pravin K. 2017. "Pathshala: The Next Generation of American Jains." *South Asian Times*, August 7. Accessed on November 12, 2017: http://thesouthasiantimes.info/news-Pathshala_The_Next_Generation_of_American_Jains-180593-art-books-37.html.

Shah, Shardule. 2009. "Brahmacharya and Celibacy." *Young Minds*, June 1. Accessed January 19, 2018: https://youngminds.yja.org/brahmacharya-and-celibacy-4689fc4cd240.

Shāntā, N. 1997. *The Unknown Pilgrims: The Voice of the Sādhvīs. The History, Life and Spirituality of the Jaina Women Ascetics*. Translated by Mary Rogers. New Delhi: Sri Satguru Publications.

Sharif, Adnan. 2013. "We Need More Organ Donation from Ethnic Minorities." *The BMJ* 347: 22.

Sharma, Lalit. 2015. "Rajasthan High Court Bans Jain Ritual of Fasting unto Death." *Hindustan Times*, August 10. Accessed September 1, 2015: www.hindustantimes.com/india/rajasthan-high-court-bans-jain-ritual-of-fasting-unto-death/story-uKTA8106hb51s3jgVEMNKP.html.

Sharma, P.V. 1992. "Medicine in Buddhist and Jaina Traditions." In *History of Medicine in India (From Antiquity to 1000 A.D.)*, edited by P.V. Sharma, 117–35. New Delhi: Indian National Science Academy.

Sherwin, Susan. 2010. "Feminist Ethics and In Vitro Fertilization." In *Biomedical Ethics*, 7th ed., edited by David DeGrazia, Thomas A. Mappes, and Jeffrey Brand-Ballard, 553–59. New York: McGraw-Hill.

Sikdar, J.C. 1964. *Studies in the Bhagawatīsūtra*. Prakrit Jain Institute Research Publications Series, vol. 1. Muzaffarpur: Research Institute of Prakrit, Jainology and Ahimsa.

———. 1974. *Jaina Biology*. L.D. Series 111. Ahmedabad, India: L.D. Institute of Indology.

———. 1975. "The World of Life According to the Jaina Literature." *Sambodhi* 4 (1): 9–20.

Singh, Ram Bhushan Prasad. 1975. *Jainism in Early Medieval Karnataka (c. A.D. 500–1200)*. Delhi: Motilal Banarsidass.

Singhvi, L.M. 2002. "The Jain Declaration on Nature." In *Jainism and Ecology: Nonviolence in the Web of Life*, edited by Christopher K. Chapple, 217–24. Cambridge, MA: Harvard University Press for the Center for the Study of World Religions, Harvard Divinity School.

Smith, Martin. 2012. "Brain Death: Time for an International Consensus." *British Journal of Anesthesia* 108 (1): i6–i9.

———. 2015. "Brain Death: The United Kingdom Perspective." *Seminars in Neurology* 35 (2): 145–51.

Sogani, Kamal Chand. 1967. *Ethical Doctrines in Jainism*. Jīvarāja Jaina Granthamālā, no. 19. Sholapur, India: Lalchand Hirachand Doshi, Jaina Saṃskṛti Saṃrakshaka Sangha.

———. 2016. "Ethics and Mysticism in Jaina Yoga Spirituality." In *Yoga in Jainism*, edited by Christopher K. Chapple, 155–81. New York: Routledge.

Soni, Jayandra. 1991. "*Dravya*, *Guṇa* and *Paryāya* in Jaina Thought." *Journal of Indian Philosophy* 19: 75–88.

———. 2000. "Basic Jaina Epistemology." *Philosophy East and West* 50 (3): 367–77.

———. 2003. "Kundakunda and Umāsvāti on *Anekânta-vāda*." In *Essays in Jaina Philosophy and Religion*, edited by Piotr Balcerowicz, 25–35. Lal Sundarlal Jain Research Series, vol. 20. Delhi: Motilal Banarsidass.

———. 2007. "*Upayoga*, According to Kundakunda and Umāsvāti." *Journal of Indian Philosophy* 35 (4): 299–311.

———. 2016. "Yoga in the *Tattvārthasūtra*." In *Yoga in Jainism*, edited by Christopher K. Chapple, 29–36. New York: Routledge.

Soni, Luitgard. 2014. "Jaina Modes of Dying in Ārādhanā Texts." *International Journal of Jaina Studies* 10 (2): 1–14.

Sreenivasan, Gopal. 2007. "Health Care and Equality of Opportunity." *Hastings Center Report* 37 (2): 21–31.

Stirrat, Gordon M., and Robin Gill. 2005. "Autonomy in Medical Ethics after O'Neill." *Journal of Medical Ethics* 31 (3): 127–30.

Stookey, Christopher. 2015. "Christopher Stookey: A Gentle Way to Die." November. Accessed January 27, 2018: www.deathwithdignity.org/stories/christopher-stookey-gentle-way/.

Stork, Hélène. 1992. "Mothering Rituals in Tamilnadu: Some Magico-Religious Beliefs." In *Roles and Rituals for Hindu Women*, edited by Julia Leslie, 89–105. Delhi: Motilal Banarsidass.

Stuart, Mari J. 2014. "Mendicants and Medicine: Āyurveda in Jain Monastic Texts." *History of Science in South Asia* 2 (1): 63–100.

Tabaie, Sheida. 2017. "Stopping Female Feticide in India: The Failure and Unintended Consequence of Ultrasound Restriction." *Journal of Global Health* 7 (1): 010304.

Tabarrok, Alexander. 2013. "The Global Organ Shortage: Economic Causes, Human Consequences, Policy Responses." *The Independent Review* 18 (2): 296–98.

Tater, Sohan R. 2009. *The Jaina Doctrine of Karma and the Science of Genetics*. New Delhi: Readworthy.

Tatia, Nathmal. 1951. *Studies in Jaina Philosophy*. Banaras, India: Jain Cultural Research Society.

———, trans. 2011. *That Which Is: A Classic Jain Manual for Understanding the True Nature of Reality*. New Haven, CT: Yale University Press.

ten Have, Henk A.M.J. 2012. "Potter's Notion of Bioethics." *Kennedy Institute of Ethics Journal* 22 (1): 59–82.

Teno, Joan M., Sandra Licks, Joanne Lynn, Neil Wenger, Alfred F. Connors Jr., Russell S. Phillips, et al. 1997. "Do Advance Directives Provide Instructions That Direct Care?" *Journal of the American Geriatrics Society* 45 (4): 508–12.

Tukol, T.K. 1976. *Sallekhanā Is Not Suicide*. L.D. Series 55. Ahmedabad, India: L.D. Institute of Indology.

Tulsī, Ācārya. 1994. *Transmutation of Personality through Preksha Meditation*. Ladnun, India: Jain Vishva Bharati.

———. 1998. *The Vision of a New Society*. Churu, India: Adarsh Sahitya Sangh Prakashan.

"Uniform Determination of Death Act." 1980. National Conference of Commissioners on Uniform State Laws. Accessed January 4, 2018: www.uniformlaws.org/HigherLogic/System/DownloadDocumentFile.ashx?DocumentFileKey=341343fa-1efe-706c-043a-9290fdcfd909.

Upadhye, A.N., ed. 1960. *Svāmi-Kumāra's Kārttikeyānuprekṣā (Kattigeyāṇuppekkhā): An Early Treatise on Jaina Doctrines, Especially Anuprekṣās*. Agas, India: Śrī Parama-Śruta Prabhāvaka Maṇḍala, Śrīmad Rājacandra Āśrama.

"USDA Publishes 2016 Animal Research Statistics—7% Rise in Animal Use." 2017. *Speaking of Research*. n.d. Accessed August 16, 2017: https://speakingofresearch.com/2017/06/19/usda-publishes-2016-animal-research-statistics-7-rise-in-animal-use/.

Vallely, Anne. 2002a. *Guardians of the Transcendent: An Ethnography of a Jain Ascetic Community*. Toronto: University of Toronto Press.

———. 2002b. "From Liberation to Ecology: Ethical Discourses among Orthodox and Diaspora Jains." In *Jainism and Ecology: Nonviolence in the Web of Life*, edited by Christopher K. Chapple, 193–216. Cambridge, MA: Harvard University Press for the Center for the Study of World Religions, Harvard Divinity School.

———. 2004. "The Jain Plate: The Semiotics of the Diaspora Diet." In *South Asians in the Diaspora: Histories and Religious Traditions*, edited by Knut A. Jacobsen and P. Pratap Kumar, 3–22. Leiden, The Netherlands: Brill.

———. 2008. "Moral Landscapes: Ethical Discourses among Orthodox and Diaspora Jains." In *A Reader in the Anthropology of Religion*, 2nd ed., edited by Michael Lambek, 560–72. Malden, MA: Blackwell.

———. 2011. "Ancestors, Demons and the Goddess: Negotiating the Animate Cosmos of Jainism." In *Health and Religious Rituals in South Asia: Disease, Possession and Healing*, edited by Fabrizio M. Ferrari, 64–77. New York: Routledge.

———. 2014. "Being Sentiently with Others: The Shared Existential Trajectory among Humans and Nonhumans in Jainism." In *Asian Perspectives on Animal Ethics: Rethinking the Nonhuman*, edited by Neil Dalal and Chloë Taylor, 38–55. New York: Routledge.

———. 2020. "Vulnerability, Transcendence, and the Body: Exploring the Human/Nonhuman Animal Divide within Jainism." *Society and Animals* 28: 550–66.

Varelius, Jukka. 2006. "The Value of Autonomy in Medical Ethics." *Medicine, Health Care and Philosophy* 9 (3): 377–88.

Varṇī, Jinendra. 2012–14/1970–73. *Jainendra Siddhānta Kośa*. Four volumes. Delhi: Bharatiya Jnanpith.

Verheijde, Joseph L., and Mohamed Y. Rady. 2014. "The Lack of Scientific Evidence in Clinical Practice Guideline in Brain Death Determination: Implications for Organ Donation and Transplantation." *Indian Journal of Critical Care Medicine* 18 (9): 555–57.

Warren, Mary Anne. 2010. "On the Moral and Legal Status of Abortion." *Biomedical Ethics*, 7th ed., edited by David DeGrazia, Thomas A. Mappes, and Jeffrey Brand-Ballard, 468–75. New York: McGraw-Hill.

Weintraub, Karen. 2016. "20 Years after Dolly the Sheep Led the Way—Where Is Cloning Now?" *Scientific American*, July 5. Accessed July 28, 2018: www.scientificamerican.com/article/20-years-after-dolly-the-sheep-led-the-way-where-is-cloning-now/.

White, David Gordon. *The Alchemical Body: Siddha Traditions in Medieval India*. Chicago: University of Chicago Press.

Whitney, William Dwight. 1885. *The Roots, Verb-Forms and Primary Derivatives of the Sanskrit Language*. Leipzig: Breitkopf and Härtel.

Wijdicks, Eelco F.M., Panayiotis N. Varelas, Gary S. Gronseth, and David M. Greer. 2010. "Evidence-Based Guideline Update: Determining Brain Death in Adults—Report of the Quality Standards Subcommittee of the American Academy of Neurology." *Neurology* 74 (23): 1911–18.

Wiles, Royce. 2006. "The Dating of the Jaina Councils: Do Scholarly Presentations Reflect the Traditional Sources? In *Studies in Jaina History and Culture: Disputes and Dialogues*, edited by Peter Flügel, 61–85. New York: Routledge.

Wiley, Kristi L. 1999. "Gotra Karma: A Contrast in Views." In *Approaches to Jaina Studies: Philosophy, Logic, Rituals, and Symbols*, edited by N.K. Wagle and Olle Qvarnström, 113–30. Toronto: University of Toronto, Centre for South Asian Studies.

———. 2000a. "Aghātiyā Karmas: Agents of Embodiment in Jainism." PhD diss., University of California, Berkeley.

———. 2000b. "Colors of the Soul: By-products of Activity or Passions?" *Philosophy East and West* 50 (3): 348–66.

———. 2002. "The Nature of Nature: Jain Perspectives on the Natural World." In *Jainism and Ecology: Nonviolence in the Web of Life*, edited by Christopher K. Chapple, 35–59. Cambridge, MA: Harvard University Press for the Center for the Study of World Religions, Harvard Divinity School.

———. 2003. "The Story of King Śreṇika: Binding and Modifications of *Āyu Karma*." In *Jainism and Early Buddhism: Essays in Honor of Padmanabh S. Jaini, Part 1*, edited by Olle Qvarnström, 337–58. Fremont, CA: Asian Humanities Press.

———. 2006a. "*Ahiṃsā* and Compassion in Jainism." In *Studies in Jaina History and Culture: Disputes and Dialogues*, edited by Peter Flügel, 438–55. New York: Routledge.

———. 2006b. "Five-Sensed Animals in Jainism." In *A Communion of Subjects: Animals in Religion, Science, and Ethics*, edited by Paul Waldau and Kimberley Patton, 250–55. New York: Columbia University Press.

———. 2008. "Early Śvetāmbara and Digambara Karma Literature: A Comparison." In *Jaina Studies*, Papers of the 12th World Sanskrit Conference, vol. 9, edited by Colette Caillat and Nalini Balbir, 43–59. Delhi: Motilal Banarsidass.

———. 2009. *The A to Z of Jainism*. Lanham, MD: Scarecrow Press.

———. 2011. "The Significance of *Adhyavasāya* in Jain Karma Theory." *International Journal of Jaina Studies* 7 (3): 1–26.

———. 2012. "Supernatural Powers and Their Attainment in Jainism." In *Yoga Powers: Extraordinary Capacities Attained through Meditation and Concentration*, edited by Knut A. Jacobsen, 145–94. Leiden, The Netherlands: Brill.

———. 2016. "Karmic Bondage and Kaṣāyas: A Re-examination of 'Umāsvāti's Jainism.'" In *Studies in Umāsvāti and his Tattvārthasūtra: Papers Presented at an International Seminar Organized by the B.L. Institute of Indology*, edited by G.C. Tripathi and Ashok Kumar Singh, 71–93. Delhi: Bhogilal Leherchand Institute of Indology.

———. 2021. Personal communication via email, February 7.

Williams, Robert. 1963. *Jaina Yoga: A Survey of the Mediaeval Śrāvakācāras*. London: Oxford University Press.

"WMA Declaration of Sydney on the Determination of Death and the Recovery of Organs." 2017. World Medical Association, February 15. Accessed March 11, 2018: www.wma.net/policies-post/wma-declaration-of-sydney-on-the-determination-of-death-and-the-recovery-of-organs/.

Wu, Diana A., Christopher J. Watson, J. Andrew Bradley, Rachel J. Johnson, John L. Forsythe, and Gabriel C. Oniscu. 2017. "Global Trends and Challenges in Deceased Donor Kidney Allocation." *Kidney International* 91 (6): 1287–99.

Wu, Juan. 2017. "Parallel Stories in the *Āvaśyakacūrṇi* and the Mūlasarvāstivāda *Vinaya*: A Preliminary Investigation." *Journal of the American Oriental Society* 137 (2): 315–47.

Wujastyk, Dominik. 1984. "The Spikes in the Ears of the Ascetic: An Illustrated Tale in Buddhism and Jainism." *Oriental Art* 30 (2): 189–94.

———. 2004. "Medicine and Dharma." *Journal of Indian Philosophy* 32 (5/6): 831–42.

Yanow, Morton Leonard. 2000. "Responding to Intractable Terminal Suffering (Letter to the Editor)." *Annals of Internal Medicine* 133 (7): 560.

Ye, Jinpei, Nicola Bates, Despina Soteriou, Lisa Grady, Clare Edmond, Alex Ross, et al. 2017. "High Quality Clinical Grade Human Embryonic Stem Cell Lines Derived from Fresh Discarded Embryos." *Stem Cell Research & Therapy* 8: article 128.

Yeates, James W. 2010. "Death Is a Welfare Issue." *Journal of Agricultural and Environmental Ethics* 23 (3): 229–41.

Zwilling, Leonard, and Michael J. Sweet. 1993. "The First Medicalization: The Taxonomy and Etiology of Queerness in Classical Indian Medicine." *Journal of the History of Sexuality* 3 (4): 590–607.

———. 1996. "'Like a City Ablaze': The Third Sex and the Creation of Sexuality in Jain Religious Literature." *Journal of the History of Sexuality* 6 (3): 359–84.

Zydenbos, Robert J. 1999. "Jainism as the Religion of Nonviolence." In *Violence Denied: Violence, Non-violence and the Rationalization of Violence in South Asian Cultural History*, edited by Jan E.M. Houben and Karel R. Van Kooij, 185–210. Brill's Indological Library, vol. 16. Leiden, The Netherlands: Brill.

———. 2000. "Divinity in Jainism." In *Jain Doctrine and Practice: Academic Perspectives*, edited by Joseph T. O'Connell, 69–94. Toronto: University of Toronto, Centre for South Asian Studies.

Zysk, Kenneth G. 1991. *Asceticism and Healing in Ancient India: Medicine in the Buddhist Monastery*. New York: Oxford University Press.

# INDEX

Founded in 1893,
UNIVERSITY OF CALIFORNIA PRESS
publishes bold, progressive books and journals on topics in the arts, humanities, social sciences, and natural sciences—with a focus on social justice issues—that inspire thought and action among readers worldwide.

The UC PRESS FOUNDATION
raises funds to uphold the press's vital role as an independent, nonprofit publisher, and receives philanthropic support from a wide range of individuals and institutions—and from committed readers like you. To learn more, visit ucpress.edu/supportus.